Skin Cancer Management

Deborah F. MacFarlane

Editor

Skin Cancer Management

A Practical Approach

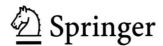 Springer

Editor
Deborah F. MacFarlane, MD, MPH
Professor of Dermatology
  and Plastic Surgery
The University of Texas MD Anderson
  Cancer Center
Houston, TX, USA

ISBN 978-0-387-88494-3   e-ISBN 978-0-387-88495-0
DOI 10.1007/978-0-387-88495-0
Springer New York Dordrecht Heidelberg London

Library of Congress Control Number: 2009931796

Printed on acid-free paper

Springer is part of Springer Science+Business Media (www.springer.com)

To the memory of my father, Francis P. MacFarlane, who encouraged both my quest to become a physician and to write.

Foreword

The editor of *Skin Cancer Management: A Practical Approach,* Dr. Deborah MacFarlane, gathers experts in selected techniques related to the assessment and management of skin cancer and has them critically review the existing literature in light of their considerable experience delivering care. The authors make recommendations for the best way to perform procedures. The tables provided in each chapter then become a manual of how to perform these procedures, and may in time be adopted by the wider universe of dermatologists as the standard of performance. The detailed descriptions of technique and treatment pearls lead the novice through the sequence of events in a way that instills confidence in their ability to safely perform the procedure. An example of the painstaking explanations is found in Chapter 5, Intralesional and Perilesional Treatment of Skin Cancers. The reader is advised to place eye protection on the patient and those performing the injection of methotrexate into a keratoacanthoma with a central crust. Rest assured that there will be a spray or stream of methotrexate emitted from the crusted area. Having eye protection will prevent methotrexate from accidentally getting into someone's eye.

Since we all learn to assimilate new information by taking action on the recommendations that we read, it would be a good idea for the physician to create, where relevant, a checklist for each procedure in the text. The checklist can be given to the office staff to set up the equipment for the procedure. This step-wise approach may also help orient and train new office staff. For infrequently performed procedures, the physician may review the checklist with the office assistant prior to performing the procedure. This same clarity and easily read format ensures that this book will be of use to a variety of medical personnel faced with treating skin cancers.

Another learning tool used to great advantage in the text is the presentation of illustrative cases with ample clinical photographs. Dermatologists have a refined visual memory of cases. When a patient with a similar problem presents for care, the dermatologist's recall reaction sends him/her scurrying off to find the memorable case report. Among the many memorable cases for the reader of this book to recall are examples of complications and their management. Dr. Humphreys recommends conservative debridement of nonviable tissue in a failed flap. The traditional way of managing flap necrosis is to allow an eschar to develop and separate. Having managed a few cases of compromised facial flaps in this way, I can attest to the discomfort of the patient suffering the odorific assault of waiting for the process to come to completion. The practical implications of Dr. Humphrey's recommendation to debride devascularized tissue are enormous. There is less potential for cellulitis from infection arising in the necrotic tissue. The patient is more comfortable.

The clinician-friendly distillation of complex matters is noteworthy. An excellent example is the recommendation to those challenged by which imaging study to perform for a head and neck NMSC. Shah et al. simply state begin with computerized tomography unless perineural invasion is suspected in which case MRI is best. For the dermatologist who orders fewer than six imaging studies a year, this recommendation dispels the magic of the alphabet soup of imaging studies. Demystifying complex issues helps us all to deliver better care. *Skin Cancer Management: A Practical Approach* is a step along the path toward conceiving and performing randomized trials comparing treatments with "manualized" procedures. I congratulate the authors and the editor, Dr. Deborah MacFarlane, for the clarity they bring to the treatment of skin cancer.

Chicago, Illinois   June K. Robinson

Preface

The concept behind this book was to provide something eminently practical, to address some of the questions I, and others, have encountered over the years, but haven't readily found answers for. I wanted experts in their fields to put on paper the pearls of their wisdom, to give us the laser settings, the recipes for anesthesia, which are often only quickly referred to in lectures. I wanted to address topics that as physicians we don't always feel readily comfortable with, for example, when and how to refer certain patients on to other colleagues. I wanted answers for some of the more unusual questions we might come across, for instance, for how long does a facial prosthesis last?

As dermatologists we are strongly visually oriented and it was my desire to present as much data as possible in a visual mode, with figures, case histories, and tables, along with a synopsis of the most pertinent, recent literature. All too often in surgery we tend to concentrate on excellent outcomes. However, in surgery, as in life, it is from analyzing our mistakes that we truly progress. For this reason, complications and their management are discussed in detail in each chapter.

Having trained both in surgery and dermatology, I have always been especially interested in bridging the boundaries between specialties. Hence the chapter on radiologic imaging of skin cancers, which took months to write as we had to first find a common language before we set about actually communicating ideas and then marrying clinical presentations with radiologic images. Similarly, I wished to know in detail what actually happened when I sent a patient to radiation oncology. Additionally, I wanted a chapter that would conveniently address all the intra- and perilesional medications that could be used to treat skin cancers; something I had not been able to find in the literature and I wanted recipes and techniques for these.

It is my overall hope that this book will be of use not just to dermatologists, but to all those medical personnel who come into contact with what is increasingly a cause for worldwide concern.

Houston, TX, USA   Deborah F. MacFarlane

Acknowledgements

I would like to thank the many fine surgeons, too numerous to list, whom I have had the honor of training with over the years.

I am especially appreciative of Dr. Leonard Goldberg, who taught me the finer points of dermatologic surgery, but most importantly, showed me every day how to treat patients with equal parts of compassion, humor, and respect.

I am indebted to my friends and colleagues who patiently tolerated my quest for unique book chapters and generously shared their valuable knowledge and experience.

I would be remiss not to thank my patients who have taught me some of the most important lessons of my life and to them I am deeply grateful.

Lastly, I am grateful for the loyal support of my husband Michael and daughter Lara.

Houston, TX, USA   Deborah F. MacFarlane

Contents

Contributors

Nicole M. Annest, MD, MS Staff Physician, Kaiser Permanente, Mohs Surgical Unit, Department of Dermatology, Lafayette, CO, USA

Christopher J. Arpey, MD Professor, Department of Dermatology, University of Iowa Hospitals and Clinics, Iowa City, IA, USA

Matthew T. Ballo, MD Associate Professor and Medical Director, Radiation Oncology Outreach, Department of Radiation Oncology, MD Anderson Cancer Center, University of Texas, Houston, TX, USA

John A. Carucci, MD, PhD Chief, Department of Dermatology, Weill Medical College of Cornell, Mohs Micrographic and Dermatologic Surgery, New York, NY, USA

Laura T. Cepeda, MD Haley Dermatology Group, Dermatologist and Mohs Surgeon, Fairhope, AL, USA

Susannah Collier, MD Laser and Dermatologic Surgery Center, Chesterfield, MO, USA

Tejas Desai, DO Division of Dermatology, Fellow, Mohs Micrographic Surgery, Loma Linda University, Loma Linda, CA, USA

Gloria F. Graham, MD Clinical Associate Professor, Department of Dermatology, Wake Forest University School of Medicine, Winston-Salem, NC, USA

George Hruza, MD Laser and Dermatologic Surgery Center, Chesterfield, MO, USA

Tatyana Humphreys, MD Professor, Director of Cutaneous Surgery, Department of Dermatology, Thomas Jefferson University, Philadelphia, PA, USA

Brooke A. Jackson, MD Medical Director, Assistant Clinical Professor, Department of Dermatology, Skin Wellness Center of Chicago, Northwestern Memorial Hospital, Chicago, IL, USA

David R. Lambert, MD Clinical Associate Professor, Division of Dermatology, The Ohio State University, Columbus, OH, USA

Mollie A. MacCormack MD Chief, Procedural Dermatology, Department of Dermatology, Lahey Clinic, Burlington, MA, USA

Deborah F. MacFarlane, MD, MPH Professor, Departments of Dermatology and Plastic Surgery, The University of Texas MD Anderson Cancer Center, Houston, TX, USA

Jennifer L. MacGregor, MD Department of Dermatology, Columbia University Medical Center, New York, NY, USA

Susan L. McGovern, MD, PhD Department of Radiation Oncology, MD Anderson Cancer Center, Houston, TX, USA

Gary D. Monheit, MD Department of Dermatology and Ophthalmology, Total Skin and Beauty Dermatology Center, University of Alabama, Birmingham, AL, USA

Dariush Moussai, MD Postdoctoral Fellow, Department of Dermatology, Weill Medical College of Cornell, New York, NY, USA

David J. Najarian, MD Assistant Clinical Professor of Dermatology, Department of Dermatology, University of Medicine and Dentistry of New Jersey, Robert Wood Johnson Medical School, Somerset, NJ, USA

Mark F. Naylor, MD Dermatology Associates of San Antonio, San Antonio, TX, USA

Jane Onufer, MD Assistant Professor, Department of Diagnostic Radiology, The University of Texas, M.D. Anderson Cancer Center, Houston, TX, US

Allan R. Oseroff, MD, PhD [†] Chairman, Department of Dermatology, Roswell Park Cancer Institute and State University of New York at Buffalo, Buffalo, NY, USA

Chad L. Prather, MD Clinical Assistant Professor, Department of Dermatology, Louisiana State University School of Medicine, New Orleans, LA, USA

Ronald P. Rapini, MD Professor and Chair, Department of Dermatology, MD Anderson Cancer Center, University of Texas Medical School, Houston, TX, USA

Désirée Ratner, MD Professor of Dermatology, Director of Dermatology Surgery, Department of Dermatology, Columbia University Medical Center, New York, NY, USA

June K. Robinson, MD Professor of Clinical Dermatology, Department of Dermatology, Northwestern University, Feinberg School of Medicine, Chicago, IL, USA

Amy S. Ross, MD Palm Harbor Dermatology, Mohs Surgeon, Palm Harbor, FL, USA

Richard K. Scher, MD, FACP Professor of Dermatology, Head, Section for Diagnosis and Treatment of Nail Disorders, Department of Dermatology, University of North Carolina, Chapel Hill, NC, USA

Komal Shah, MD Assistant Professor, Department of Diagnostic Radiology, M.D. Anderson Cancer Center, The University of Texas, Houston, TX, USA

Daniel Mark Siegel, MD, MS Clinical Professor of Dermatology, Director, Procedural Dermatology Fellowship, Department of Dermatology, Downstate Health Science Center at Brooklyn, State University of New York, Brooklyn, NY, USA

Thomas Stasko, MD Associate Professor of Medicine, Department of Dermatology, Vanderbilt University Medical Center, Nashville, TN, USA

Abel Torres, MD, JD Professor of Dermatology/Internal Medicine, Loma Linda Department of Dermatology, University School of Medicine, Loma Linda, CA, USA

Stephen B. Tucker, MD Clinical Professor of Dermatology, Department of Dermatology, University of Texas Health Science Center at Houston, Houston, TX, USA

Nathalie Zeitouni, MD Department of Dermatology, Roswell Park Cancer Institute, State University of New York, Buffalo, NY, USA

Fiona Zwald, MD, MRCPI Assistant Professor, Department of Dermatology, Director of Transplant Dermatology, Emory University, Atlanta, GA, USA

Chapter 1
Biopsy Techniques and Interpretation

Deborah F. MacFarlane and Ronald P. Rapini

The performance of a skin biopsy is an intrinsic part of the initial management of a patient suspected of having a skin cancer.[1,2] This first chapter will therefore begin with a discussion of the various skin biopsy techniques most commonly used in the diagnosis of skin cancer and their clinical indications. This will be followed by a frank discussion of the interpretation of biopsy results. Discussion of other biopsy techniques such as curettage and sentinel lymph node biopsy will be dealt with elsewhere (Chapters 6 and 15, respectively).

Biopsy Technique

Pre-Op

Before performing a biopsy, it is important to have taken a medical history and performed a physical exam. The presence of potential problems such as coagulopathies, drug allergies including lidocaine allergies, artificial joints, and heart valves should be ascertained (Chapter 8). Most biopsy procedures can be safely performed in patients on warfarin, heparin, clopidogrel bisulfate, aspirin, and non-steroidal anti-inflammatory drugs if sufficient care is taken and hemostatic agents are available. The risks and benefits of the biopsy should be explained and consent obtained.

Site Preparation and Anesthesia

The site should next be cleansed with an antiseptic such as isopropyl alcohol, povidone-iodine, or chlorhexidine, for example. Local anesthesia is best performed with a 30-gauge needle used to slowly infiltrate a buffered lidocaine solution.[3] Most physicians utilize 1% lidocaine with 1:100,000 epinephrine. A buffered lidocaine solution can be less painful, and for larger procedures the 0.5% lidocaine solution reduces the possibility of toxicity that may occur when large amounts of lidocaine are used. One common dilution is 9 parts of 0.5% lidocaine with 1:200,000 epinephrine to one part of the standard available sodium bicarbonate solution. With such a dilute concentration of epinephrine, one does not need to worry about potential interactions between epinephrine and beta-blockers for instance, and patients do not experience the tachycardia that sometimes occurs with a stronger epinephrine solution.

Hemostasis

For biopsy sites that are not sutured, styptic agents are often used. Ferric subsulfate (Monsel's solution) may pigment the tissue, complicating histologic interpretation and aluminum chloride hexahydrate (Drysol) is preferable. The styptic is applied on a cotton-tipped swab with pressure to the biopsy site and held in place for several seconds and reapplied if necessary. Another alternative in a freely bleeding biopsy site is to apply a piece of hemostatic sponge, such as Gelfoam, and to bandage the site.[4] Larger wounds may require electrocoagulation for hemostasis prior to wound closure (Chapter 10).

D.F. MacFarlane (ed.), *Skin Cancer Management,* DOI 10.1007/978-0-387-88495-0_1,
© Springer Science+Business Media, LLC 2010

Shave Biopsy

In this technique the superficial layer of the skin is sampled and it is therefore minimally invasive and usually not associated with significant scarring. It can be used in the diagnosis of superficial skin cancers such as actinic keratoses (AK), squamous cell carcinoma in situ (SCCIS), and basal and squamous cell carcinomas (BCC and SCC). One disadvantage of this technique is that tumor existing deep to the plane of the shave can be missed (see Table 1.1).[5]

Table 1.1 Biopsy techniques

Biopsy type	Lesion
Shave	AK, BCC, SCC
Saucerization	Pigmented lesions, SCC
Punch	SCCIS to check for invasion
Incisional	Melanoma in situ to check for invasion
Wedge	Ulcerated SCC
Excisional	Atypical nevi, melanoma

Reproduced from Rapini (1994) with permission from Elsevier.

Equipment

A number 15 blade, toothed forceps, hemostatic agent, cotton-tipped applicator, gauze, and bandage. Please note that a razor blade may also be substituted for a number 15 blade.[6]

Technique

After cleansing the area, the local anesthetic is slowly infiltrated to raise a wheal. The skin is stabilized using the first and second fingers of the non-dominant hand, then the belly of the blade is held against the skin in a horizontal position and a gentle sawing motion is used to slowly separate the specimen and some surrounding skin from its base (Fig. 1.1). The specimen should include full-thickness epidermis and superficial dermis. Forceps may be used to gently hold the specimen toward the end of the procedure. If the specimen is especially small and/or thin, a drop of India ink can be placed on it before transfer to the container. This will reduce the possibility of it being

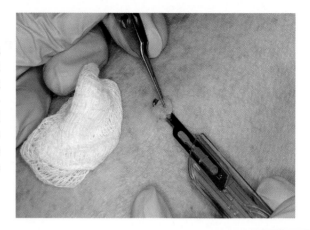

Fig. 1.1 Shave biopsy

lost and will in no way interfere with pathologic interpretation.[7] The specimen is then transferred to the specimen container using the wooden end of the cotton-tipped applicator, sparing the forceps from being immersed in formalin. Artifactual changes occur if the specimen is not immediately and continually immersed in the formalin.[8]

Hemostasis is achieved; the biopsy site is then dressed with an application of antibiotic ointment or petrolatum and covered with a dressing, which is changed daily for approximately 1 week until the area has healed.

Complications

Hypopigmentation and cutaneous depression may occur if the biopsy is deep.

Saucerization

In a saucerization biopsy, a razor blade is bent into a U-shape to obtain a deeper specimen. This is indicated for the biopsy of lesions reaching the upper to mid-dermis such as SCC, atypical nevi, and superficial melanoma.

Equipment

A Gillette super blue razor blade and the same equipment as used with the shave biopsy.

Technique

After cleansing and infiltrating the area as previously described, the razor blade is bent into a U-shape and held between the first two fingers of the dominant hand. A sawing motion is used to obtain the biopsy (Fig. 1.2). Hemostasis and aftercare are as previously described.

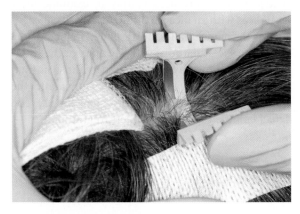

Fig. 1.2 Saucerization biopsy. Note hair is taped down to facilitate biopsy

Punch Biopsy

Punch biopsy is useful for providing information about the depth of tumor invasion as, depending on the size of punch used, it can reach subcutaneous tissue. A 3-mm punch is standard, but 6- and 8-mm punches may be used for removing larger lesions. A 2-mm punch is most often used for cosmetically sensitive areas such as the face, but may be harder to process in the lab and may give an inadequate sample for diagnostic purposes, especially for melanocytic neoplasms.

Equipment

Sterile punch, scissors, toothed forceps, suture.

Technique

Prepare and anesthetize the skin as previously described. Next, stabilize the skin by stretching it taut between the first and second fingers of the nondominant hand and perpendicular to the relaxed skin tension lines, creating an oval defect, which can be more easily sutured. Holding the punch between the first two fingers of the dominant hand, place the punch on the area to be biopsied so that all edges of the punch are in contact with the skin. Rotate the punch between the fingers pressing down at the same time until there is a loss of resistance and the subcutaneous plane is reached (Fig. 1.3a, b). Next remove the punch and gently lift the specimen; divide its base and place it in the bottle of formalin. If forceps are used, avoid "crush" artifact by squeezing the specimen as this will cause cellular distortion and complicate histological interpretation.[8]

For esthetic and sometimes hemostatic purposes, the biopsy site may be sutured with 6-0 interrupted epidermal sutures on the face and 5-0 interrupted sutures on the body. The suture can be removed at 7–10 days depending on the site.

Biopsy Care

The biopsy site should be cleansed with water daily and covered with an antibiotic ointment and an occlusive dressing. The incidence of contact

Fig. 1.3 (a) Punch biopsy. Note that punch is perpendicular to relaxed skin tension lines. (b) Punch biopsy specimen is gently handled with toothed forceps to prevent crush artifact

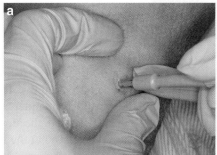
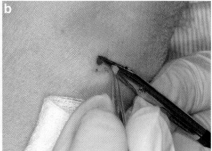

dermatitis is fairly high with certain antibiotics and this should be taken into consideration. Leaving the wound open to air or allowing it to dry will slow re-epithelialization and may not optimize the final appearance.[9]

Incisional Biopsy

The incisional biopsy is used when a larger specimen is needed for examination, such as with large pigmented lesions where total excision is not easily achieved.[8]

Equipment

Sterilized instruments including a #15 scalpel, toothed forceps, scissors, suture, and gauze.

Technique

Prepare and anesthetize the skin as previously described. Holding the scalpel perpendicular to the skin, make a fusiform incision through the middle of the lesion down to the subcutaneous tissue (Fig. 1.4). Remove the specimen and suture the wound.

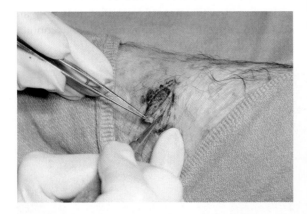

Fig. 1.4 Incisional biopsy of a suspected melanoma

Complications

Wound infection, hematoma, dehiscence, scar, and pigmentation change.

Wedge Biopsy

Wedge biopsies are used mainly to examine ulcer tissue—as with an ulcerated squamous cell cancer—and, as the name implies, are designed to include the normal tissue at the edge with the apex of the triangle pointed into the affected tissue. Thus, normal and affected tissue are sampled together and the resulting specimen is therefore pie-shaped. The defect can then be sutured or left to granulate.

Complications

Bleeding, infection, scar, pigmentation change.

Excisional Biopsy

Excisional biopsies are defined as extending completely around the clinically apparent lesion, extending to fat, and not necessarily intended to remove the entire lesion. If the intent is to remove the entire lesion, then it is more correctly called an "excision," since the term "biopsy" means that the intent is not to remove the entire lesion. Excisional biopsies are performed for atypical nevi or when melanoma is suspected, for example.[10]

Technique

The borders should be marked before the excision (Fig. 1.5). Once the area has been prepped and anesthetized as above, the specimen can be removed in a fusiform manner including subcutaneous tissue.[11,12] To aid the dermatopathologist, a suture should be placed at the 12 o'clock position to orient the lesion with respect to the patient's body. This is

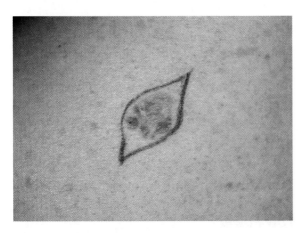

Fig. 1.5 A border is outlined around a suspected melanoma prior to excisional biopsy

cannot be overemphasized. A log-book should list the date, patient's name, biopsy site and result, and plan. As biopsy results are received, patients should be notified of these results, which should be notated in the log book along with whether the plan has been accomplished. If the biopsy is lost, it is necessary to inform the patient of the situation and to discuss whether or not to re-biopsy the lesion site. There is no credible legal defense if a skin cancer later develops at or near the site of a lesion that had been previously biopsied, the specimen lost, and the patient never informed of the situation.[7]

only necessary for larger lesions if the surgeon wants to know more precisely where involved margins are present. For smaller excisions, or those where the entire area would be excised anyway if margins are involved, detailed orientation may not be needed. It is advisable to place this suture before excising the specimen to avoid misorientation.

Complications

Bleeding, hematoma, infection, scar.

Biopsy Log

It is the physician's responsibility to track the biopsy and a protocol must be established within the practice. The importance of a biopsy log

Interpretation of Results

In general, biopsies obtained by skin punch and elliptical excision provide better specimens than shave or tangential biopsies, as punches and ellipses are more likely to sample deeper dermis or subcutaneous tissue. There are general advantages and disadvantages to each biopsy type (see Table 1.2).

The least helpful type is that obtained by curettage. The many fragments are often difficult to process and the pathologist has to reconstruct the lesion mentally. In some instances curettage may be helpful and it is then preferable for the clinician to shave the bulk of the lesion, send this to pathology, and then to curette the base, discarding the curetting.

Elliptical excisions, both incisional and excisional, are preferred for the complete removal of dysplastic nevi and malignant skin cancers.

Table 1.2 Advantages and disadvantages of punch, shave, and excisional biopsies

Punch	Shave	Ellipse
+ Better depth	– Often too superficial	+ Best depth
– Maximum 8-mm width	+ Easier to remove wider lesions	– Difficult closing wide lesions
– More scarring (unless sutured)	– Less scarring (unless deep shave)	– Most scarring
– More equipment	– Least equipment	– Most equipment
– Slower	+ Fastest	– Slowest
– Little skill needed	+ Little skill needed	– More skill needed

+ advantage; – disadvantage
Reproduced from Rapini (1994) with permission from Elsevier.

Tissue Orientation and Margin Evaluation

The first step in examination of a skin biopsy specimen consists of gross cutting and orientation of the specimen referred to as "grossing."[13] All pathology reports need to contain a description of the gross examination and should specify the orientation of the specimens so that the margins seen on the slides can be appropriately determined. In addition, the report should state whether all the tissue was embedded ("in toto"), or if "representative sections" were embedded.

Various decisions may be made at grossing and for this reason the process is performed by a physician or a trained pathology assistant. One decision is to determine if representative sections are to be made, just which tissue will be examined, and which will be discarded. Another grossing question to consider is whether or not to bisect punch biopsy specimens. If punches are bisected, and assuming the clinician placed the most specific changes in the center, then the initial sections are more likely to exhibit the desired histological changes. Sometimes, however, the two bisected pieces may become fragmented, difficult to orientate, or even lost. In addition, important sections may be discarded in the process of "facing" where initial incomplete sections are removed from the paraffin block and discarded until the block becomes smooth, providing complete sections. In contrast, a larger unbisected punch specimen may be easier to handle, but initial sections may be non-specific, and deeper levels may be needed.

Various tissue orientation errors can occur. Sectioning the surface of a punch specimen will result in a round specimen with epidermis present around most of the edges, and curling of a thin shave biopsy specimen will produce a section with epidermis on opposite sides. Tangential sectioning may give the false impression of hyperkeratosis, hypergranulosis, acanthosis, an apparent increase of melanocytes and basal cells, or perhaps even a pseudomalignancy.[14]

Reporting of Surgical Margins

Some pathologists like to state on the report that re-excision is indicated. However, this may place the clinician in a bind, feeling that they have to either follow this suggestion or explain why they do not in the chart. Other clinicians may appreciate this advice.

It is preferable, though not always practical, for pathologists to measure precisely in millimeters how close a tumor is to the margin, than to use terms such as tumor "near," "adjacent to," or "approximating the margin."

Fundamental Slide Interpretation

Low Power

Initially, the number of sections can be examined by holding the glass slide up to the light without the microscope. Next, low-power microscopy should be used to scan the slide; indeed, many cases can be diagnosed with low power alone. It is important to examine all sections or at least to look at each type of section that is different grossly.

Develop a Method for Examining Skin Specimens

It is important to develop a method for systematically examining skin sections. Some dermatopathologists will start in the dermis and later examine epidermal changes, while others will start in the stratum corneum and proceed down to the subcutaneous tissue. While observation of the architectural pattern will allow for preliminary diagnosis, it is also important to view cytologic detail such as mitoses and pleomorphism with high power. When looking at a clinical lesion, one should try to imagine what it would look like under the microscope. Similarly, when looking at a pathology specimen, one should imagine what the lesion would look like clinically. A differential diagnosis is then considered by focusing on individual histologic changes together.

Knowing the Clinician

Since many clinicians often have customary treatment habits, it is often possible for the dermatopathologist to guess who performed the biopsy or excision. The best clinicians modify their treatment based on the clinical circumstances. The following are extreme examples presented with the hope that some readers may recognize a pattern and, if applicable, maybe modify their behavior.

Too Small a Sample

Some clinicians send curettage fragments or shave biopsy specimens in more than 95% of the specimens they submit. Pieces of epidermis are submitted when there is clinical suspicion of dermal tumor. It is useful for the dermatopathologist to know if the biopsy procedure was followed by electrodesiccation and curettage, for instance, because then it is not necessary for them to comment on margin involvement. In this way confusion can be avoided if the patient gets another opinion from another physician who is unaware that the lesion has been destroyed.

Too Aggressive a Sample

Other clinicians may be too aggressive in the size of the specimen they submit for diagnosis. One instance of this would be the excision to adipose tissue of seborrheic keratoses. Another example would be the excision of a suspected melanoma with 1–3-cm margins, which is later found to be benign.

Two-Step Management

Some clinicians always perform a biopsy and then have the patient return for a subsequent visit. There are instances where one should biopsy first rather than initiate treatment at the first visit, for instance in the case of a facial lentigo maligna. However there are other instances, such as a patient with nevoid basal cell nevus syndrome, where it is expedient and cost-effective to initiate treatment in one step when possible.

Too Little or Too Much Information

It is important to include all relevant history or diagnosis on the laboratory requisition slip. Extensive differential diagnoses are not helpful.

Know Your Laboratory

It may be helpful for clinicians to recognize certain characteristics of their dermatopathology laboratory.

One Diagnosis Only

Some pathologists may provide one specific diagnosis and rarely comment on other possible diagnoses. For some of these pathologists, there may be little doubt about the diagnosis of a Spitz nevus. For others, the possibility of a melanoma is considered with less dogmatic certainty.

Too Many Diagnoses

Some pathologists may not give a specific diagnosis, instead providing a descriptive one such as: "perivascular and spongiotic dermatitis." While these pathologists will often not elaborate further, others may at least give a differential diagnosis.

Summary

In conclusion, it behooves the clinician to understand the various biopsy techniques and to be aware of the clinical indications for each type. In the interest of patient care, accurate communication between the clinician and the dermatopathologist is important. It is also helpful for clinicians to recognize certain characteristics of the dermatopathology laboratory they use.

References

1. Rapini RP. Obtaining a skin biopsy and interpreting the results. *Dermatol Clin.* 1994;12:83–91.
2. Olbricht S. Biopsy techniques and basic excisions. In: Bolognia JL, Jorizzo JL, Rapini RP, eds. *Dermatology.* 2nd ed. London: Elsevier; 2008:2209–2225.
3. Stewart JH, Cole GW, Klein JA. Neutralized lidocaine with epinephrine for local anesthesia. *J Dermatol Surg Oncol.* 1989;15:1081–1083.
4. Armstrong RB, Nickhols J, Pachance J. Punch biopsy wounds treated with Monsel's solution or a collagen matrix: a comparison of healing. *Arch Dermatol.* 1988;122:546–549.
5. Ackerman B. Shave biopsies: the good and right, the bad and wrong. *Am J Dermatopathol.* 1983;5:211–212.
6. Harvey DT, Fenske NA. The razor blade biopsy technique. *Dermatol Surg.* 1995;21:345–347.
7. Silvers DN. The "lost" skin biopsy: how to prevent it. *Cutis.* 1999;64:355–356.
8. Ackerman AB. Biopsy why, where, when, how. *J Dermatol Surg.* 1975;1:21–23.
9. Eaglstein WH. Moist wound healing with occlusive dressings: a clinical focus. *Dermatol Surg.* 2001;27:175–181.
10. Salopek TG, Slade J, Marghoob AA, et al. Management of cutaneous malignant melanoma by dermatologists of the American Academy of Dermatology. I. Survey of biopsy practices of pigmented lesions suspected as melanoma. *J Am Acad Dermatol.* 1995;33:441–450.
11. Dunlavey E, Leshin B. The simple excision. *Dermatol Clin.* 1998;16:49–64.
12. Zitelli JA. Tips for a better ellipse. *J Am Acad Dermatol.* 1990;2:101–103.
13. Rapini RP. Comparison of methods for checking surgical margins. *J Am Acad Dermatol.* 1990;123:288–294.
14. Rapini RP. Pitfalls of Mohs micrographic surgery. *J Am Acad Dermatol.* 1990;22:681–686.

Chapter 2
Topical Therapies for Nonmelanoma Skin Cancers

Abel Torres and Tejas Desai

Introduction and Background

As the incidence of nonmelanoma skin cancer (NMSC) continues to rise, topical therapies will be used with increasing frequency. Topical therapies are currently being utilized as primary or adjunctive means of treating an array of NMSCs. Although surgical therapies, such as Mohs Micrographic Surgery (MMS), remain the mainstay for tumor removal, topical therapy provides an alternative treatment modality for some skin cancer patients as well as serving as a useful adjunct to surgery. Topical therapies may also increase overall efficacy by treating subclinical lesions and identifying asymmetrical growth of NMSCs. In some patients, such as high-risk surgical candidates, they can be used to avoid surgery altogether or to minimize the extent of surgery. Topical therapies may also be helpful in a diagnostic manner. In instances where biopsy sites are equivocal, topical therapies may facilitate tumor identification prior to surgery.

Transplant patients who suffer from multiple NMSCs may benefit from topical therapies. In patients who have problems with scarring, in general, topical therapies may be preferable to other methods of treatment for NMSCs.

The most commonly employed topical therapies include imiquimod, 5-fluorouracil (5-FU), and diclofenac. Each agent has a different pharmacologic action and may be used in various settings. In this chapter, the authors will discuss the aforementioned drugs and their application in such situations as adjunctive therapy and in the transplant population for instance. (Refer to Chapter 17 for further details.) Drawing from their own myriad of experience with each topical therapy for NMSCs, they will provide tips to optimize treatment outcome.

Imiquimod

Mechanism of Action

Imiquimod is a type of imidazoquinolone, a class of immuno-enhancing drugs that mobilize several cytokines having antiviral and tumoricidal properties.[1] This cytokine recruitment occurs due to a highly intricate process involving the innate and adaptive immune response through cell surface receptors named toll-like receptors (TLR), located on macrophages, Langerhans cells (LC), and dendritic cells. TLR activation also causes a host of secondary effects at the molecular and cellular levels that are not fully understood.[2] It is beyond the scope of this chapter to explain the voluminous information that exists regarding the mechanism of action of imiquimod and the reader is advised to seek out the references in this regard.[3–23] Imiquimod's complex mechanism of action may be represented by Fig. 2.1.[8]

Side Effect Profile

Side effects of imiquimod may be local and/or systemic in nature. Common local reactions include

D.F. MacFarlane (ed.), *Skin Cancer Management*, DOI 10.1007/978-0-387-88495-0_2,
© Springer Science+Business Media, LLC 2010

Fig. 2.1 Schematic of imiquimod's primary mechanism of action. Imiquimod upregulates the Th1-lymphocyte-mediated immune response, releasing a host of cytokines that are tumoricidal in nature. In addition, the Th2 immune response is blocked by the actions of IL-4. Reprinted with permission from Gaspari AA and Sauder DN[8]

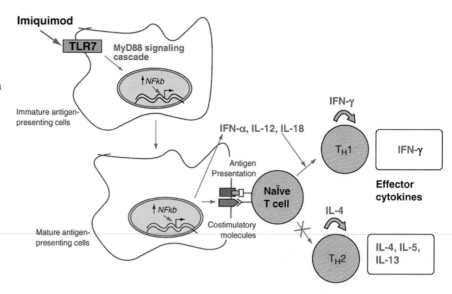

erythema, erosion, pain of differing levels, and ulceration in severe cases[24] (Fig. 2.2). Dyschromia, namely hyperpigmentation and hypopigmentation, is not uncommon, although usually mild due to postinflammatory changes. A vitiligo-like hypopigmentation has been reported on several occasions, but whether this is a local or systemic immunologic response remains to be explained.[25–28] Rare local reactions that have been reported include drug-induced pemphigus involving the vulva and aphthous ulcers, presumably caused by various proinflammatory cytokines such as IFN-α and TNF-α.[29–32] Acute urinary retention and eruptive epidermoid cysts are reported nonimmunologic

effects of imiquimod.[33,34] Since imiquimod is an immunostimulant of TH_1 cell-mediated immunity, exacerbation of preexisting conditions that are mediated by this part of the immune system may theoretically occur. Multiple studies reporting a worsening of psoriasis following imiquimod application have been noted.[35–37] Moreover, exacerbation of atopic dermatitis and HLAB-27 spondyloarthropathy have also been observed after imiquimod therapy.[38,39] Systemic symptoms have also been reported with the use of imiquimod. These likely occur when proinflammatory cytokines enter the systemic circulation, but could also be the result of an individual hypersensitivity response to these cytokines. Albeit uncommon, these systemic signs and/or symptoms are likened to a "flu-like" illness, including malaise, fatigue, anorexia, weight loss, diarrhea, postural hypotension, and elevated erythrocyte sedimentation rate.[40] Upon discontinuation of imiquimod these systemic symptoms usually abate quickly.

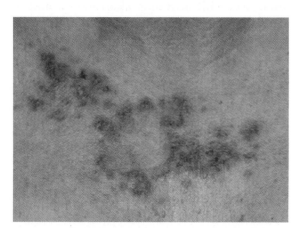

Fig. 2.2 An acceptable reaction after imiquimod use. Note the subclinical areas represented by the satellite erythematous regions

5-Fluorouracil

Mechanism of Action

5-FU is a structural analog of thymine that competes for enzymes with normal metabolites such as uracil.[12] It is eventually incorporated into ribonucleic acid (RNA), and inhibits deoxyribonucleic acid (DNA) formation by covalent bonding that blocks thymidylate synthetase.[12] This ultimately results in cell death since protein synthesis is halted. No immunomodulatory mechanisms have been identified, but one has to wonder if the intense inflammation caused by 5-FU contributes to tumor regression, or whether the release of antigens by destroyed tumor cells results in an accompanying immunologic response to the metabolic effect.

Side Effect Profile

Like imiquimod, 5-FU may cause intense erythema, erosions, and ulceration depending on the dose and schedule (0.5–5%). There is always potential for problems with wound healing on areas of the body such as the lower extremity should extensive ulceration occur. However, 5-FU most likely depends on the presence or absence of proliferating cells in NMSCs and sun damage, and not on the body's ability to mount an immune response. True allergic contact dermatitis to 5-FU is rare, and is more commonly triggered by a preservative or vehicle compounded within the cream.[41–46]

Systemic responses to topical 5-FU are rare but have been known to occur in patients with variable deficiency of dihydropyrimidine dehydrogenase, an enzyme critical for metabolism.[47–50] The French Summary of Product Characteristics (SPC) on topical 5-FU states that while absorption of drug by intact skin is very low, absorption by damaged skin is higher.[51] One should reconsider applications of 5-FU to large body surface areas, since damaged skin could theoretically result in increased absorption with possible systemic effects.

Of note, no phase II trials have been performed for topical 5-FU.[52] Once the initial safety of the study drug has been confirmed in Phase I trials, Phase II trials are performed on larger groups (*n* = 20–300) and are designed to assess how well the drug works, as well as to continue Phase I safety assessments in a larger group of volunteers and patients.[52] However, Phase III trials have been conducted to demonstrate its efficacy on multiple occasions.

Diclofenac

Mechanism of Action

Topical diclofenac is a nonsteroidal anti-inflammatory drug (NSAID) primarily used to treat actinic keratoses. The main target of NSAIDs seems to be the inhibition of cyclooxegnase-2 (COX-2), which is overexpressed in several epithelial tumors and catalyzes the synthesis of prostaglandins.[53] In addition to having anti-inflammatory activities, diclofenac may inhibit neoplastic cell proliferation by inducing apoptosis.[53] Pathways such as bcl2 and caspase-8 are similar to the ones seen in imiquimod-induced apoptosis.

Side Effect Profile

Numerous reports of allergic contact dermatitis to topical diclofenac have been observed.[54–56] These eczematous eruptions occurred as a result of diclofenac itself and less with the vehicle or preservative. One case involved a marked photoallergy from topical use as well.[57] The importance of clinical suspicion is imperative since an eczematous dermatitis may mimic local reactions induced by topical diclofenac.

Topical Therapy for Actinic Keratoses— The Loma Linda Experience

Monotherapy for Actinic Keratoses

Actinic keratoses are induced by ultraviolet light radiation (UVR), and, in some cases, appear to develop directly into full-blown squamous cell carcinomas (SCCs).[58] Topical therapies including imiquimod, 5-FU, and diclofenac may offer some advantages over traditional modalities. Several major trials demonstrating the clinical efficacy of each topical treatment as monotherapy for AKs have been well studied.[59–78] Table 2.1 summarizes the authors' approach for each topical therapy. Figure 2.3 illustrates the concept of field therapy.

Table 2.1 Topical agents for actinic keratoses

5% Imiquimod	5-Fluorouracil	Diclofenac
– Apply as field therapy over a cosmetic unit such as one cheek or forehead (approx. 25 cm^2) until the skin retains a shiny appearance.	– Apply 0.5–5% formulation as field therapy in the same manner as for imiquimod (Fig. 2.3).	– Apply as field therapy (similar to imiquimod and 5-FU) twice-daily to any part of the body for 90 days.
– Start application 3x/weekly for 4 weeks.	– Apply twice-daily to treat face and scalp for 3 weeks, and up to 4 weeks for the trunk and extremities.	– The side effect profile is more favorable than the other topicals, but its efficacy is inferior.
– If no response after 2 weeks, dosing may be increased to once-daily until an acceptable reaction occurs and treat for 4 weeks (Fig. 2.2).	– If the reaction becomes brisk, titration to once-daily or every other day may be required.	– May be used for patients with contraindications to other topical therapies, patient preference, or if unable to follow-up as recommended.
– After a 4-week treatment, monitor for residual lesions.	– Keratolytics may be added to reach beyond the depth of a thick lesion.	– Contact or irritant dermatitis may be more common and should be monitored.
– Repeat treatment if lesions are still persistent after a 4-week rest period post-treatment.	– Large body surface area application is discouraged due to potential risk of absorption on damaged skin.	
– If no response even after daily dosing, treatment should continue through 16 weeks per package insert.	– Topical steroids may be used to calm the treated area since the mechanism does not solely depend on the inflammatory response.	
– For hypertrophic lesions, keratolytics or retinoids may be added to aid penetration.	– Topical anesthetics are not regularly implemented since pain can help to titrate therapy and to avoid contact sensitization.	
– A thorough history and physical is important to screen for preimmunologic conditions that are cell mediated and could be exacerbated.	– Infection may be assessed in the same manner for imiquimod.	
– Topical steroids are not used to reduce inflammation since they may inhibit imiquimod's mechanism of action.		
– The regular use of topical antibiotics is not encouraged unless infection is diagnosed.		
– Infection may be present if the area feels worse than it looks or there is purulence or signs of cellulitus.		

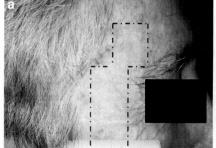 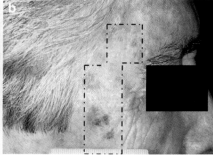

Fig. 2.3 Field therapy depicting the presence of hidden AKs. (**a**) Baseline AK lesion count of 5, (**b**) but after imiquimod therapy commenced, 10 visible lesions appeared in the area treated

Imiquimod vs. 5-Fluorouracil for AKs

One study compared the efficacy of imiquimod (three times per week for 4 weeks), 5% 5-FU (twice-daily for 4 weeks), and cryosurgery (20–40 s per lesion) for treating actinic keratoses.[79] Twenty-five patients were randomized to treatment with imiquimod, 5-FU, or cryosurgery, and displayed 68, 96, and 85% initial clearance, respectively.[79] However, after a 12-month follow-up, a higher rate of recurrent and new lesions was seen in the 5-FU and cryosurgery arms.[79] Furthermore, imiquimod-treated lesions showed greater histologic clearance.[79] In addition, the imiquimod-treated group was judged to have the best cosmetic outcomes.[79] The study concluded that although imiquimod did not clear AK lesions as well as 5-FU or cryosurgery initially, sustained clearance over time was greater.

A more recent article compared the clinical efficacy between imiquimod (twice weekly for 16 weeks) and topical 5-FU (twice-daily for 2–4 weeks) applied as field therapy.[80] Five percent 5-FU was more effective than imiquimod in exposing what were presumed to be subclinical AK lesions, reducing the final count (total AK count declined during the 24-week study by 94% vs. 66%, $p < 0.05$), achieving complete clearance (incidence of 84% vs. 24% by week 24, $p < 0.01$), and attaining clearance rapidly.[80] Tolerability was similar except erythema, initially significantly higher with 5-FU than imiquimod, then resolved rapidly and was significantly lower than imiquimod by week 16.[80]

Finally, a meta-analysis examined 10 different studies comparing topical 5-FU and imiquimod with various treatment doses and schedules.[81] Results suggested that imiquimod may have higher efficacy than 5-FU for AK lesions located on the face and scalp.[81]

The authors practice a case-based approach for each patient with AK lesions. In obvious situations, any patient who cannot tolerate one topical medication, for various reasons, may benefit from the other. It is important to obtain a pertinent medical history with respect to cellular immunity. As described before, imiquimod has induced exacerbation of preexisting dermatoses (i.e., psoriasis) and even systemic conditions (i.e., spondyloarthropathy).[35–37] In these cases, topical 5-FU may be a better option. On the other hand, it has been demonstrated that 5-FU may increase gene mutations, with an unclear implication of the risk of carcinogenesis.[66] Although the mechanism and its significance need to be further investigated, this encourages the authors to use imiquimod when it is a viable option.

From an efficacy standpoint, the authors find 5-FU and imiquimod to have similar short-term efficacy after corresponding treatment protocols. Our experience is similar to studies that suggest imiquimod maintains clearance longer than its counterparts for AKs.[66]

Imiquimod and 5-FU Combination Therapy

Combination therapy involving the use of topical 5-FU and imiquimod has been used successfully to optimize therapy. Each topical treatment has a different mechanism of action, thereby affecting AK lesions uniquely. Thus, imiquimod and 5-FU may be utilized to complement each other. This is analogous to the use of different chemotherapeutic agents for the treatment of cancer in order to maximize outcomes. In one study, patients applied 5-FU in the morning and imiquimod each night to their lesions daily for 1 week each month over the course of 3 months.[82] The study concluded that this combination was a relatively more rapid and convenient form of therapy compared to each medication alone.[82] The authors' approach to combination therapy is described in Table 2.2.

Table 2.2 Combination therapy for actinic keratoses

Combination therapy with imiquimod and 5-FU is intended for patients that fail monotherapy or have numerous lesions.
Two suggested regimens
1. Separate: Start with a course of imiquimod daily for 1 month immediately followed by a course of 5-FU twice-daily for 1 month.
2. Concurrent: Start alternating daily treatment with imiquimod and 5-FU until a sustained inflammatory response for 1 month is observed.

Combination Therapy with Cryotherapy

AK lesions may not completely clear with topical treatments alone. Topical therapy may be used in conjunction with cryosurgery and serve to clear residual AK lesions. The opposite technique may be performed as well, by starting with topical therapy first, then destroying remaining lesions with liquid nitrogen. One randomized trial has demonstrated the use of 0.5% 5-FU subsequent to cryotherapy to be more statistically significant than using liquid nitrogen therapy alone for the head and neck.[83] Another open-label study depicted the advantages of applying 0.5% 5-FU prior rather than after cryotherapy, with significant decreases from the baseline number of AK lesions.[84] On a comparable level, topical diclofenac used sequentially with cryotherapy has been shown to reduce the number of AK lesions more effectively than cryosurgery alone.[85] The authors' approach to combination therapy with cryosurgery is described in Table 2.3.

Table 2.3 Combining topical therapy with cryosurgery for actinic keratoses

Even when failing to clear lesions, topical therapies may highlight lesions to a more confined distribution, facilitating cryosurgery.
Two suggested regimens:
Treat hypertrophic lesions with liquid nitrogen followed 1–2 weeks later with monotherapy with either imiquimod or 5-FU for 1 month or diclofenac for 90 days.
Treat with initial monotherapy with either imiquimod, 5-FU, or diclofenac followed by liquid nitrogen to residual lesions. (Caveat: If lesions are clinically suspicious or persist after both monotherapy and liquid nitrogen, consider a biopsy to rule out invasive SCC.)

Cost and Treatment Choice for AKs

While the authors focus on the clinically ideal treatment, they realize that cost will always be a limiting factor when treating AKs and impacts direct patient care and compliance. On a strict cost basis, diclofenac is the most inexpensive and imiquimod is the costliest to treat AK lesions.[86]

Diclofenac may be the most economical but not the most clinically effective. It has been postulated that 5% 5-FU is the most cost-effective topical agent and should be used as a first-line therapy for clearance of AK lesions.[87] Yet, what also has to be considered is the cost of failed therapy. Since many authors have observed sustained clearance with imiquimod, it may be more economical than 5-FU if repeated treatments are required. Similarly, pharmaceutical companies often provide discount coupons/cards that can help minimize the cost differential, and this should be considered when making cost a central factor in decision-making. Ultimately the clinical picture should guide the decision-making process.

Topical Therapy and Nonmelanoma Skin Cancer—The Loma Linda Experience

BCC Monotherapy

Imiquimod

Currently, imiquimod 5% is approved by the US Federal Drug Administration (FDA) for the treatment of biopsy-confirmed, primary superficial basal cell carcinomas (BCCs) in immunocompetent adults, with a maximum tumor diameter of 2.0 cm, located on the trunk (excluding anogenital skin), neck, or extremities (excluding hands and feet).[88] Imiquimod may be more desirable when surgical methods are medically less appropriate and patient follow-up can be reasonably assured, imiquimod is also FDA-indicated.[88] Imiquimod in other treatment settings may be considered as an off-label application and is not FDA approved. Yet, several studies have shown that lesions larger than 2 cm, above the neck lesions, and nodular BCCs can be effectively treated with imiquimod.[89–98] Moreover, multiple trials have established imiquimod's clinical efficacy for superficial and nodular BCCs, and to a lesser degree more aggressive BCC varieties (Figs. 2.4 and 2.5).[89–98] As with AK lesions, the authors do not advocate one schedule over another and simply present the data and our experience to help the provider prescribe imiquimod for their patients in the most effective manner.

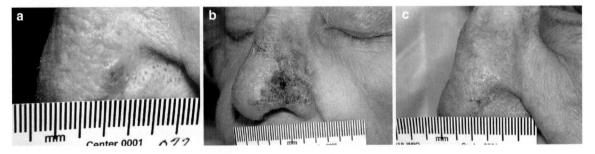

Fig. 2.4 (**a**) A nodular BCC (**b**) treated with imiquimod (**c**) showing complete clinical and histologic devolution. However, we do not treat nodular BCC with imiquimod as monotherapy. We pretreat nodular types with imiquimod prior to surgery, but sometimes clearance may be achieved. We view this as a serendipitous event

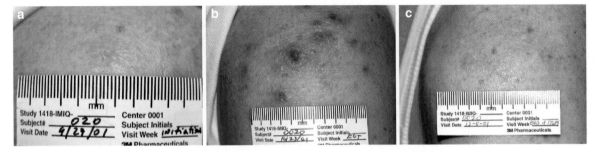

Fig. 2.5 (**a**) Imiquimod treatment for superficial BCC on the left upper arm. (**b**) Note the intense reactionary radius that extends up to the left upper shoulder. Clinically, this is not observed prior to treatment. (**c**) Note that although a biopsy may have appeared to remove the entire superficial BCC on clinical examination, imiquimod may nonetheless incite a robust reaction, which we hypothesize is because of remaining cellular atypia that cannot be detected with the naked eye

The package insert states that imiquimod cream should be applied to the lesion including a 1-cm margin five times per week for 6 weeks prior to normal sleeping hours and left on the skin for at least 8 h.[88] In a study looking at 5% imiquimod cream as an adjunct modality to Mohs Micrographic Surgery for the treatment of basal cell carcinoma, Torres noted results were similar for patients using imiquimod five times weekly for 4 and 6 weeks.[98] Thus, the authors instruct patients to apply imiquimod five times per week for at least 4 weeks, aiming for 6 weeks if patients are able to tolerate the medication.[98] The package label recommendation is emphasized. See Table 2.4 for the authors' approach to BCC monotherapy.

A question frequently raised by clinicians is how do we assure that tumor has been completely removed after using topical imiquimod? In reality, this is no different than knowing if tumor has been removed after any treatment. There is a probability that tumor can recur even after excision, and the prudent course is always to clinically follow the patient for evidence of recurrence. The negative predictive value for imiquimod treatment has been reported to be 88.9–93% in various trials.[92,97,99] This may be defined as the probability of a negative clinical assessment confirmed as being histologically free of tumor, suggesting that most clinicians would be able to determine if a treated superficial BCC has responded appropriately to imiquimod. Longer follow-up periods may be warranted to decrease the amount of false-positive evaluations while observing for evidence of recurrence. It has been our experience that no perfect follow-up time period exists, and the key is to assure that follow-up occurs.

Table 2.4 Topical therapies for nonmelanoma skin cancers

	BCC	SCC
5% Imiquimod	– Apply 5x/weekly as field therapy for at least 4 weeks, aiming for 6 weeks if tolerable. – If no response after 2 weeks, daily dosing may be implemented. – Sometimes twice-daily dosing is required to incite a reaction, but caution should be taken, decreasing to daily or 5x/weekly once signs of an initial response ensue. – If clinical response has occurred but residual tumor is left behind, consider further treatment. – A 4-week wait period can be allowed to pass before a clinical evaluation for residual tumor. – If tumor seems to be evident, then we encourage a biopsy or procedural therapy. – If the clinical assessment is ambiguous, then the option is given to the patient to re-biopsy or follow-up after 4-weeks for re-evaluation. – For BCCs other than superficial types, we do not routinely recommend monotherapy, unless a patient is bedridden, terminal or unable to tolerate a procedure (Fig. 2.4). – Warn patients with extensive, adjacent photodamage to expect severe reactions from epidermal field carcinogenesis (Fig. 2.5).	– For SCCs other than superficial in situ types, we do not routinely recommend monotherapy, unless a patient is bedridden, terminal or unable to tolerate a procedure. – Surgery should remain the mainstay for treatment for all SCC types, including Bowen's disease, KAs, and superficial or invasive SCCs. – The main goal of monotherapy is to shrink the tumor prior to surgery. – Apply 5x/week to daily dosing from 4 up to 16 weeks planning for a need to extend therapy to 16 weeks since SCCs may take longer for the immune response to occur. – The patient should follow up intermittently during the 16 weeks to monitor for clinical improvement. – Regular topical use for treating KAs is not encouraged due to conflicting clinical and histopathologic diagnosis.
5% 5-Fluorouracil	– It is FDA approved regardless of site. – Extensive studies evaluating efficacy are lacking. – Used by authors if there are apparent contraindications to imiquimod. – The recommended dose is twice-daily for 3–6 weeks up to 10–12 weeks, in the amount sufficient to cover the lesion as per package insert.	– For SCCs other than superficial types, we do not routinely recommend monotherapy, unless a patient is bedridden, terminal or unable to tolerate a procedure. – The authors typically reserve its use as an adjunct to surgery for all SCC types, including Bowen's disease, KAs, and superficial or invasive SCCs. – Bowen's disease is the prototypical SCC type. 5-FU may be considered for monotherapy when surgery is not the best option for a patient. – For Bowen's disease, twice-daily dosing for up to 10–12 weeks is recommended. – Regular topical use to treat KAs is not encouraged due to conflicting clinical and histopathologic diagnosis.

5-Fluorouracil

If a physician is going to use 5-FU for the treatment of superficial BCCs, then the recommended dose and strength according to the FDA labeling is 5% applied twice-daily in an amount sufficient to cover the lesions.[100] Treatment should be continued for at least 3–6 weeks. Therapy may be required for as long as 10–12 weeks before the lesions are obliterated.[100]

Refer to Table 2.4 for the authors' approach to the treatment of BCC with 5-FU.

SCC Monotherapy

There is growing evidence topical agents may serve as noninvasive treatment for SCC, including

Bowen's disease, but neither imiquimod nor 5-FU have an FDA indication for this use. Topical treatments may benefit patients with large bowenoid lesions that may be ill defined or extend beyond the clinical margin. Likewise, inoperable, invasive SCC may sometimes be treated with topical therapy to minimize morbidity or as palliative treatment. Generally, surgery should remain the mainstay of treatment for SCC, especially in light of the increased risk of metastasis and perineural invasion with SCC. However, a few clinical trials and a host of case reports have demonstrated efficacy with imiquimod and topical 5-FU.

Imiquimod

The authors approach to the treatment of SCC with imiquimod is described in Table 2.4. Our treatment goal is a minimum of 4 weeks up to 16 weeks, although 20-week regimens have been utilized.[101]

The authors err on the side of caution when treating SCCs with imiquimod. We reserve imiquimod and other topical treatments for those that cannot tolerate surgery or for those where we use it as adjunctive preparation prior to surgery. Since Bowen's disease may exemplify subclinical extension beyond clinical margins, these lesions tend to be ill defined. Imiquimod as well as other topical treatments may redefine the true clinical margins under most circumstances, sometimes clearing tumor completely. The authors consider complete clearance as a fortuitous incident, with the main goal being to shrink the tumor before surgery. Part of our reasoning for this approach is that we have seen residual SCC with perineural invasion in some patients who appeared to have significant clinical clearance following imiquimod use.

5-Fluorouracil

Topical 5-FU is not FDA indicated for the treatment of SCC, but has been used with varying treatment success. The authors prefer to use topical 5-FU for the treatment of SCC in combination with a surgical modality. Bowen's disease is one type of SCC for which we would consider using 5-FU as monotherapy when surgery is not the best option for the patient. We find that invasive SCC responds to 5-FU poorly, but can be effective in clearing up AK lesions and SCC in situ surrounding invasive SCCs, thus making the subsequent surgery much less cumbersome for the patient.

Combination Topical Therapy

Topical combination therapy with 5-FU and imiquimod has been used for Bowen's disease in patients who have failed monotherapy with either treatment.[102] It has been our experience that lesions on extremities and digits have the propensity to be thicker, where topical treatments may be more difficult to penetrate. It seems the effects of 5-FU are enhanced in the presence of several cytokines induced by imiquimod, producing a synergistic reaction whose mechanisms are not fully understood.[102]

Topical Therapy as a Surgical Adjunct to NMSC

Preoperative Topical Therapy

The authors prefer to use imiquimod or 5-FU preoperatively to help reduce the size of the surgical defect and thus repair (Table 2.5). Although Mohs Micrographic Surgery may approach cure rates up to 99%, incomplete removal can occur (see Chapter 11 for further details). Imiquimod has been used as adjuvant treatment following incomplete MMS for large, mixed type BCCs.[103]

The authors investigated the mean reduction in tumor size after using imiquimod prior to MMS.[99] Subjects applied imiquimod five times weekly for 2, 4, or 6 weeks in this double-blind, randomized, placebo-controlled study.[99] The 4- and 6-week treatment groups demonstrated statistically significant reductions in pretreatment versus post-treatment tumor target areas and surgical wound sizes. Yet, they also found cure rates were equal for both the 4-and 6-week treatment groups at

Table 2.5 Preoperative topical therapies as surgical adjuncts for NMSCs

5% Imiquimod	5% 5-Fluorouracil
– Goal is to facilitate excision by reducing tumor load/size and complete clearance is a fortuitous incident.	– Goal is to facilitate excision by reducing tumor load/size and the patient should be aware of this.
– May be used to clean up actinic and in situ changes adjacent to invasive SCC or BCC, helping to better delineate the neoplasm.	– Used if there is a contraindication to imiquimod for debulking of tumor.
– Dosing schedule is similar to treating superficial BCC as monotherapy.	– May be used to clean up actinic and in situ changes adjacent to invasive SCC or BCC, helping to better delineate the neoplasm.
– A wait of 2–4 weeks is encouraged before MMS or excision so inflammation may subside and the excised tissue can be better evaluated histologically.	– When treating invasive SCC, it is important to confirm the location prior to surgery since the skin lesions may at times appear to have clinically resolved.

approximately 66%. Thus, presurgical adjunctive therapy with imiquimod resulted in elimination of surgery in two-thirds of the patients, or a reduction in the extent of surgery in the remaining poor responders (Fig. 2.6).

If there is a contraindication to imiquimod, then topical 5-FU may be considered to reduce tumor size. Anecdotally, before imiquimod was available, the authors used 5-FU for the preoperative treatment of SCC. The logic behind this is SCC often occurs in sun-damaged skin with a background of actinic keratoses. SCC in situ and superficial forms of SCC may also be difficult to differentiate from AK. The authors found that often the entire SCC cleared with 5-FU use, but even when the SCC did not clear, a substantial part of the AK and/or SCC in situ component resolved making the final surgery smaller and easier. It is important to confirm the location of the SCC when using this approach so that surgery can be performed in the appropriate area. The authors emphasize to patients that this is adjunctive, and surgery is recommended to ensure the tumor has been removed appropriately.

Intraoperative Topical Therapy

It has been reported that 30–47% of NMSCs located on the head and neck that were treated with electrodesiccation and curettage (ED&C) are associated with residual tumor.[104–106]

It is the authors' experience that using imiquimod with curettage without electrodesiccation for nodular and/or superficial BCC patients may induce at least equivalent cure rates to curettage and electrodesiccation with better cosmetic results.[107] In this study, 57 nodular and superficial BCCs were curetted without electrodesiccation. A week later, imiquimod 5% cream was initiated once-daily five times per week for 6 weeks. At 1-year follow-up, 0 of the 57 BCCs treated had clinical recurrences. Cosmetic results were deemed to be very good to excellent, and depicted superior cosmetic outcomes when compared to curettage and electrodesiccation.[107] See Table 2.6 for the authors' approach. Figure 2.7 compares the cosmetic results of curettage with electrodesiccation and curettage with imiquimod cream. In addition, electrodesiccation has a potential for interaction with implantable

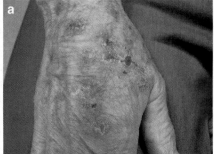 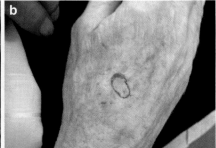

Fig. 2.6 (**a**) A biopsy proven SCC with surrounding actinic damage. After pretreatment with 5-FU, the area was considerably debulked for MMS. (**b**)The *circle* represents the SCC site

Table 2.6 Intraoperative topical therapies as surgical adjuncts for NMSCs

Curettage followed by imiquimod may facilitate tumor clearance and improve overall cosmesis and cure rate
Curettage without electrodesiccation may serve as a vehicle for maximal imiquimod penetration to help remove remaining cellular atypia.
Curettage without electrodesiccation is performed, then the patient waits for 1 week, followed by imiquimod 5x/weekly for 6 weeks, titrating up or down as discussed for monotherapy for superficial BCCs.
The patient may return for a clinical evaluation 4 weeks after completing imiquimod.
The same rules apply as if it were being used as monotherapy, performing a re-biopsy if the BCC appears to be present, or clinical observation if tumor presence or absence is ambiguous to interpret.
This procedure is not recommended for SCCs, since they may portend more aggressive behavior unless the patient is deemed a candidate for electrodesiccation and curettage.

cardiac and neurologic devices.[108–110] Patient satisfaction is much higher postoperatively when using imiquimod rather than electrodesiccation. The cost of the latter approach is a consideration when choosing the appropriate treatment modality. The average cost of curettage and imiquimod cream is greater than treatment with excision if patients use each imiquimod packet once.[111] In practice, most patients apply multiple applications from each packet, which substantially decreases the cost of this treatment and in many cases makes it less expensive than excision.[111]

Postoperative Topical Therapy

There is scant data to prove if postoperative use of imiquimod or 5-FU prevents recurrence, however, in theory it would seem logical that use of these topicals may serve to benefit patients with tumors that have high chance of recurrence. In addition, imiquimod or 5-FU treatment may address discontinuous growth patterns and perineural spread susceptible to recurrence after surgery. It is our opinion that imiquimod may facilitate the clearance of remaining tumor in high-risk lesions successfully due to its unique immunomodulatory mechanism.

Unusual Situations/Complications/ Variations

Problematic Areas

Lips

Diclofenac is an FDA-approved treatment for AK lesions of the lip.[77] Cure rates with 90 days of diclofenac have been shown to be similar when applied to skin after a 30-day follow-up.[112] Furthermore, the tolerability profile of diclofenac would appear to lend itself well, especially when treatment decisions involve cosmetic appearance during and subsequent to therapy.[112] An isolated study also illustrated that topical diclofenac after 6 weeks of therapy may improve this condition with minimal adverse events.[113]

Topical 5-FU has been used to treat isolated lip AKs as well as diffuse actinic damage of the lower lip.[114] Although it produced considerable

Fig. 2.7 (**a**) Curettage with imiquimod consistently appears to induce pink, flat scars that tend to fade quickly. (**b**) Electrodesiccation and curettage may cause atrophic or hypertrophic cicatrices, depending on a patient's skin type

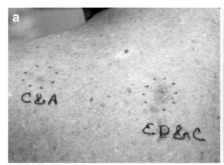
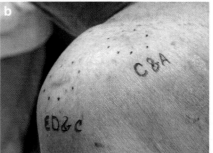

temporary discomfort, final results in one study proved excellent, with recurrences in only 2 of 12 patients.[114] The mean length of therapy was 12 days applying topical 5-FU every other day up to once-daily, and patients were clear up to an average of 22 months. Actinic cheilitis has also been treated with imiquimod three times weekly for 4–6 weeks.[115] All 15 patients showed clinical clearing of their actinic damage at 4 weeks after discontinuation of imiquimod. Sixty percent of patients experienced a moderate to marked increased local reaction consisting of increased erythema, induration, erosions, or ulcerations, which in some cases continued through the period of therapy.[115]

The authors contend that topical therapies have an important role in the treatment of lip AKs and actinic cheilitis. Although topicals may result in uncomfortable side effects during treatment, they may help avoid more aggressive forms of therapy such as carbon dioxide laser ablation. In addition, topical therapies may "biologically image" and discern malignant lesions from more benign varieties, especially in this area at high risk for metastasis. These medications may obviate the need for biopsies if clinical success ensues after their use. The authors' suggested approach in this regard is described in Table 2.7.

Eyelids

Eyelid BCCs have been treated with success with imiquimod on numerous occasions according to smaller published studies.[116–118] We have treated two patients with eyelid lesions that at 5 years out have shown no recurrence. However, this is an off-label use and the safety profile would have to be further investigated before we could advocate the regular use of imiquimod for eyelid lesions.

Avoiding the use of 5-FU near the eye, especially the conjunctiva, may be wise since multiple cases of ectropion have been reported.[119–121] Other ocular side effects include a transient keratitis, erythema, and irritation.[122] As a result, we do not promote the use of 5-FU on or near the conjunctival margin, medial, or lateral canthi. The degree of irritation may be exaggerated in these areas, and cicatricial ectropion has been reported.[119]

Table 2.7 Pearls for topical treatment of lip AKs/actinic cheilitis

5% Imiquimod	5-Fluorouracil
– Initially, twice-weekly application is employed.	– 5% formulation is used every other day, then increased gradually to daily after a week, and finally twice-daily after 2 weeks as tolerated.
– Careful and slow titration increasing to daily treatment may be required if no evident reaction occurs after 1–2 weeks.	– Once the patient develops a reaction, it is recommended the patient stays with that regimen or steps down to the prior dosing scheme to prevent a severe dermatitis and possibly subsequent discontinuation.
– If any type of response is experienced, then the patient is highly encouraged to continue with that schedule or the previous schedule.	– An antiviral agent may be prescribed to prevent herpes labialis, if there is a history of HSV but is not an absolute.
– An antiviral agent may be prescribed to prevent herpes labialis, if there is a history of HSV but is not an absolute.	– Strong clinical suspicion for a more invasive process is imperative, especially if persistent after several treatment cycles.
– If lesion is persistent after several treatment cycles, suspect a more invasive process.	– If after 4 weeks of therapy there is no reaction, the topical agent can be switched to imiquimod or diclofenac.
– If after 4 weeks of therapy there is no reaction, the topical agent can be switched to 5-FU or diclofenac.	– If no response with either medication, treatment is discontinued and procedural therapy is recommended such as surgical excision or MMS.
– If no response with either medication, treatment is discontinued and procedural therapy is recommended such as surgical excision or MMS.	

Penis

No randomized trials exist to determine the true value of imiquimod for Bowen's disease of the penis. However, multiple cases have been treated with imiquimod and various dose regimens have been implemented.[123–125] Bowenoid papulosis has been successfully treated with imiquimod, illustrating the medication's antiviral properties.[126] In some instances, a penectomy may have been prevented with the use of topical imiquimod for an invasive SCC.[127] Our experience has been that topical imiquimod has been moderately efficacious for SCC in situ lesions of the penis, including erythroplasia of Queyrat and bowenoid papulosis. We find that topical imiquimod prior or subsequent to surgery should be tried as an adjunct, although not FDA approved, for SCC in situ of the penis to prevent more invasive procedures that would not allow maximal sparing of tissue. The authors do not advocate the use of imiquimod as monotherapy for invasive SCC of the penis since locoregional spread or worse may occur as a result of the extensive blood supply. Although, Schroeder et al. depicted complete resolution of SCC in situ of the penis, a case-by-case assessment should be made before any patient receives imiquimod as the sole treatment for SCC in situ of the penis.[128]

Basal Cell Nevus Syndrome

Imiquimod has been used to treat many patients with Gorlin's syndrome and/or multiple acquired BCCs. The BCCs described in these studies were usually not only superficial but also included nodular and morpheaform types.[129–131] The authors have had success in a patient with a similar presentation (Fig. 2.8).

Transplant Patients

The treatment of NMSC in immunosuppressed patients has become a hot topic since the advent of imiquimod. This immunosuppression category includes chiefly organ transplantation recipients, but may include any patient that may be undergoing chemotherapy for various reasons (i.e., lymphoma). Some studies have observed up to a 2:1 ratio of SCC/BCC for organ transplant patients.[132] Although the concept of utilizing an immune booster to treat NMSC in patients that are immunosuppressed may seem counterintuitive, there lies growing evidence for a possible role of imiquimod in this group.[133–136] Ideally, if imiquimod were to be approved as monotherapy, it would benefit patients by obviating the undesirable effects of acitretin or multiple surgeries. Combination therapy of imiquimod and topical 5-FU has shown clinical efficacy in an open-label study.[135]

Currently, imiquimod is not FDA-approved for AK, SCC, or BCC in immunosuppressed patients.[89] The authors' current preference is to use topical 5-FU in this population since there is likely less risk of immune system interference; but results of a double-blinded European multicenter

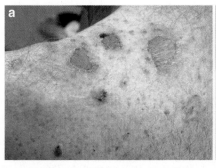
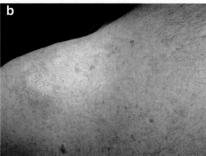

Fig. 2.8 (**a**) Multiple acquired superficial BCCs of the left posterior shoulder. These BCCs resolved after imiquimod 5x/weekly application for 6 weeks. (**b**) The residual pink, flat scar may erroneously cause false positive readings. We recommend close follow-up and observe for recurrence. These pink areas usually fade with time

trial suggest imiquimod should also be a viable option in these patients who often desperately need intervention.[137]

At present the authors would limit the extent of exposure to imiquimod when treating a transplant recipient. In a recent survey of dermatologists' treatment practices in organ transplant recipients, nearly half of the responders had used imiquimod as monotherapy for NMSCs in this patient population.[138]

Delayed Mohs Micrographic Surgery

For surgical candidates with BCCs whose MMS procedure is delayed (i.e., scheduling conflicts, travel, insurance issues), the authors employ imiquimod during the wait period (Table 2.8). The authors treat SCCs with some reservation, depending on the quality of the tumor. Although NMSCs are slowly evolving tumors, we feel that the benefits of treating with imiquimod outweigh the alternative of doing nothing. The behavior of untreated NMSCs may be unpredictable and pose potential risk of increasing in size or worse. When the patient is ready for MMS, the authors observe for residual disease, and often find the tumor has considerably decreased in size or even cleared.

Table 2.8 Pearls for using topical therapies when MMS is delayed

Patients with scheduling conflicts, travel, or insurance issues may use either topical agent in the same manner as recommended for preoperative use until they can return for surgery.
When the patient is ready for surgery, careful inspection for residual disease is performed using the prior confirmation of the pretreatment lesion site.
Even when the tumor appears to be cleared, a frozen biopsy may be helpful on the day of MMS to confirm tumor removal.
The biopsy may also help ensure the patient has used the topical adequately and tumor has cleared.

The Skip Area Controversy

Another issue often raised by physicians is whether skip areas will occur after presurgical treatment with imiquimod or 5-FU. In other words, can the topical therapy destroy only parts of the tumor so as to make it appear clinically resolved, when in fact it is now broken up into subclinical islands of tumor? To answer this question, the authors treated 72 BCCs with imiquimod, then performed MMS, followed by post-treatment biopsies.[139] The biopsies and MMS were performed regardless of whether tumor appeared clinically resolved post-treatment. Accuracy of the biopsies and MMS was established through the use of pretreatment plastic templates localizing the anatomic sites and tattooing of the treatment site. In this double-blind, randomized, placebo-controlled trial there were no statistically significant increases in skip areas in the treatment versus placebo arm. Five skip areas were identified in the placebo group, and one skip area was noted in the imiquimod arm. Thus, there does not seem to be any greater risk of leaving behind untreated BCC by topical pretreatment prior to surgery. The authors have not performed a similar study with 5-FU in the pretreatment of SCC. However, a review of more than 40 patients treated by the authors in this manner did not reveal any higher incidence of recurrence or complications in those tumors.

Summary

Topical therapies, including immunomodulators, provide a useful addition to the list of agents used to treat skin cancers and it behooves the physician to be conversant with their modes of action. As the incidence of NMSC continues to rise, further advances can be expected in immunomodulatory therapies.

References

1. Stanley MA. Imiquimod and the imidazoquinolones: mechanism of action and therapeutic potential. *Clin Exp Dermatol*. 2002 Oct;27(7):571–577.
2. Schon MP, Schon M. TLR7 and TLR8 as targets in cancer therapy. *Oncogene*. 2008 Jan;27(2):190–199.
3. Barnetson RC, Satchell A, Zhuang L, et al. Imiquimod induced regression of clinically diagnosed superficial basal cell carcinoma is associated with early infiltration by CD4

T cells and dendritic cells. *Clin Exp Dermatol.* 2007 Feb;29:639–643.

4. Wolf IH, Kodama K, Cerroni L, et al. Nature of inflammatory infiltrate in superficial cutaneous malignancies during topical imiquimod treatment. *Am J Dermatopathol.* 2007 Jun;29(3):237–241.

5. Stary G, Bangert C, Tauber M, et al. Tumoricidal activity of TLR7/8-activated inflammatory dendritic cells. *J Exp Med.* 2007 Jun;204(6):1441–1451.

6. Urosevic M, Dummer R, Conrad C, et al. Disease-independent skin recruitment and activation of plasmacytoid predendritic cells following imiquimod treatment. *J Nat Can Inst.* 2005 Aug;97(15):1143–1153.

7. Quatresooz P, Pierard GE. Imiquimod-responsive basal cell carcinomas and factor XIIIa-enriched dendrocytes. *Clin and Exp Derm.* 2003 Aug;28(Suppl 1):27–29.

8. Gaspari AA, Sauder D. Immunotherapy of basal cell carcinoma: evolving approaches. *Dermatol Surg.* 2003;29:1027–1034. Review PMID: 12974699, Wiley-Blackwell.

9. Torres A, Storey L, Anders M, et al. Microarray analysis of aberrant gene expression in actinic keratosis: effect of the Toll-like receptor-7 agonist imiquimod. *Br J Dermatol.* 2007;157:1132–1147.

10. Metcalf SA, Crowson N, Naylor M, et al. Imiquimod as an antiaging agent. *JAAD.* 2007 Mar;56(3):422–425.

11. Smith K, Hamza S, Germain M, et al. Does imiquimod histologically rejuvenate ultraviolet radiation-damaged skin? *Derm Surg.* 2007;33:1419–1429.

12. Wolverton SE. *Comprehensive Dermatologic Drug Therapy.* 1st ed. Philadelphia: Saunders Elsevier; 2001: 529–530.

13. Schon MP, Schon M. The small antitumoral immune response modifier imiquimod interacts with adenosine receptor signaling in a TLR7- and TLR8-independent fashion. *J Invest Dermatol.* 2006 Jun;126(6):1338–1347.

14. Schon MP, Schon M. Immune modulation and apoptosis induction: two sides of the antitumoral activity of imiquimod. *Apoptosis.* 2004 May;9(3):291–298.

15. Brouty-Boye D, Zetter BR. Inhibition of cell motility by interferon. *Science.* 1980;208:516–518.

16. Yoshida A, Anand-Apte B, Zetter BR. Differential endothelial migration and proliferation to basic fibroblast growth factor and vascular endothelial growth factor. *Growth Factors.* 1996;13:57–64.

17. Shousong C, Kun L, Toth K, et al. Persistent induction of apoptosis and suppression of mitosis as the basis for curative therapy with S-1, and oral 5-fluorouracil prodrug in a colorectal tumor model. *Clin Cancer Res.* 1999;5:267–274.

18. Fujita M, Kuwano K, Kunitake R, et al. Endothelial cell apoptosis in lipopolysaccharide-induced lung injury in mice. *Int Arch Allergy Immunol.* 1998;117:202–208.

19. Riedel F, Gotte K, Bergler W, et al. Expression of basic fibroblast growth factor protein and its down-regulation by interferons in head and neck cancer. *Head Neck.* 2000;22:183–189.

20. Reddy KB, Hocevar BA, Howe PH. Inhibition of G1 phase cyclin dependent kinases by transforming growth factor beta 1. *J Cell Biochem.* 1994;56:418–425.

21. Majewski S, Marczak M, Mlymarczyk B, et al. Imiquimod is a strong inhibitor of tumor cell-induced angiogenesis. *Int J Dermatol.* 2005;44:14–19.

22. Li VW, Li WW. Antiangiogenesis in the treatment of skin cancer. *J Drugs Dermatol.* 2008;7(Suppl 1):17–24.

23. Sidky Y, Borden E, Weeks C, et al. Inhibition of murine tumour growth by an interferon inducing imidazoquinolinamine. *Cancer Res.* 1992;52:3528–3533.

24. Medonca CO, Yates VM. Permanent facial hypopigmentation following treatment with imiquimod cream. *Clin Exp Dermatol.* 2006;31:721.

25. Al-Dujaili Z, Hsu S. Imiquimod-induced vitiligo. *Dermatol Online J.* 2007 May 1;13(2):10.

26. Brown T, Zirvi M, Cotsarelis G, et al. Vitiligo-like hypopigmentation associated with imiquimod treatment of genital warts. *J Acad Dermatol.* 2005;52(4):715–716.

27. Senel E, Seckin D. Imiquimod-induced vitiligo-like depigmentation. *Indian J Dermatol Venereol Leprol.* 2007 Nov–Dec;73(6):423.

28. Stefanki C, Nicolaidu E, Hadjivassilou M, et al. Imiquimod-induced vitiligo in a patient with genital warts. *J Eur Acad Dermatol Venerol.* 2006 Jul;20(6):755–756.

29. Campagne G, Roca M, Martinez A. Successful treatment of a high-grade intraepithelial neoplasia with imiquimod, with vulvar pemphigus as a side effect. *Eur J Obst Gynecol Reprod Bio.* 2003;109:224–227.

30. Chakrabarty AK, Mraz S, Geisse JK, et al. Aphthous ulcers associated with imiquimod and the treatment of actinic cheilitis. *JAAD.* 2005 Feb;52(2 Suppl 1):35–37.

31. Lin R, Ladd DJ Jr, Powell DJ, et al. Localized pemphigus foliaceus induced by topical imiquimod treatment. *Arch Dermatol.* 2004 Jul;140(7):889–890.

32. Mashiah J, Brenner S. Possible mechanisms in the induction of pemphigus foliaceus by topical imiquimod treatment. *Arch Dermatol.* 2005 Jul;141(7):908–909.

33. Marty CL, Randle HW, Walsh JS. Eruptive epidermoid cysts resulting from treatment with imiquimod. *Dermatol Surg.* 2005 Jul;31(7 Pt 1):780–782; discussion 782–783.

34. McQuillan O, Higgins SP. Acute urinary retention following self-treatment of genital warts with imiquimod 5% cream. *Sex Transm Infect.* 2004 Oct;80(5):419–420.

35. Fanti PA, Dika E, Vaccari S, et al. Generalized psoriasis induced by topical treatment of actinic keratosis with imiquimod. *Int J Dermatol.* 2006 Dec;45(12):1464–1465.

36. Gilliet M, Conrad C, Geiges M, et al. Psoriasis triggered by toll-like receptor 7 agonist imiquimod in the presence of dermal plasmacytoid dendritic cell precursors. *Arch Dermatol.* 2004 Dec;140(12):1490–1495.

37. Rajan N, Langtry JA. Generalized exacerbation of psoriasis associated with imiquimod cream treatment of superficial basal cell carcinomas. *Clin Exp Dermatol.* 2006 Jan;31(1):140–141.

38. Benson E. Imiquimod: potential risk of an immunostimulant. *Australas J Dermatol.* 2004 May;45(2):123–124.

39. Taylor CL, Maslen M, Kapembwa M. A case of severe eczema following use of imiquimod 5% cream. *Sex Transm Infect.* 2006 Jun;82(3):227–228.

40. Hanger C, Dalrymple J, Hepburn D. Systemic side effects from topical imiquimod. *NZ Med J.* 2005 Oct;118(1223):1–4.

41. De Berker D, Marren P, Powell SM, et al. Contact sensitivity to the stearyl alcohol in Efudix® cream (5-fluorouracil). *Contact Dermatitis*. 1992;26:138.

42. Farrar CW, Bell HK, King CM. Allergic contact dermatitis from propylene glycol in Efudix®. *Contact Dermatitis*. 2003;48:345.

43. Goette DK, Odom RB. Allergic contact dermatitis to topical fluorouracil. *Arch Dermatol*. 1977;113:1058–1061.

44. Meijer BUGA, de Waard-van der Spek FB. Allergic contact dermatitis because of topical use of 5-fluorouracil (Efudix® cream). *Contact Dermatitis*. 2007;57:58–60.

45. Tennstedt D, Lachapelle JM. Allergic contact dermatitis to 5-fluorouracil. *Contact Dermatitis*. 1987;35:124–125.

46. Yesudian PD, King CM. Allergic contact dermatitis from stearyl alcohol in Efudix® cream. *Contact Dermatitis*. 2001;45:313–314.

47. Harris BE, Carpenter JT, Diasio RB. Severe 5-fluorouracil toxicity secondary to dihydropyrimidine dehydrogenase deficiency. *Cancer*. 1991;68(3):499–501.

48. Johnson MR, Hageboutros A, Wang K, et al. Life threatening toxicity in a dihydropyrimidine dehydrogenase-deficient patient after treatment with topical 5-fluorouracil. *Clin Cancer Res*. 1999;5:2006–2011.

49. Takimoto CH, Lu Z-H, Zhang R, et al. Severe neurotoxicity following 5-fluorouracil-based chemotherapy in a patient with dihydropyrimidine dehydrogenase deficiency. *Clin Cancer Res*. 1996;2:477–481.

50. Tuchman M, Stoeckeler JS, Kiang DT, et al. Familial pyrimidinemia and pyrimidinuria associated with severe fluorouracil toxicity. *N Engl J Med*. 1985;313(4):245–249.

51. "Efudix®". In: "Dictionnaire Vidal" OVP Editions du Vidal, Paris, Thérapeutique dermatologique, Médecine-Sciences Flammarion, 2001:694.

52. Guidance for Industry, Investigators, and Reviewers Exploratory IND Studies U.S. Department of Health and Human Services. Food and Drug Administration. Center for Drug Evaluation and Research (CDER). http://www.fda.gov/cder/guidance/index.htm. Accessed Jan 9, 2009.

53. Fecker LF, Stockfleth E, Nindl I, et al. The role of apoptosis in therapy and prophylaxis of epithelial tumours by nonsteroidal anti-inflammatory drugs (NSAIDS). *Br J Dermatol*. 2007 May;156(Suppl 3):25–33.

54. Kerr OA, Kavanagh G, Horn H. Allergic contact dermatitis from topical diclofenac in Solaraze gel. *Contact Dermatitis*. 2002 Sep;47(3):175.

55. Kleyn CE, Bharati A, King CM. Contact dermatitis from 3 different allergens in Solaraze® gel. *Contact Dermatitis*. 2004;51(4):215–216.

56. Valsecchi R, Pansera B, Leghissa P, et al. Allergic contact dermatitis of the eyelids and conjunctivitis from diclofenac. *Contact Dermatitis*. 1996 Feb;34(2):150–151.

57. Kowalzick L, Ziegler H. Photoallergic contact dermatitis from topical diclofenac in Solaraze gel. *Contact Dermatitis*. 2006 Jun;54(6)348–349.

58. Ridky TW. Nonmelanoma skin cancer. *J Am Acad Dermatol*. 2007 Sep;57(3):484–502.

59. Alomar A, Bichel J, McRae S. Vehicle-controlled, randomized, double-blind study to assess safety and efficacy of imiquimod 5% cream applied once daily 3 days per week in one or two courses of treatment of actinic keratoses on the head. *Br J Dermatol*. 2007;157:133–141.

60. Jorizzo J, Dinehart S, Matheson R, et al. Vehicle controlled, double blind, randomized study of imiquimod 5% cream applied 3 days per week in one or two courses of treatment for actinic keratoses on the head. *J Am Acad Dermatol*. 2007 Aug;57(2):265–268.

61. Hadley G, Derry S, Moore R. Imiquimod for actinic keratosis: systematic review and meta-analysis. *J Invest Dermatol*. 2006;126:1251–1255.

62. Korman N, Moy R, Ling M, et al. Dosing with 5% imiquimod cream 3 times per week for the treatment of actinic keratosis. *Arch Dermatol*. 2005 Apr;141:467–473.

63. Lebwohl M, Dinehart S, Whiting D, et al. Imiquimod 5% cream for the treatment of actinic keratosis: results from two phase III, randomized, double-blind, parallel group, vehicle-controlled trials. *J Am Acad Dermatol*. 2004 May;50(5):714–721.

64. Persuad AN, Shamuelova E, Sherer D, et al. Clinical effect of imiquimod 5% cream in the treatment of actinic keratosis. *JAAD*. 2002 Oct;47(4):553–556.

65. Salasche SJ, Levine N, Morrison L. Cycle therapy of actinic keratoses of the face and scalp with 5% topical imiquimod cream: an open-label trial. *J Am Acad Dermatol*. 2002 Oct;47(4):571–577.

66. Stockfleth E, Meyer T, Benninghoff B, et al. A randomized, double blind, vehicle-controlled study to assess 5% imiquimod cream for the treatment of multiple actinic keratoses. *Arch Dermatol*. 2002 Nov;138:1498–1502.

67. Szeimes R, Gerritsen MJ, Gupta G, et al. Imiquimod 5% cream for the treatment of actinic keratosis: results from a phase III, randomized, double-blind, vehicle-controlled, clinical trial with histology. *J Am Acad Dermatol*. 2004 Oct;51(4):547–555.

68. Gupta AK, Weiss JS, Jorizzo JL. 5-fluorouracil 0.5% cream for multiple actinic or solar keratoses of the face and anterior scalp. *Skin Therapy Lett*. 2001 Jun;6(9):1–4.

69. Jury CS, Ramraka-Jones VS, Gudi V, et al. A randomized trial of topical 5% 5-fluorouracil (Efudix cream) in the treatment of actinic keratoses comparing daily with weekly treatment. *Br J Dermatol*. 2005 Oct;153(4):808–810.

70. Loven K, Stein L, Furst K, et al. Evaluation of the efficacy and tolerability of 0.5% fluorouracil cream and 5% fluorouracil cream applied to each side of the face in patients with actinic keratosis. *Clin Ther*. 2002 Jun;24(6):990–1000.

71. Robbins, P. Pulse therapy with 5-FU in eradicating actinic keratoses with less than recommended dosage. *J Drugs Dermatol*. 2002;1:25–30.

72. Simmonds WL. Double-blind investigation comparing a 1% vs 5% 5-fluorouracil topical cream in patients with multiple actinic keratoses. *Cutis*. 1973;12:615–617.

73. Weiss J, Menter A, Hevia O, et al. Effective treatment of actinic keratosis with 0.5% fluorouracil cream for 1,2, or 4 weeks. *Cutis*. 2002 Aug;70(Suppl 2):22–29.

74. Fariba I, Ali A, Hossein SA, et al. Efficacy of 3% diclofenac gel for the treatment of actinic keratoses: a randomized, double-blind, placebo controlled study. *Indian J Dermatol Venerol Leprol*. 2006 Sep–Oct;72(5):346–349.

75. Gebauer K, Brown P, Varigos G. Topical diclofenac in hyaluron gel for the treatment of solar keratoses. *Australas J Dermatol*. 2003 Feb;44(1):40–43.

76. Nelson C, Rigel D, Smith S, et al. Phase IV, open-label assessment of the treatment of actinic keratosis with 3. 0% diclofenac sodium topical gel (Solaraze). *J Drugs Dermatol*. 2004 Jul–Aug;3(4):401–407.

77. Pirard D, Vereecken P, Melot C, et al. Three percent diclofenac in 2.5% hyaluron gel in the treatment of actinic keratoses: a meta-analysis of the recent studies. *Arch Dermatol Res*. 2005 Nov;297(5):185–189.

78. Rivers JK, Arlette J, Shear N, et al. Topical treatment of actinic keratoses with 3.0% diclofenac in 2.5% hyaluronan gel. *Br J Dermatol*. 2002 Jan;146(1):94–100.

79. Krawthcenko N, Roewert-Huber J, Ulrich M, et al. A randomized study of topical 5% imiquimod vs. topical 5-fluorouracil vs cryosurgery in immunocompetent patients with actinic keratoses: a comparison of clinical and histological outcomes including 1 year follow up. *Br J Dermatol*. 2007;157 (Suppl 2):34–40.

80. Tanghetti E, Werschler WP. Comparison of 5% 5-fluorouracil cream and 5% imiquimod cream in the management of actinic keratoses on the face and scalp. *J. Drugs Dermatol*. 2007 Feb;6(2):144–147.

81. Gupta AK, Davey V, Mcphail H. Evaluation of the effectiveness of imiquimod and 5-fluorouracil for the treatment of actinic keratosis: critical review and meta-analysis of efficacy studies. *J Cutan Med Surg*. 2005 Oct;9(5):209–214.

82. Price NM. The treatment of actinic keratoses with a combination of 5-fluorouracil and imiquimod creams. *J Drugs Dermatol*. 2007 Aug;6(8):778–781.

83. Jorizzo J, Weiss J, Furst K, et al. Effect of a 1-week treatment with 0.5% topical fluorouracil on occurrence of actinic keratosis after cryosurgery: a randomized, vehicle-controlled clinical trial. *Arch Dermatol*. 2004 Jul;140(7):813–816.

84. Jorizzo J, Weiss J, Vamvakias G. One-week treatment with 0.5% fluorouracil cream prior to cryosurgery in patients with actinic keratoses: a double blind, vehicle-controlled, long-term study. *J Drugs Dermatol*. 2006 Feb;5(2):133–139.

85. Berlin J, Rigel D. A prospective double-arm, multicenter, open-label phase IV evaluation of the use of diclofenac sodium 3% gel in the treatment of AK lesions postcryosurgery. *J Am Acad Dermatol*. 2007 Jan P2303 poster presentation.

86. Gold MH. Pharmacoeconomic analysis of the treatment of multiple actinic keratoses. *J Drugs Dermatol*. 2008 Jan;7(1):23–25.

87. Kircik L, Earl M. Pharmacoeconomic evaluation of 5-fluorouracil for the treatment of actinic keratosis. *J Am Acad Dermatol*. 2007 Jan P2301 poster presentation

88. "Imiquimod" www.drugs.com, last updated December 11, 2008.

89. Beutner KR, Geisse JK, Helman D, et al. Therapeutic response of basal cell carcinoma to the immune response modifier imiquimod 5% cream. *J Am Acad Dermatol*. 1999 Dec;41(6):1002–1007.

90. Eigentler TK, Kamin A, Weide BM, et al. A phase III, randomized, open label study to evaluate the safety and efficacy of imiquimod 5% cream applied thrice weekly for 8 and 12 weeks in the treatment of low-risk nodular basal cell carcinoma. *J Am Acad Dermatol*. 2007 Oct;57(4):616–621.

91. Ezughah FI, Dawe RS, Ibbotson SH, et al A randomized parallel study to assess the safety and efficacy of two different dosing regimens of 5% imiquimod in the treatment of superficial basal cell carcinoma. *J Dermatolg Treat*. 2008;19(2):111–117.

92. Geisse J, Caro I, Lindholm J, et al. Imiquimod 5% cream for the treatment of superficial basal cell carcinoma: results from two phase III, randomized, vehicle-controlled studies. *J Am Acad Dermatol*. 2004 May;50(5):722–733.

93. Huber A, Huber JD, Skinner RB, et al. Topical imiquimod treatment for nodular basal cell carcinomas: an open label series. *Dermatol Surg*. 2004;30:429–430.

94. Marks R, Gebauer K, Shumack S, et al. Imiquimod 5% cream in the treatment of superficial basal cell carcinoma: results of a multicenter 6-week dose-response trial. *J Am Acad Dermatol*. 2001 May;44(5):807–813.

95. Schiessl C, Wolber C, Tauber M, et al. Treatment of all basal cell carcinoma variants including large and high-risk lesions with 5% imiquimod cream: histological and clinical changes, outcome, and follow-up. *J Drugs Dermatol*. 2007 May;6(5):507–513.

96. Schulze HJ, Cribier B, Requena L, et al. Imiquimod 5% cream for the treatment of superficial basal cell carcinoma: results from a randomized vehicle-controlled phase III study in Europe. *Br J Dermatol*. 2005 May;152(5):939–947.

97. Shumack S, Robinson J, Kossard S, et al. Efficacy of topical 5% imiquimod cream for the treatment of nodular basal cell carcinoma. *Arch Dermatol*. 2002 Sep;138:1165–1171.

98. Torres A, Niemeyer A, Berkes B, et al. 5% imiquimod cream and reflectance-mode confocal microscopy as adjunct modalities to Mohs micrographic surgery for treatment of basal cell carcinoma. *Dermatol Surg*. 2004 Dec;30(12 Pt 1):1462–1469.

99. Sterry W, Ruzicka T, Herrera E, et al. Imiquimod 5% cream for the treatment of superficial and nodular basal cell carcinoma: randomized studies comparing low-frequency dosing with and without occlusion. *Br J Dermatol*. 2002;147(6):1227–1236.

100. "5-fluorouracil" www.drugs.com, last updated December 11, 2008.

101. Smitha P, Raghavendra R, Sripathi H, et al. Successful use of imiquimod 5% cream in Bowen's disease. *Indian J Dermatol Leprol*. 2007 Nov–Dec;73(6):423–425.

102. Ondo Al, Mings SM, Pestak RM, et al. Topical combination therapy for cutaneous squamous cell carcinoma in situ with 5-fluorouracil cream and imiquimod cream in patients who have failed topical monotherapy. *J Am Acad Dermatol*. 2006 Dec;55(6):1092–1094.

103. Thissen MR, Kuijpers DI, Krekis GA. Local immune modulator (imiquimod 5% cream) as adjuvant treatment after incomplete Mohs micrographic surgery for large, mixed type basal cell carcinoma: a report of 3 cases. *J Drugs Dermatol*. 2006 May;5(5):461–464.

104. Salasche SJ. Curettage and electrodessication in the treatment of midfacial basal cell epithelioma. *J Am Acad Dermatol*. 1983;8:496–503.

105. Silverman MK, Kopf AW, Gladstein AH, et al. Recurrence rates of treated basal cell carcinomas, part 4: x-ray therapy. *J Dermatol Surg Oncol*. 1992;18:549–554.

106. Suhge d'Aubermont PC, Bennett RG. Failure of curettage and electrodessication for removal of basal cell carcinoma. *Arch Dermatol*. 1984;120:1456–1460.

107. Rigel DS, Torres AM, Ely H. Imiquimod 5% cream following curettage without electrodessication for basal cell carcinoma: preliminary report. *J Drugs Dermatol*. 2008;7(Suppl 1):15–16.

108. Nercessian OA, Wu H, Nazarian D, et al. Intraoperative pacemaker dysfunction caused by the use of electrocautery during a total hip arthroplasty. *J Arthroplasty*. 1998;13:599–602.

109. Levine PA, Balady GJ, Lazar HL, et al. Electrocautery and pacemakers: management of the paced patient subject to electrocautery. *Ann Thoracic Surg*. 1986;41:313–317.

110. Snow JS, Kalenderian D, Clasacco JA, et al. Implanted devices and electromagnetic interference: case presentations and review. *J Invasive Cardiol*. 1995;7:25–32.

111. Neville JA, Williford PM, Jorizzo JL. Pilot study using topical imiquimod 5% cream in the treatment of nodular basal cell carcinoma after initial treatment with curettage. *J Drugs Dermatol*. 2007 Sep;6(9):910–914.

112. Nelson CG, Spencer J, Nelson CG Jr. A single-arm, open label efficacy and tolerability study of diclofenac sodium 3% gel for the treatment of actinic keratosis of the upper and lower lip. *J Drugs Dermatol*. 2007 July;6(7):712–717.

113. Ulrich C, Forschner T, Ulrich M, et al. Management of actinic cheilitis using diclofenac 3% gel: a report of six cases. *Br J Dermatol*. 2007 May;156(Suppl 3):43–46.

114. Epstein E. Treatment of lip keratoses (actinic cheilitis) with topical fluorouracil. *Arch Dermatol*. 1977 July;113:906–908.

115. Smith KJ, Germain M, Yeager J, et al. Topical 5% imiquimod for the therapy of actinic cheilitis. *JAAD*. 2002 Oct;47(4):497–501.

116. Biasi MA, Giammaria D, Balestrazzi E. Immunotherapy with imiquimod 5% cream for eyelid nodular basal cell carcinoma. *Am J Ophthalmol*. 2005 Dec;140(6):1136–1139.

117. Choontanom R, Thanos S, Busse H, et al. Treatment of basal cell carcinoma of the eyelids with 5% topical imiquimod: a 3-year follow-up study. *Graefes Arch Clin Exp Ophthalmol*. 2007 Mar;245:1217–1220.

118. Leppala J, Kaarniranta K, Uuusitalo H, et al. Imiquimod in the treatment of eyelid basal cell carcinoma. *Acta Ophthalmol Scand*. 2007 Aug;85(5):566–568.

119. Galentine P, Sloas H, Hargett N, et al. Bilateral cicatricial ectropion following topical administration of 5-fluorouracil. *Ann Ophthalmol*. 1981 May;13(5):575–577.

120. Hecker D, Hacker SM, Ramos-Caro FA, et al. Temporary ectropion due to topical fluorouracil. *Cutis*. 1994 Mar;53(3):137–138.

121. Lewis JE. Temporary ectropion due to topical fluorouracil. *Int J Dermatol*. 1997 Jan;36(1):79.

122. Poothullil AM, Colby KA. Topical medical therapies for ocular surface tumors. *Semin Ophthalmol*. 2006 Jul–Sep;21(3):161–169.

123. Danielsen AG, Sand C, Weisman K. Treatment of Bowen's disease of the penis with imiquimod 5% cream. *Clin Exp Dermatol*. 2003 Nov;28(Suppl 1):7–9.

124. Micali G, Nasca MR, Tedeschi A. Topical treatment of intraepithelial penile carcinoma with imiquimod. *Clin Exp Dermatol*. 2003 Nov;28(Suppl 1):4–6.

125. Orengo I, Rosen T, Guill C. Treatment of squamous cell carcinoma in situ of the penis with 5% imiquimod cream: a case report. *J Am Acad Dermatol*. 2002 Oct;47(4):225–228.

126. Goorney BP, Polori R. A case of Bowenoid Papulosis of the penis successfully treated with topical imiquimod cream 5%. *Int J STD AIDS*. 2004 Dec;15(12):833–835.

127. Bernstein DI, Spruance SL, Arora SS, et al. Evaluation of imiquimod 5% cream to modify the natural history of herpes labialis: a pilot study. *Clin Infect Dis*. 2005 Sep 15;41(6):808–814. Epub 2005 Aug 10

128. Schroeder TL, Sengelmann RD. Squamous cell carcinoma in situ of the penis successfully treated with imiquimod 5% cream. *J Am Acad Dermatol*. 2002 Apr;46(4):545–548.

129. Ferreres JR, Macaya A, Jucgla A, et al. Hundreds of basal cell carcinomas in a Gorlin-Goltz syndrome patient cured with imiquimod 5% cream. *J Eur Acad Dermatol Venereol*. 2006 Aug;20(7):877–878.

130. Micali G, Lacarrubba F, Nasca MR, et al. The use of imiquimod 5% cream for the treatment of basal cell carcinoma as observed in Gorlin's syndrome. *Clin Exp Dermatol*. 2003 Nov;28(Suppl 1):19–23.

131. Stockfleth E, Ulrich C, Hauschild A, et al. Successful treatment of basal cell carcinomas in a nevoid basal cell carcinoma syndrome with topical 5% imiquimod. *Eur J Dermatol*. 2002 Nov–Dec;12(6):569–572.

132. Vereecken P, Monsieur E, Petein M, et al. Topical application of imiquimod for the treatment of high-risk facial basal cell carcinoma in Gorlin syndrome. *J Dermatolog Treat*. 2004 Apr;15(2):120–121.

133. Kovach BT, Stasko T. Use of topical immunomodulators in organ transplant recipients. *Dermatol Ther*. 2005;18:19–27

134. Prinz BM, Hafner J, Dummer R, et al. Treatment of Bowen's disease with imiquimod 5% cream in transplant patients. *Transplantation*. 2004;77(5):790–791.

135. Smith KJ, Germain M, Skelton H. Squamous cell carcinoma in situ (Bowen's disease) in renal transplant patients treated with 5% imiquimod and 5% 5-fluorouracil therapy. *Dermatol Surg*. 2001;27(6):561–564.

136. Vidal D, Alomar A. Efficacy of imiquimod 5% cream for basal cell carcinoma in transplant patients. *Clin Exp Dermatol*. 2004;29(3):237–239.

137. Ulrich C, Stockfelth E. Safety and efficacy of imiquimod 5% cream applied once daily 3 days per week for the treatment of actinic keratoses in immunosuppressed organ transplant recipients-results of a double blinded, European multicentre study. *J Am Acad Dermatol*. 2007 Jan P2304 poster presentation.

138. Clayton AS, Stasko T. Treatment of nonmelanoma skin cancer in organ transplant recipients: review of responses to a survey. *J Am Acad Dermatol*. 2003 Sep;49(3):413–416.

139. Torres A, Marra D, Desai TD, et al. Imiquimod 5% cream does not induce tumor skip areas in the topical treatment of basal cell carcinoma. Unpublished data.

Chapter 3
Chemical Peels for Precancerous Skin Lesions

Gary D. Monheit and Chad L. Prather

The use of chemoexfoliating agents to peel the epidermis and superficial dermis dates as far back as ancient Egypt, where sour milk baths were once used to soothe the skin. History has recorded the use of such chemicals as salt, sulfur, and various animal oils to exfoliate the skin for therapeutic and cosmetic purposes.[1] The modern era of chemoexfoliation began in the early twentieth century, with phenol used as a peeling agent for post-acne scarring.[2] Various strengths and combinations of phenol were originally applied, but severe facial scarring and cardiac toxicity limited the safety of phenol peels until the early 1960s when Baker and Gordon began to advocate the safe use of the formula still utilized today (Table 3.1).[3]

Table 3.1 The Baker-Gordon phenol formula

88% liquid phenol, USP	3 ml
Tap water	2 ml
Septisol liquid soap	8 drops
Croton oil	3 drops

Between 1940 and 1970, other exfoliating agents such as sulfur, resorcinol paste, salicylic acid, and solid carbon dioxide were popularized. These were often combined to cause a deeper dermal injury than could be achieved with any single agent alone. One such formulation that still enjoys widespread use, Jessner's solution, is composed of a combination of resorcinol, lactic acid, and salicylic acid in ethanol (Table 3.2).

Table 3.2 Jessner's solution

Resorcinol	14 g
Salicylic acid	14 g
85% lactic acid	14 g
95% ethanol (q.s.a.d.)	100 ml

In the 1950s and 1960s, trichloracetic acid (TCA) became a popular agent for superficial, medium, and deep chemical peeling. Low concentrations of TCA were found to cause light peeling, and more highly concentrated solutions of TCA were used to achieve greater peel depths. Yet 50% and higher concentrations of TCA commonly led to scarring and pigmentary complications. Such adverse effects directed a search for peeling agents and protocols that approached the efficacy of phenol and highly concentrated TCA, but demonstrated a higher level of patient safety with fewer complications. Brody first combined solid CO_2 ice with 35% TCA, which produced a deeper resurfacing procedure than low concentrations of TCA alone, but demonstrated fewer side effects than highly concentrated TCA.[4] This was soon followed by the Monheit combination of Jessner's solution and 35% TCA, and later the Coleman combination of glycolic acid and 35% TCA (Table 3.3).[5,6]

Over the past 30 years, myriad chemical formulations and peeling protocols have entered the market, mainly for the purposes of rejuvenating skin and reversing cutaneous photodamage. Although chemical peeling has a lengthy history, it remains one of the most common procedures performed today by dermatologists, and indeed

D.F. MacFarlane (ed.), *Skin Cancer Management*, DOI 10.1007/978-0-387-88495-0_3,
© Springer Science+Business Media, LLC 2010

Table 3.3 Agents used for medium-depth chemical peeling

Agent	Comment
40–50% TCA	Not recommended
Combination 35% TCA + solid CO$_2$ (Brody)	The most potent combination
Combination 35% TCA + Jessner's (Monheit)	The most popular combination
Combination 35% TCA + 70% glycolic acid (Coleman)	An effective combination
88% phenol	Rarely used

Table 3.4 Classification of chemical peeling methods

Superficial—Very Light	Low potency formulations of glycolic acid or other alpha-hydroxy acid
	10–20% TCA (weight-to-volume formulation)
	Jessner's solution (light application)
	<20% salicylic acid
	70% glycolic acid (must be neutralized)
	Jessner's solution (vigorous application)
Superficial—Light	25–30% TCA
	20–30% Salicylic acid
	Solid CO$_2$ slush
Medium-depth	88% phenol
	35–40% TCA
	Jessner's + 35% TCA
	70% glycolic acid + 35% TCA
	Solid CO$_2$ + 35% TCA
Deep	Unoccluded or occluded Baker-Gordon phenol peel
	TCA in concentrations >50%

* This classification represents an oversimplification. The depth of injury actually varies along a continuum according to method of application. However, it is helpful when discussing the various options with patients.

has enjoyed a resurgence in popularity over the past several years.[7] Salicylic acid, glycolic acid, Jessner's solution, lactic acid, resorcinol, TCA, phenol, and many other formulations are regularly employed for improving acne; for reversing actinic damage in the form of precancerous lesions, fine rhytides, and hyperpigmentation; and for rejuvenating the texture and appearance of aged or damaged skin.

Classification

Like all resurfacing modalities, chemical peeling entails the iatrogenic creation of a cutaneous wound. The peeling agent is essentially a chemical escharotic that damages the epidermal and dermal layers of the skin for therapeutic purposes. When properly performed, the partial wound of controlled depth will remove the damaged or precancerous epidermal and dermal layers and allow collagen remodeling and re-epithelialization from adjacent follicles, generating healthier skin. Diverse acidic and basic chemical agents are used to produce varying effects, though there are differences in their ability to destroy the cellular and non-cellular components of the epidermis and dermis. Their level of penetration, capacity for destruction, and degree of inflammation determine the depth, efficacy, and final result of the chemical peel.

Conceptually, chemical peels are best classified into very light, light, medium-depth, and deep categories (Table 3.4). Light superficial peels remove the stratum corneum portion of the epidermis only.

Since they do not destroy the viable cells of the epidermis, necrosis does not occur. However, inflammation may occur, and through exfoliation the epidermis may thicken and demonstrate qualitative regenerative changes. Destruction of the viable epidermis at any level below the stratum corneum defines a light chemical peel. Since regeneration of the epidermis must occur, a portion of epidermal actinic damage may be treated. However, the basal layer of the epidermis is not reliably and consistently reached with a light peel. For this reason, light peels are not the peels of choice for treating precancerous lesions. Full-thickness destruction of the epidermis and partial or full-thickness destruction of the papillary dermis constitutes a medium-depth peel.[8] For the treatment of actinic damage and precancerous lesions, the medium-depth chemical peel is considered the practitioner's peel of choice, as it demonstrates the greatest measure of efficacy without compromising an adequate degree of safety. Finally, a deep chemical peel is defined by destruction through the papillary dermis and into the mid-reticular dermis. Importantly, destruction at this depth begins to approach the level where the stem cells of the hair bulge, which serve as the reservoir for re-epithelialization, reside. Destruction by any means—chemical, mechanical, thermal, or other—deeper than the level of the hair bulge leaves no local source of epithelium, and may result in both prolonged healing and scarring. The margin of safety for deep chemical peels is compromised; thus only the well-qualified and experienced physician should use this modality of destruction and resurfacing.

The above classification of chemical peeling by depth has been validated by experience and has proven useful for selecting the appropriate approach for a particular degree of photoaging based on the desired level of cutaneous penetration. Mild, moderate, or severe actinic damage may thus be treated with agents that act very superficially, superficially, at a medium-depth, or deeply.

Indications

While very light and light peels may improve conditions such as acne and skin texture, and deep peels may help improve moderate rhytides and acne scarring, the chief indication for medium-depth chemical

peels is the reversal of actinic changes such as photo-damage, mild rhytides, precancerous actinic lesions such as actinic keratoses and Bowen's disease, and pigmentary dyschromias (Figs. 3.1, 3.2, 3.4, 3.5; Table 3.5).[9] When performed properly, medium-depth peels have a favorable benefit/risk profile for the reversal of actinic damage, including precancerous actinic keratoses. Solitary actinic keratoses are best treated by cryotherapy or other means. Yet when a large area beyond a few solitary lesions must be treated with a "field" approach, a medium-depth chemical peel ranks as a favorable choice. Though topical chemotherapy may be applicable, it is a prolonged treatment program with significant morbidity such as erythema, edema, scabbing, and crusting over a 6-week period. The medium peel is a single treatment with recovery within 1 week. Multiple actinic keratoses, or actinic keratoses on a background of significant solar damage, respond very well to medium-depth peels. Typically there is a clearance of existing

Table 3.5 Major indications for medium-depth chemical peels

Destruction of premalignant epidermal lesions—actinic keratoses
Resurfacing moderate to advanced photoaged skin (Glogau levels II, III)
Improving pigmentary dyschromias
Improving mild acne scars
Blending laser, dermabrasion, or deep chemical peeling in photoaged skin (transition from treated to non-treated area)

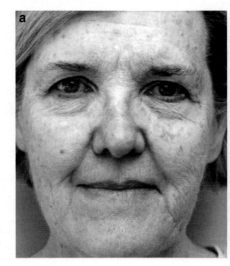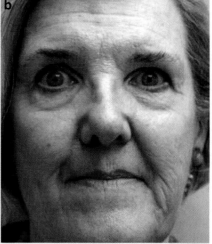

Fig. 3.1 (**a**) A 65-year-old female with rhytides and pigmentary dyschromia prior to medium-depth chemical peel. (**b**) Four weeks after Jessner's/35% TCA combination peel, with improvement in fine rhytides and dyschromia

Fig. 3.2 (**a**) A 63-year-old male with facial actinic damage and multiple actinic keratoses prior to medium-depth chemical peel. (**b**) Four weeks after Jessner's/35% TCA combination peel, with improvement in actinic damage and resolution of actinic keratoses

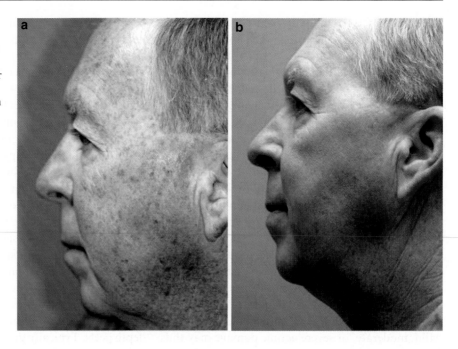

lesions and a delay in new lesion formation for several months to several years. The procedure is particularly well suited for the male with actinic keratoses that have required repeated removal with either cryosurgery or 5-fluorouracil chemoexfoliation. The entire face can be treated as a unit; or a subfacial cosmetic unit such as the forehead, temples, cheeks, or chin can be treated independently. Both active lesions and as-yet-undetected growths will be removed as the epidermis is sloughed. Advantages for the patient include a short recovery period—normally 7–10 days, with little post-healing erythema so the patient can return to work after the skin has healed. The medium-depth peel is a reliable treatment for full epidermal destruction and can be combined with cryosurgery and/or dermasanding for thicker resistant solitary lesions. Though photodynamic therapy has been used with less down time, it is less effective for destruction and prevention of actinic keratoses than the medium-depth chemical peel.

Contraindications

Several contraindications exist when choosing a medium-depth chemical peel for the treatment of actinic damage and precancerous keratoses rather than photodynamic therapy, dermabrasion, or topically applied medications such as 5-fluorouracil, imiquimod, or diclofenac (Table 3.6). As patient compliance during the recovery period is essential to avoiding permanent negative sequelae, a medium-depth peel should not occur in the setting of a poor physician–patient relationship. Likewise, a frank

Table 3.6 Contraindications to medium-depth chemical peeling

Absolute
Poor physician–patient relationship
Unrealistic expectations
Poor general health and nutritional status
Isotretinoin therapy within the last 6 months
Complete absence of intact pilosebaceous units on the face
Active infection or open wounds (such as herpes, excoriations, or open acne cysts)

Relative
Medium-depth or deep resurfacing procedure within the last 3–12 months
Recent facial surgery involving extensive undermining, such as a rhytidectomy
History of abnormal scar formation or delayed wound healing
History of therapeutic radiation exposure
History of certain skin diseases (such as rosacea, seborrheic dermatitis, atopic dermatitis, psoriasis, and vitiligo) or active retinoid dermatitis

discussion of what the peel can and cannot accomplish is necessary, and unrealistic expectations on the part of the patient must be recognized if present. Furthermore, poor general health and nutritional status will compromise wound healing and should also dissuade a consideration of a medium-depth chemical peel. Moreover, isotretinoin therapy within the previous 6 months has been associated with increased risk of scarring[10], and a chemical peel should be delayed until the patient is beyond 6 months of finishing a course of isotretinoin. Topical tretinoin, while not associated with an increased risk of scarring, will allow a greater depth of penetration. It is our practice to discontinue topical retinoids 2 weeks prior to a medium-depth chemical peel. Additionally, the presence of active infections or open wounds such as herpes simplex vesicles, excoriations, or open acne cysts should postpone the treatment until such conditions resolve. All patients with a history of herpes simplex virus I of the facial area should be premedicated with an antiviral agent such as acyclovir or valacyclovir and remain on prophylactic therapy for 10 days (Valtrex 500 mg BID × 10 days).

While not absolute contraindications, patients with overly sensitive, hyperreactive, or koebnerizing skin disorders such as atopic dermatitis, seborrheic dermatitis, psoriasis, or contact dermatitis may find their underlying disease exacerbated by a chemical peel. In particular, patients with rosacea typically develop an exaggerated inflammatory response to the peeling agents, which serves as a trigger factor for symptoms. A history of keloid formation should be screened for prior to chemical peeling. Likewise, patients with a recent history of extensive or major facial surgery, or those who have recently had a medium-depth peel in the preceding months should be evaluated closely with regard to risks and benefits. The collagen-remodeling phase of wound healing due to prior treatments is still underway in such patients, and an altered wound healing response may occur. Another important relative contraindication is a history of radiation therapy to the proposed treatment area. An absence of pilosebaceous units should serve as a harbinger that the area does not have the reserve capacity of follicular epidermal cells with which to repopulate.

Another consideration that may serve as a relative contraindication for medium-depth chemical

Table 3.7 Fitzpatrick's classification of skin types

Skin Type	Color	Reaction to Sun
I	Very white or freckled	Always burns
II	White	Usually burns
III	White to olive	Sometimes burns
IV	Brown	Rarely burns
V	Dark brown	Very rarely burns
VI	Black	Never burns

peeling is a higher Fitzpatrick skin type (Table 3.7). While Fitzpatrick skin types I and II are at low risk for post-resurfacing hyperpigmentation or hypopigmentation, types III through VI are at greater risk for these complications.[11] The authors will readily peel Fitzpatrick skin types I–III, cautiously peel types IV and V, and rarely or never peel type VI due to the high risk of permanent hypopigmentation. If concern exists over the possibility of permanent post-procedural pigmentary alteration, a test spot in an inconspicuous area such as under the chin or behind the ear may be performed to assess long-term cutaneous response.

Though purely epidermal precancerous growths such as actinic keratoses respond well to medium-depth chemical peels, cancerous growths that extend into the dermis do not respond fully. Basal cell carcinomas, squamous cell carcinomas, and malignant melanoma will not be sufficiently destroyed and will recur. Also, squamous cell carcinoma in situ and malignant melanoma in situ may extend through the pilosebaceous apparatus into the dermis beyond the reach of a medium chemical peel. All invasive carcinomas should be treated surgically.

Advantages

The advantages of chemical peeling as compared to other modalities used to treat precancerous lesions include a low cost, the ease of a single application, the ability to be performed in a routine treatment setting without the need for specialized equipment, and a reliable efficacy. The cost of most chemicals used for medium-depth peeling is far more economical than any laser treatment, photodynamic therapy, or topical medication used to treat actinic keratoses. Furthermore, only a single treatment session with a healing time of 7–10 days is required, rather than the several weeks to a few months required with topical medications such as 5-fluorouracil, imiquimod, or diclofenac. Additionally, chemical peeling may be performed in any office setting with routine dermatological supplies such as 2 × 2- or 4 × 4-inch gauze pads and cotton-tipped applicators, and does not require special equipment like that necessary with laser treatment or photodynamic therapy. And chemical peels are reliably efficacious. When performed properly on the correctly chosen patient, a medium-depth peel will usually produce sustained clearing of most precancerous lesions for a period of several months to several years. And, of course, chemical peeling gives the added cosmetic benefit of improving the appearance of photoaging skin.

Current Products Available

The original chemical of choice for a medium-depth peel was 50% trichloroacetic acid. It was felt to achieve acceptable results in ameliorating fine wrinkles, actinic damage, and preneoplastic keratoses. However, since TCA in strengths of 40% or higher was found to be more likely fraught with complications, particularly scarring, it has fallen out of favor as a single agent chemical peel.[12] The agents currently used most often for medium-depth chemical peeling include products combined with 35% TCA into three different regimens: (1) Jessner's solution with 35% trichloroacetic acid, (2) 70% glycolic acid with 35% TCA, and (3) solid carbon dioxide with 35% TCA. All three combinations have proven effective and safer than the use of 50% trichloroacetic acid alone.

The advantage of preceding 35% TCA with a lighter peeling chemical is that the TCA application and frosting are better controlled, so that the "hot spots" seen with higher concentrations of TCA, which can produce dyschromias and scarring, are not a significant problem. The authors' preference of Jessner's solution followed by 35% TCA is a relatively simple and safe combination. It is most effective for mild-to-moderate photoaging including pigmentary changes, lentigines, and epidermal growths

such as actinic keratoses, seborrheic keratoses, sebaceous hyperplasia, dyschromias, and fine rhytides. The authors' preferred medium-depth peel is dependent on three components for therapeutic effect: (1) degreasing, (2) Jessner's solution, and (3) 35% TCA. The amount of each agent applied determines the effectiveness of this peel. The variables can be adjusted according to the patient's skin type and the areas of the face being treated. It is thus the workhorse of peeling and resurfacing in our practices as it can be individualized for most patients we see.

Patient Selection

The most important factors to consider prior to performing a chemical peel for precancerous lesions are skin type and degree of photoaging. It is of utmost importance that the physician understands the patient's skin and its ability to withstand this damage, as patients with extensive photodamage require stronger peeling agents and often repeated applications of medium-depth peeling solutions to obtain therapeutic results. In general, Fitzpatrick skin types I and II, which often have the greatest degree of actinic damage and precancerous changes, also have the least risk for hypopigmentation or reactive hyperpigmentation after a medium-depth peel. Patients with type III through VI skin, however, have a greater risk for post-peel pigmentary hyper- or hypopigmentation and may need pre- and post-treatment with both sunscreen and bleaching to prevent these complications.[13]

Both the Glogau and Monheit systems of assessing photodamage are useful in matching the depth of chemical peel necessary in a particular patient.[13] The Glogau system (Table 3.8) categorizes the severity of photodamage into groups I through IV, representing mild, moderate, advanced, and severe photodamaged skin. These categories are devised to assist in guiding therapeutic intervention. Glogau categories II and III benefit most from medium-depth chemical peeling. Monheit and Fulton (Table 3.9) have also devised a system of quantifying photodamage using numerical scores that correspond with indicated rejuvenation programs.[14] A score of 10–14 in this system, as typically seen with precancerous lesions or a history of skin

Table 3.8 Glogau photoaging classification

Group I—Mild (typically age 28–35)	Little wrinkling or scarring
	No keratoses
	Requires little or no make-up
Group II—Moderate (age 35–50)	Eary wrinkling; mild scarring
	Sallow color with early actinic keratoses
	Little make-up
Group III—Advanced (age 50–65)	Persistent wrinkling or moderate acne scarring
	Discoloration with telangiectases and actinic keratoses
	Wears make-up always
Group IV—Severe (age 60–75)	Wrinkling: photo aging, gravitational, and dynamic
	Actinic keratoses with or without skin cancer or servere acne scars
	Wears make-up with poor coverage

cancer, calls for medium-depth chemical peeling. The patient may be shown his or her degree of photodamage during the consultation and the necessity for an individual peeling program.

Informed Consent

A thorough pre-treatment discussion is imperative. It allows the opportunity to discuss the risks and benefits, as well as to educate the patient on the expected time frame and course of recovery. It also allows the surgeon to assess the patient's goals and expectations so that the procedure is performed only on appropriate candidates. Those who are not willing to tolerate an acute event followed by 7–10 days of desquamation and 3–4 weeks of erythema are best served by other treatments. The patient must fully understand the potential benefits, limitations, and risks of the procedure; and an informed consent must be signed. Pre-treatment photographs are also highly recommended to allow for post-treatment comparison.

Setup

All necessary reagents for a Jessner's + 35% TCA medium-depth peel may be obtained in bulk for multi-application use from leading dermatologic suppliers.

The standard setup includes a facial cleanser such as Septisol, acetone, Jessner's solution, TCA, cotton-tipped applicators, 2 × 2- and 4 × 4-inch gauze pads, and cool-water soaks for patient comfort (Fig. 3.3).

> When ordering TCA, one must ensure that the strength of the acid is as intended by the physician. While both weight-to-weight and volume-to-volume methods of calculating acid concentration may be used, the authors prefer the even more common method of weight-to-volume calculations. When changing vendors or ordering new products, the distributor's method of calculation should be confirmed so as to avoid application of a more highly concentrated or less highly concentrated than intended product.

Patient Preparation

All patients with a history of oral or facial herpes simplex virus infection should be pre-treated with anti-herpetic agents such as acyclovir or valacyclovir to prevent herpetic activation during the post-peel period. Since a negative history of HSV does not always correspond with actual prior exposure, and since anti-viral medications are extremely safe, it is prudent to place all patients undergoing medium-depth peels on a post-procedural course of medication.

Table 3.9 Monheit index of photoaging

Texture changes	Points				Score
Wrinkles (% of potential lines)	1	2	3	4	
	<25%	<50%	<75%	<100%	
Cross-hatched line (% of potential lines)	1	2	3	4	
	<10%	<20%	<40%	<60%	
Sallow color	1	2	3	4	
	Dull	Yellow	Brown	Black	
Leathery appearance	1	2	3	4	
Crinkly (thin & parchment)	1	2	3	4	
Pebbly (deep whitish nodules)	2	4	6	8	
(% of face)	<25%	<50%	<75%	<100%	
Lesions	**Points**				**Score**
Freckles-mottled skin (# present)	1	2	3	4	
	<10	<25	<50	>100	
Lentigines & Seborrheic Keratoses (Size)	2	4	6	8	
	<5 mm	<10 mm	<15 mm	>20 mm	
Telangiectasia-erythema flush (# present)	1	2	3	4	
	<5	<10	<15	>15	
Actinic Keratoses and Seborrheic Keratoses (# present)	2	4	6	8	
	<5	<10	<15	>15	
Skin cancers (# present-now or by history)	2	4	6	8	
	1 ca	2 ca	3 ca	>4 ca	
Senile comedones (in cheek bone area)	1	2	3	4	
	<5	<10	<20	>20	
				Total Score	

Corresponding Rejuvenation Program	
Score	**Needs**
1–4	Skin care program with tretinoin, glycolic acid peels
5–9	Same plus Jessner's peels; pigmented lesion laser and/or vascular laser
10–14	Same plus medium peels—Jessner's/TCA peel; skin fillers and/or Botox
15 or more	Above plus laser resurfacing

All anti-herpetic agents act by inhibiting viral replication in the intact epidermal cell, such that the skin must be re-epithelialized before the agent has its full effect. Thus the anti-viral agent must be continued after a medium-depth peel for at least 10 days.

Routine anti-viral agents are not necessary in light or superficial chemical peeling, as the injury pattern usually is not enough to activate the herpes simplex virus.

Analgesia and Sedation

Medium-depth peels may be performed without anesthesia, with preceding topical anesthesia, with local nerve blocks, with mild preoperative sedation or anxiolytic medications, or a combination of any of the above (see Chapter 9 for further details). For full-face peels in anxious patients, it is useful to give preoperative sedation (diazepam 5–10 mg orally) along with mild analgesia in the form of meperidine 50 mg (Demerol—Winthrop, New York) and a mild sedative such as hydroxyzine hydrochloride 25 mg

Fig. 3.3 A standard setup includes a facial cleanser such as Septisol, acetone, Jessner's solution, 35% TCA, cotton-tipped applicators, and 2 × 2- and 4 × 4-inch gauze pads

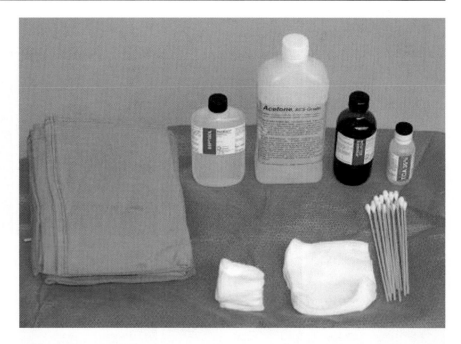

intramuscularly (Vistaril—Lorec, New York). The discomfort from this peel is not long lasting, so short-acting anxiolytics and analgesics are all that are necessary.[11]

Application Technique

The removal of sebum, scale, and thickened stratum corneum is particularly important for even penetration of the solution.

> Vigorous cleansing and degreasing of the skin prior to application of the active peeling agent are an essential and often overlooked step in the peeling protocol.

The face is first washed with an anti-bacterial cleanser in glycerin (Septisol—Vestal Laboratories, St. Louis, MO) applied with 4 × 4-inch gauze pads, then rinsed with water. Acetone is then applied with 4 × 4-inch gauze pads to remove residual oils and debris. The skin is thus debrided of loose stratum corneum and excessive scale. The necessity for thorough degreasing in order to achieve reliable and even penetration cannot be over emphasized. Prior to application of the active peeling agent, one should assess the thoroughness of degreasing. If oil or scale

is felt, the degreasing step should be repeated. Particular attention should be focused on the hairline and nose. This then will give an even peel over the entire face.

Next, Jessner's solution is evenly applied, either with cotton-tip applicators or 2 × 2-inch gauze pads (Table 3.10). Jessner's solution alone constitutes a very light peel, and thus will open the epidermal barrier for a more even and more deeply penetrating TCA application. Only one coat of Jessner's solution is usually necessary to achieve a light, even frosting with a background of erythema. The expected frosting is much lighter than that produced by the TCA. The face is treated in sequential segments

Table 3.10 Jessner's + TCA medium-depth chemical peel procedure

1. The skin should be cleansed thoroughly with Septisol to remove oils.
2. Acetone is used to further debride oil and scale from the surface of the skin.
3. Jessner's solution is applied with 2 × 2-inch gauze in an even coating, region by region.
4. 35% TCA is applied with cotton-tipped applicators until a light frost appears.
5. Cool saline compresses are applied for patient comfort.
6. Post-peel regimen begun with 0.25% acetic acid soaks and a mild emollient cream.

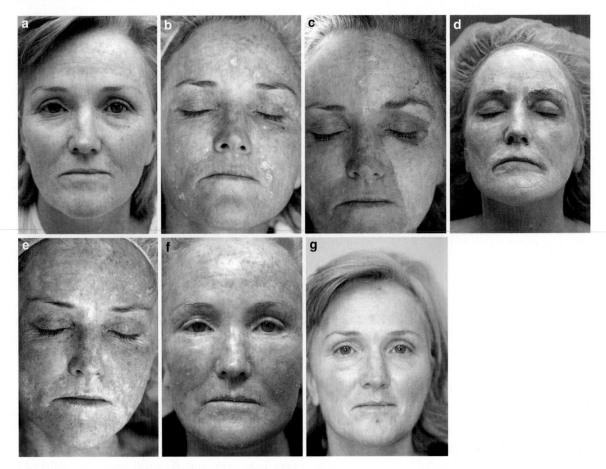

Fig. 3.4 (**a**) A 48-year-old female just prior to medium-depth chemical peel with Jessner's/35% TCA combination peel for multiple actinic keratoses and actinic damage. (**b**) After cleansing with Septisol and acetone and application of Jessner's solution, 35% TCA has been applied directly to actinic keratoses as evidenced by focal frosting of the lesions. (**c**) 35% TCA is applied regionally in a stepwise manner, allowing time for evidence of frosting. Level II frosting is achieved. (**d**) Level II frosting after full-face application. (**e**) Five minutes after completion of TCA, frosting has significantly decreased. (**f**) Three days later. (**g**) Thirteen days later. Note focal residual healing of actinic keratoses on forehead and mental crease

progressing inferiorly from the hairline. Even strokes are used to apply the solution to the forehead, each cheek, the nose, and the chin. The perioral area should follow, and the eyelids are treated last, creating the same erythema with blotchy frosting.

As with the application of Jessner's, cosmetic units of the face are then peeled sequentially with TCA from forehead to temple to cheeks, and finally to the cutaneous lips and eyelids (Fig. 3.4a–g). The 35% weight-to-volume TCA is applied evenly with one to four cotton-tipped applicators rolled over different areas with lighter or heavier doses of the acid. Four well-soaked cotton-tipped applicators are used with broad strokes over the forehead

and the medial cheeks. Two mildly soaked cotton-tipped applicators can be used across the lips and chin, and one damp cotton-tipped applicator on the eyelids. The amount of acid delivered is thus dependent upon both the saturation of an individual cotton-tipped applicator and the number of cotton-tipped applicators used. In this manner, the application is titrated according to the cutaneous thickness of the treated area.

The white frost from the TCA application, which represents the keratocoagulated endpoint, should appear on the treated area within 30 s to 2 min after application. An even application should eliminate the need for a second or a third pass, but if

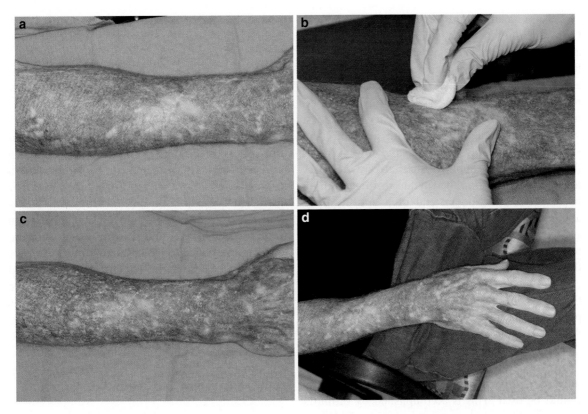

Fig. 3.5 (**a**) A 74-year-old male with a history of numerous non-melanoma skin cancers presents for a chemical peel of numerous actinic keratoses on his arms. (**b**) Following application of Jessner's solution, 25% TCA is applied. (**c**) Frosting is apparent. (**d**) At follow-up 1 month later

frosting is incomplete or uneven, the solution should be reapplied to these areas. TCA takes longer to frost than a deep phenol peel, but less time than the superficial peeling agents do.

> After a single application of TCA to an area, the surgeon should wait at least 3–4 min to ensure that frosting has reached its peak before considering further application.

The thoroughness of application can then be analyzed, and a touch-up, or less commonly another pass, can be applied as needed. Areas of poor frosting should be retreated carefully with a thin application of TCA.

The physician should seek to achieve a level II to level III frosting. Level II frosting is defined as white-coated frosting with a background of erythema.[15] A level III frosting, which is associated with penetration to the reticular dermis, is solid white enamel frosting with no background of erythema. A deeper level III frosting should be restricted only to areas of heavy actinic damage and thicker skin. Most medium-depth chemical peels should strive to obtain no more than a level II frosting. This is especially true over eyelids and areas of sensitive skin. Those areas with a greater tendency to scar formation, such as the zygomatic arch, the bony prominences of the jawline, and chin, should only receive up to a level II frosting. Over-coating trichloroacetic acid with multiple passes or highly saturated cotton-tipped applicators will increase its penetration, so that a second or third application will create further damage. One must be extremely careful to re-treat only areas where the amount of solution taken up was not adequate or the skin is much thicker. One should never overcoat a fully frosted area.

Certain facial features require special attention. Careful feathering of the solution into the hairline and around the rim of the jaw and brow conceals the line of demarcation between peeled and non-peeled areas. The perioral area has fine, radial rhytides that require a complete and even application of solution over the lip skin to the vermilion border. This is best accomplished with the help of an assistant who stretches and fixates the upper and lower lips as the peel solution is applied. Alternatively, the TCA may be applied along the rhytide to the vermilion border with the wooden end of a cotton-tipped applicator. It should be noted that deeper furrows such as expression lines will not be eradicated by a medium-depth peel and thus should be treated like the remaining skin.

Thickened keratoses should stand in contrast to the frosted background since they do not pick up peel solution evenly and thus do not frost evenly. Additional applications rubbed vigorously into these lesions may be needed for penetration.

Eyelid skin must be treated delicately and carefully. A damp, rather than saturated, applicator should be used. This is accomplished by draining the excess TCA on the cotton tip against the rim of the bottle or onto a dry gauze pad before using it for application. The patient should be positioned with the head elevated at 30° and the eyelids closed.

> Be cautious when peeling periocularly. Dry cotton-tipped applicators should be used at the lateral and medial ocular commissures to prevent spread of acid by capillary action of tears.

The applicator is then rolled gently on the lids and periorbital skin within 2–3 mm of the lid margin. Never leave excess peel solution on the lids, because the solution can roll into the eyes.

The patient will experience an immediate burning sensation as the TCA is applied, but this subsides as frosting is completed. A circulating fan may be placed beside the patient for comfort. Cool saline or water compresses also offer symptomatic relief for a peeled area. The compresses are placed over the face for 5–6 min after the peel until the patient is comfortable. The burning subsides fully by the time the patient is ready to be discharged. At that time, most of the frosting has faded and a brawny desquamation is evident.

Post-procedure

Postoperatively, edema, erythema, and desquamation are expected. With periorbital peels and even forehead peels, eyelid edema can be severe enough to close the lids. For the first 2–4 days, the patient is instructed to soak four times a day with 0.25% acetic acid compresses made of one tablespoon white vinegar in one pint of warm water. A bland emollient is applied to the desquamating areas after soaks. After 4 days, the patient can shower and clean gently with a mild facial cleanser. The erythema intensifies as desquamation becomes complete within 4–5 days. Thus, healing is completed within 7–10 days. At this time the bright red color has faded to pink and has the appearance of a sunburn. This erythema may be covered by cosmetics and will fade fully within 2–3 weeks.

Complications

While medium-depth chemical peels are generally safe when appropriately performed, complications do exist. The most common are prolonged erythema, infection, pigmentary alteration, and scarring.

Seven to ten days of desquamation and erythema are to be expected, yet prolonged erythema occasionally occurs. This is common in patients with an underlying diagnosis of rosacea, where the chemical peel serves as a trigger for inflammation. The event is limited, however, and should resolve within several weeks to a few months. Erythema associated with pain should prompt consideration of and investigation for an infection, particularly with herpes simplex virus. All patients with a history of herpes simplex virus I of the facial area should take an anti-viral agent such as acyclovir or valacyclovir and remain on prophylactic therapy for 10 days.

Permanent hypopigmentation of Fitzpatrick skin types III–VI is a potential complication, although the risk is not as great as that seen with carbon dioxide laser resurfacing. If hypopigmentation is a concern, a test spot in an inconspicuous area such as under the chin or behind the ear and follow-up appointment are warranted prior to full-face application. Finally, scarring may occur as a result of various factors. Fifty percent and higher concentrations of TCA commonly lead to scarring, so lower concentrations should be used. Isotretinoin therapy within the previous 6 months has also been associated with an increased risk of scarring. A history of keloid formation should also be screened for prior to chemical peeling.

Summary

Chemical peeling continues to be one of the most common procedures performed today by dermatologists for improving acne, reversing actinic damage, and rejuvenating the texture and appearance of aged or damaged skin. Furthermore, the medium-depth chemical peel remains the peel of choice for the treatment of actinic damage and precancerous lesions, as it demonstrates the greatest risk/benefit ratio. While the potential for permanent complications does exist, medium-depth chemical peels remain a safe procedure for the treatment of precancerous lesions when adherence to well-established protocols occurs.

References

1. Brody HJ, Monheit GD, Resnick SS, Alt TH. A history of chemical peeling. *Dermatol Surg*. 2000;26:405–409.
2. Mackee GM, Karp FL. The treatment of post-acne scars with phenol. *Br J Dermatol*. 1952;64:456.
3. Baker TJ, Gordon HL. Chemical face peeling: an adjunct to surgical facelifting. *South Med J*. 1963;56:412–414.
4. Brody HJ. Variations and comparisons in medium depth chemical peeling. *J Dermatol Surg Oncol*. 1989;15:953–963.
5. Monheit GD. The Jessner's + TCA peel: a medium depth chemical peel. *J Dermatol Surg Oncol*. 1989;15:945–950.
6. Coleman WP, Futrell JM. The glycolic acid trichloroacetic acid peel. *J Dermatol Surg Oncol*. 1994;20:76–80.
7. 2007 American Academy of Dermatology Survey. "Majority of dermatologists are providing cosmetic services". *Skin & Allergy News*. February 2008:29.
8. Stegman SJ. A comparative histologic study of the effects of three peeling agents and dermabrasion on normal and sun-damaged skin. *Aesthetic Plast Surg*. 1982;6:123–125.
9. Glogau RG. Chemical peeling and aging skin. *J Geriatr Dermatol*. 1994;2(1):30–35.
10. Coleman WP. Dermabrasion and hypertrophic scars. *Int J Dermatol*. 1991;30(9):629–631.
11. Monheit GD. The Jessner's-trichloroacetic acid peel. *Dermatol Clin*. 1995;13(2):277–283.
12. Brody HJ. Trichloroacetic acid application in chemical peeling, operative techniques. *Plast Reconstr Surg*. 1995;2(2):127–128.
13. Monheit GD. Chemical peeling for pigmentary dyschromias. *Cosmetic Dermatol*. 1995;8(5):10–15.
14. Monheit GD. Presentation at the American Academy of Dermatology in New Orleans. March 25, 1999.
15. Rubin M. *Manual of Chemical Peels*. Philadelphia: Lippincott; 1995:120–121.

Chapter 4
Photodynamic Therapy

Nathalie C. Zeitouni, Allan Oseroff, and David J. Najarian

In general terms, photodynamic therapy (PDT) involves the use of a light source to activate a compound (photosensitizer) within malignant cells. The activated compound then transfers its energy to molecular oxygen, which works in a destructive capacity to eliminate the tumor.[1]

After more than 100 years of research, PDT is now an established form of treatment for actinic keratoses (AKs), squamous cell carcinoma in situ (SCCIS), superficial basal cell carcinoma (sBCC), and nodular basal cell carcinoma (nBCC) (Tables 4.1 and 4.2).

Several studies emphasize superior cosmesis obtainable with PDT, while some trials emphasize patient preference for PDT over other invasive modalities.[2-4] Finally, because PDT generally treats a field of skin, PDT is effective for patients presenting with multiple lesions on sun-damaged skin.

Researchers have developed several protocols for performing photodynamic therapy. In addition, published protocols vary widely from institution to institution; however, only a few of these protocols have been approved for use by major regulatory agencies, such as the US Food and Drug Administration (FDA).

This chapter is designed to serve as a practical user's guide for anyone involved in the management of skin cancer. It will emphasize techniques and treatment algorithms used at Roswell Park Cancer Institute, a pioneer in the research and development of PDT and currently a tertiary referral center for the use of PDT for skin cancer.

Photodynamic Therapy for Actinic Keratoses and Actinic Cheilitis

Patient Selection

PDT treats a field of skin and is, therefore, most appropriate for patients who present with multiple AKs on sun-damaged skin. A variety of other treatment modalities exist for the treatment of AKs, including cryotherapy, 5% imiquimod cream (Aldara), 5% 5-fluorouracil cream (Efudex), and 3% diclofenac gel (Solaraze). The risks and benefits of each are typically discussed with each patient, and the choice of treatment is made on a case-by-case basis.

A number of concerns should be weighed before initiating PDT. For example, there are contraindications to PDT that practitioners need to be aware of before prescribing treatment (Table 4.3). In addition, one must consider the type of PDT that will be utilized. In the United States, the FDA has approved the use of aminolevulinic acid (ALA). The Metvixia™ (methyl aminovulinate) PDT system for treating AKs was approved for use in the US in June 2008. In Australia, Europe, and South Africa, methyl aminolevulinic acid (MAL) is currently approved for use with a non-coherent red light source with a continuous spectrum of 570–670 nm and a total light dose of 75 J/cm^2.

Before initiating PDT, one should confirm the ability of the patient to return for multiple visits before complete clearance of AKs can be expected. For example, in clinical trials that led to FDA approval of ALA PDT for AKs, patients were treated at week 0 and week 8 if needed.[5] Upon evaluation

Table 4.1 Selected worldwide approvals for photodynamic therapy of actinic keratoses

Approving agency	Indications	Approved light source	Approved photosensitizer
US FDA	Type 1 and type 2 (non-hyperkeratotic) AKs on face and scalp	Blu-U	ALA (Levulan Kerastick)
US FDA (June 2008)	Non-hyperkeratotic AKs on the face and scalp in immunocompetent patients, after lesion debridement, when other therapies are inappropriate, by trained physicians only	570–670-nm red light	MAL (Metvixia)
Australia, South Africa, UK	Non-hyperkeratotic, non-pigmented AKs on face and scalp where other therapies are inappropriate	570–670 nm red light	MAL (Metvix)

ALA—aminolevulinate, MAL—methyl-aminolevulinate.

Table 4.2 Selected worldwide approvals for photodynamic therapy of non-melanoma skin cancer

Condition	Approving agency	Indications	Approved light source	Approved photosensitizer
Squamous cell carcinoma in situ	Australia, UK	Biopsy proven, where surgery is inappropriate	570–670 nm red light	MAL (Metvix)
		Where surgery is less appropriate	570–670 nm red light	MAL (Metvix)
Superficial basal cell carcinoma	Australia, South Africa, UK	Primary treatment where surgery is inappropriate	570–670 nm red light	MAL (Metvix)
		Only when other therapies are unsuitable due to possible treatment-related morbidity and poor cosmetic outcome; such as lesions on the mid-face and ears, lesions on sun-damaged skin, large lesions, or recurrent lesions	570–670 nm red light	MAL (Metvix)
Nodular basal cell carcinoma	Australia, South Africa, UK	Primary treatment where surgery is inappropriate	570–670 nm red light	MAL (Metvix)
		Only when other therapies are unsuitable due to possible treatment-related morbidity and poor cosmetic outcome; such as lesions on the mid-face and ears, lesions on sun-damaged skin, large lesions, or recurrent lesions	570–670 nm red light	MAL (Metvix)

MAL—methyl-aminolevulinate.

3 months after treatment, 72% of patients achieved complete clearance. Therefore, at week 12 after the first treatment, the physician should be prepared to treat non-responding AKs by alternative means or to biopsy non-responding AKs to rule out squamous cell carcinoma. Notably, approximately 90% of lesions that fail to respond to two PDT treatments are non-invasive AKs.[6]

The treatment schedule differs for MAL PDT. In clinical trials, patients received two treatments, 1 week apart.[7] Upon evaluation 3 months after the second treatment, 79–81% of patients were completely cleared. Therefore, patients treated with MAL PDT should be capable of presenting for three visits over a 3-month period, and should be prepared to receive additional treatments or biopsies at the third visit.

Before proceeding with treatment, candidates for PDT are physically examined to carefully evaluate for the presence of skin cancers in the expected field of treatment. Grade 3 (hyperkeratotic) AKs and

Table 4.3 Contraindications to the use of photodynamic therapy

1. Inability to avoid or block light exposure to skin on which the photosensitizer (e.g., ALA) has been applied for 48 h after application may cause extensive stinging, burning, and swelling (see Fig. 4.2).

2. There is a theoretical risk of excessive phototoxicity when treating patients using medicines that pre-dispose to phototoxicity, including griseofulvin, thiazide diuretics, sulfonylureas, phenothiazines, sulfonamides, and tetracyclines.

3. Patients with pre-existing photosensitivity should not be treated with PDT.

4. ALA PDT and MAL PDT are pregnancy category C according to the FDA. Therefore, ALA and MAL PDT should be given to pregnant women only if clearly needed, according to the FDA label.

5. According to FDA labels, caution is advised when considering the use of ALA and MAL PDT on nursing women, since it is unknown if ALA or its metabolites are excreted in milk. The UK Summary of Product Characteristics recommends discontinuing breast feeding for 48 h after application of Metvix cream.

6. Consider delaying PDT if expected post-treatment erythema, crusting, and edema would interfere with the patient's social plans.

7. Avoid PDT if the patient has an allergy to porphyrins or any of the ingredients of ALA or MAL. Metvixia cream contains peanut and almond oil and has a high rate of contact sensitization. Metvix contains cetostearyl alcohol, which may cause contact dermatitis, and methyl- and propyl parahydroxybenzoate (preservatives), which may cause allergic reactions. Nitrile gloves, but not vinyl or latex gloves, provide an adequate barrier to the cream.

8. Patients with acquired or inherited coagulation disorders were not included in clinical trials that led to FDA approval of ALA and MAL PDT. Consider avoiding PDT in such patients.

9. ALA and MAL PDT are contraindicated for use on the mucous membranes and the eye. Consider avoiding PDT if ALA or MAL cream could accidentally be applied to the mucous membranes or eyes.

lesions believed to represent SCCIS and sBCC may be treated with PDT and subsequently biopsied or treated by alternative means if they do not respond. Lesions suspicious for melanoma, invasive squamous cell carcinoma, and non-superficial basal cell carcinoma are biopsied and treated by other modalities.

Patient Education and Consent

Before patients are treated with PDT, they are thoroughly educated about the procedure. An education form is provided (Fig. 4.1). Patients are also asked to read and sign a consent form (Fig. 4.2).

ALA Photodynamic Therapy

Aminolevulinic acid is an intermediate in the heme synthesis metabolic pathway. When applied to skin it is somewhat selectively absorbed by skin cancer cells and converted into protoporphyrin IX. Protoporphyrin IX absorbs light in several wavelengths, including 407 nm (Soret Band) and approximately 540, 580, and 635 nm, leading to its own destruction and the generation of reactive oxygen species. These destructive molecules are believed to underlie the capacity of topically applied aminolevulinic acid to destroy the cancer cells absorbed by it.[1]

Technique of Application

ALA is applied to the skin with the Levulan Kerastick (sold by DUSA Pharmaceuticals). Levulan Kerasticks are sold as single units (for $109.50) or in cartons of 6 units (for $657.00). They are stored at 25°C. Two glass ampoules are housed within the Levulan Kerastick. One ampoule contains the vehicle, comprising ethanol, water, laureth-4, isopropyl alcohol, and polyethylene glycol. The other ampoule contains ALA HCL in a dry solid form. Ampoules are housed within a common plastic tube, and the plastic tube itself is housed within a cardboard sleeve.

The Levulan Kerastick is prepared in four steps. First, the device is held with the applicator tip pointing up. Next, the bottom ampoule containing the vehicle solution is crushed by applying finger pressure to the cardboard sleeve (Fig. 4.3a). The top ampoule containing ALA HCL is then crushed with finger pressure to the cardboard sleeve (Fig. 4.3b). Finally, holding the stick between the thumb and forefinger, it is rotated back and forth around its central axis like a baton for 3 min (Fig. 4.3c).

Immediately before applying ALA, AKs and surrounding sun-damaged skin are treated with medical-grade sandpaper (3 M Red Dot Trace Prep Catalog number 2236) to enhance ALA penetration (Fig. 4.4a, b). Alternatively, AKs and surrounding sun-damaged skin may be delipidated with an

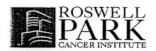

Elm & Carlton Streets
Buffalo, NY 14263
716-845-2300
www.roswellpark.org
E-mail: askrpci@roswellpark.org

connecting for life

Roswell Park Cancer Institute
Photodynamic Therapy/ Dermatology Department
Blue U Treatment with Topical Levulan

Introduction

Blue U treatment using Levulan Kerastick / Photodynamic Therapy (PDT) is a two-step investigational treatment that uses a light-sensitive drug and visible blue light.

Process of the Application of Levulan Keratick

We will photograph the treatment areas and may prep the area as ordered by your physician. We will apply Levulan Kerastick to the entire area to be treated. This application may cause mild irritation such as burning or tingling. The treatment area may be covered and protected from sunlight or bright light until treatment.

Blue U Treatment:

Treatment is performed after the physician specified Levulan application time by applying a visible blue light. This light activates the Levulan and causes destruction of the abnormal cells.

We will provide protective goggles or light shields to protect your eyes from the laser during treatment, as necessary.

The amount of discomfort varies from person to person but is likened to a burning sensation. The treatment can be stopped at any time.

The laser treatment will last for approximately 10-16 minutes.

Expected Side Effects

We expect no significant reaction to the drug, but after treatment, the treatment area may become swollen or red. There may be temporary discomfort and the treated area may peel. Cool cloths/ ice packs are applied, as needed, post treatment to decrease discomfort and swelling. Benadryl may be taken t decrease swelling. Tylenol may be taken to decrease discomfort.

The skin will be sensitive to bright light for 24-48 hours post treatment due to left over medication. Apply sun screen to protect the skin from this reaction and do not go into bright light or sunlight for 48 hours following the procedure.

QUESTIONS

If you have any problems with sunburn, fever, chills, pain, infection or anything that is unusual, please contact your nurse or physician immediately.

A National Cancer Institute-designated Comprehensive Cancer Center • A National Comprehensive Cancer Network Member

Fig. 4.1 Information sheet for patients undergoing BLU-U PDT with topical ALA

acetone scrub. Only one cosmetic field—such as the face, scalp, or extremities—is treated at a time. The applicator tip is then pressed onto AKs and surrounding sun-damaged skin until it appears uniformly wet. Care is taken not to allow ALA onto the eye or conjunctiva. Therefore, periorbital lesions are typically not treated. After the ALA appears dry—about 1–2 min later, a second application is performed with the same stick. Treated skin is then covered with a transparent dressing, such as Opsite,

ROSWELL PARK CANCER INSTITUTE
ELM AND CARLTON STREETS • BUFFALO, NY 14263

SPECIAL CONSENT TO OPERATION OR OTHER PROCEDURE

Addressograph

DATE: _____ TIME: _____ ☐ AM ☐ PM

1. **I hereby authorize** Dr. _____ and/or such assistants as may be selected and supervised by him/her as may be deemed necessary, to remedy the condition(s) which appear indicated by the diagnostic studies already performed. [Explain the nature of the condition(s) and the need to remedy such condition(s).]
   Actinic keratoses are rough scaly patches on the skin caused by excessive sun exposure. Left untreated, they may progress to skin cancer.

2. **I understand** that the following surgical, medical, and/or diagnostic procedure(s) necessary to treat my condition has (have) been explained to me by Dr. _____. I understand the nature of the procedure(s); and I voluntarily consent and authorize the procedure(s) described here.
   [Describe the procedure(s) in the language of laymen.]
   Levulan-photodynamic therapy is a two-step procedure. On Day 1, a light sensitive drug (Levulan) is applied to the actinic keratoses. On Day 2, the actinic keratoses are exposed to a blue light that may destroy them.

3. **It has been explained to me** that, during the course of the procedure(s), unforeseen conditions may be revealed that necessitate an extension of the original procedure(s) or different procedure(s) than those set forth in Paragraph 2. I therefore authorize and request that the above-named physician, and his/her assistants, perform such procedure(s), as necessary and desirable, in the exercise of professional judgment. The authorization granted under this Paragraph 3 shall extend to remedying all conditions that require treatment and are not known to Dr. _____ at the time the procedure is commenced.

4. **I have been made aware** of certain risk and consequences that are associated with the procedure(s) described in Paragraph 2. These are:
   1) Localized redness and swelling
   2) Increased or decreased pigmentation
   3) Small risk of infection

5. **I am aware** that the practice of medicine and surgery is not an exact science and I acknowledge that no guarantees or warranties have been made to me concerning the results or cure from the operation or procedure(s).

6. The following alternatives for care and treatment have been explained to me:
   1) Liquid Nitrogen
   2) Topical chemotherapy

7. **I hereby authorize** the physician(s) and Institute to preserve and use for scientific, teaching, or research and development purposes, or to dispose of, body fluids, tissues and organs collected as a necessary part of my care and treatment and I hereby relinquish all rights, title, and interest to such fluids, tissues and organs.

8. **I further consent** to the administration of such drugs, infusions, plasma or blood transfusions, or any other treatment or procedure(s) deemed necessary in the judgment of the medical staff.

9. **I further consent**, upon the request and/or authorization of the above named physician(s), to the presence of authorized sales representatives in the operating room.

I CERTIFY THAT I HAVE READ AND FULLY UNDERSTAND ALL OF THE ABOVE CONSENT.

_____   _____
Signature of Patient   Signature of Witnessing Physician
(If patient is unable to consent or is a minor, complete the following:) Patient [is a minor _____ years of age] [is unable to consent because]

_____   _____
Signature of Legal Guardian or closest relative available   Signature of Witness

Fig. 4.2 A sample consent form for photodynamic therapy of AKs using the Levulan Kerastick (18-h incubation) and the BLU-U light

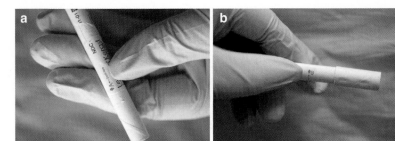

Fig. 4.3 The Levulan Kerastick is prepared in four steps. (a) First, the device is held with the applicator tip pointing up. Next, the *bottom* ampoule containing the vehicle solution is crushed by applying finger pressure to the cardboard sleeve. (b) In the third step, the *top* ampoule containing ALA HCL is crushed with finger pressure to the cardboard sleeve. (c) In the final step, holding the stick between the thumb and forefinger, it is rotated back and forth around its central axis like a baton for 3 min

Fig. 4.4 (a) To enhance the absorption of ALA, the skin may be abraded with medical-grade sandpaper (3 M Red Dot Trace Prep Catalog number 2236). (b) To enhance the absorption of ALA, the skin also may be cleansed with acetone using gauze

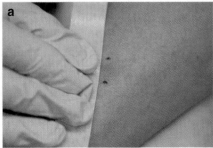
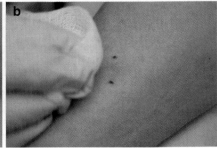

using Mastisol as the adhesive (Fig. 4.5). Finally, this dressing is covered with black duct tape to protect the treated surface from light (Fig. 4.6). The face is one cosmetic field we do not routinely occlude.

The treated skin should not be washed during this period. Moreover, a wide-brimmed hat and other protective apparel should be worn during this time. Intense sun or other light exposure should be avoided for 40 h after the application of ALA.

According to the FDA label, one should allow ALA to absorb into the skin for 14–18 h. In our practice, however, we allow ALA to absorb into the skin for 1 h (2–3 h for hyperkeratotic lesions), which enhances patient convenience. Before light exposure, AKs and surrounding skin are rinsed with normal saline and patted dry. AKs are then exposed to the BLU-U Blue Light Photodynamic Therapy Illuminator. A 1,000-s exposure provides a fluence of 10 J/cm^2. Before the light is activated, the patient

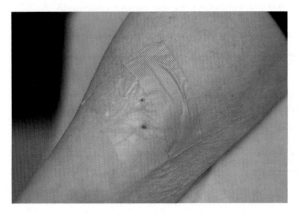

Fig. 4.5 To enhance the absorption of recently applied ALA and to prevent the spread of recently applied ALA, the skin may be covered with an Opsite dressing

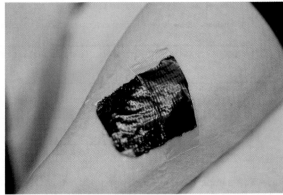

Fig. 4.6 To protect recently applied ALA from ambient light, the Opsite dressing may be covered with opaque duct tape

and all personnel in the room are provided with blue-blocking protective glasses. After the procedure, treated skin is covered with Neutrogena Ultra Sheer SPF 70 Dry-Touch Sunblock and post-PDT care instructions are given. Finally, patients are contacted by a health care professional within a week of treatment to evaluate for side effects (Fig. 4.7). See accompanying illustrative case 4.1.

Roswell Park Cancer Institute
Dermatology /PDT

PDT Post Treatment Follow up

Pt. Name:_____ MR #_____

1. Date of Treatment _____Telephone call within 3-7 days post treatment: yes   no

2. Pain level post treatment :   1 2   3   4   5 6   7 8 9 10

_____
_____
_____
_____
_____
_____

3. Signs / symptoms of infection :   yes   no

_____
_____
_____
_____
_____
_____

4. Problems post treatment :   yes   no

_____
_____
_____5. Repeat call necessary: yes
no
_____
_____
_____

6. If you are having a problem, do you know who to call?
    YES   NO   _____

_____   _____
Signature   Date

Fig. 4.7 Document used to monitor patients after PDT treatments

Illustrative Case 4.1

FW is a 66-year-old male who presented for photo-dynamic therapy of AKs.

His past medical history is remarkable for facial AKs treated in the past with cryotherapy and 5% 5-fluorouracil cream. In addition, he has had multiple cutaneous squamous cell carcinomas and basal cell carcinomas.

Physical examination revealed more than 15 AKs on the forehead, cheeks, nose, and temples (Fig. 4.8a, b).

Risks and benefits of his therapeutic options were discussed, a plan to initiate PDT treatment of his AKs was confirmed, and a consent form was signed by all parties.

At 1:40 PM, AKs were abraded with 3-M dot tape and acetone was applied. Two coats of topical ALA were then applied to the forehead, cheeks, temple, and nose, using the Levulan Kerastick. FW was

instructed to avoid sunlight and strong indoor light and return to the clinic at 2:40 PM.

At this time areas treated with ALA were rinsed with saline. Protective eyewear was distributed to FW and all caretakers, and the BLU-U light was activated with the following settings: 10 J/cm², 10 mWatts, 16-min and 20-s exposure time. FW reported no stinging and burning 2 min into treatment. At 2:54 PM, FW reported stinging, less than 1/10 on the pain scale. Treatment ended at 3:01 PM. There were no complications. Sunblock was applied. FW was instructed to return to the clinic in 6 weeks.

After a total of 12 weeks and three PDT treatments, physical examination revealed approximately 80% clearance of his AKs. A photograph documenting FW's improvement after three PDT sessions was taken (Fig. 4.9a, b). Additional PDT sessions may be required at his 6-month follow-up.

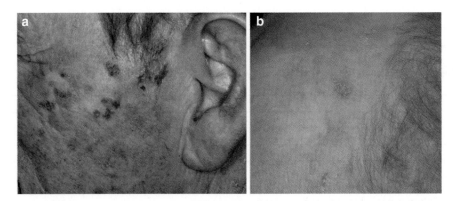

Fig. 4.8 Actinic keratoses on (a) the cheek and (b) left frontal scalp prior to PDT treatment

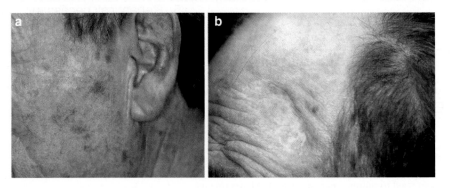

Fig. 4.9 (a, b) Improvement of AKs on the left cheek and scalp after PDT treatments

Patients are seen 4 weeks later for consideration of additional treatment of non-responding lesions. In our practice, if less than 80% of AKs have completely responded, patients are retreated with PDT. If more than 80% of AKs have completely responded, remaining AKs are treated with other modalities, such as cryotherapy. Regardless of how patients responded at 1-month follow-up, all patients are seen again at 6 and 12 months after treatment to evaluate for AK recurrence.

One clinical trial has evaluated PDT of AKs in 12 patients using BLU-U and the Levulan Kerastick with an incubation period of 1 h.[8] In this study, patients were treated once and again after 1 month. Clinical results are shown in Table 4.4.

Techniques with Off-Label Light Sources

According to the accompanying FDA label, the Levulan Kerastick is recommended for use with the BLU-U light source only. However, small studies have tested the use of other light sources in combination with ALA for the treatment of AKs.[1,9,10]

The long-pulsed dye laser (PDL, 585 nm) has been tested in combination with topical ALA[11] One research group based in Germany tested this laser in combination with a topically applied 20% ALA-HCl emulsion (produced by Medac, Hamburg, Germany). One hundred AKs on 24 patients were then treated with the PDL (18 J/cm^2 fluence, 1.5 ms pulse duration, 5 mm spot size) after a 6-h incubation period.[1] Results are shown in Table 4.4. See accompanying illustrative case 4.2.

Table 4.4 Selected clinical outcomes for PDT of actinic keratoses and actinic cheilitis

Light source (λ nm)	Photosensitizer	Incubation period	Number of treatments	Complete response rate	Notable side effects	Reference
400 BLU-U	Levulan Kerastick (ALA)	1 h	2	50% (AKs)	Erythema	5
570–670	Metvixia (MAL)	2.5–4 h	2	79–81% (AKs)	Redness, stinging, swelling, and pain frequently occur	7
585 PDL	20% oil in water emulsion of ALA (Medac, Hamburg, Germany)	6 h	1	79% (AKs)	Erythema and crusting for 10–14 days, purpura	7
595 PDL	Levulan Kerastick (ALA)	2–3 h	Up to 3	68% (AC)	Impetigo	5
580–740 non-coherent	20% oil in water emulsion of ALA (Medac, Hamburg, Germany)	6 h	1	84% (AKs)	Erythema and crusting for 10–14 days, pain	7
590–1200 IPL with 615 nm cutoff filterz	20% oil in water emulsion of ALA	4 h	2	91% (AKs)	Erythema, edema, crusting	11
630 LED	Metvix (MAL)	3 h	2	86% (AKs)	Phototoxic reactions	9

ALA—aminolevulinate, MAL—methyl-aminolevulinate.

Illustrative Case 4.2

PF is a 73-year-old male who presented for photodynamic therapy of facial and scalp AKs. PF was enrolled in a clinical trial for the treatment of AKs using ALA and the VBeam laser (pulsed dye laser 595 nm).

His AKs had been treated with cryotherapy in the past and he had no history of skin cancer.

Physical examination revealed 20 AKs on the face and scalp (Fig. 4.10).

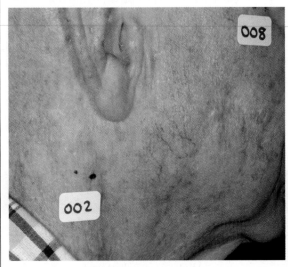

Fig. 4.10 AK (002) prior to PDT treatment

PDT treatment of his AKs was initiated according to the study protocol, and a consent form was signed by all parties. Lesions were marked, measured, and photographed. The scalp was cleansed with acetone and the face was abraded with 3-M dot tape. ALA was applied with the Levulan Kerastick at 9:45 AM. The lesions were then covered with OpSite and black tape. PF was instructed to avoid bright indoor light and sunlight. At 1:45 PM, ALA was removed with normal saline and lesions were treated with 349 pulses with the VBeam laser with the following parameters (7.5 J/cm² fluence, 6 ms pulse duration, 10 mm spot size, 30 ms cryogen cooling spray). During the procedure, PF noted significant pain with a magnitude of 8 on a scale of 1–10. PF declined offers of both topical and oral analgesics and to discontinue treatment. Post-treatment erythema without purpura was noted. Sunscreen was applied, and wound care instructions were provided.

PF received similar treatments during follow-up 1 month and 2 months later. At the third month, PF reported 85% improvement of his face and scalp skin compared with his initial presentation. Physical examination confirmed an 80% improvement compared with his initial condition (see posttreatment photograph in Fig. 4.11).

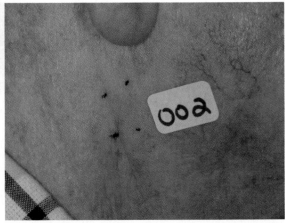

Fig. 4.11 Complete resolution of AK (002) after three PDT treatments with the pulsed-dye laser

The 595-nm PDL has been tested in combination with topical ALA for the treatment of actinic cheilitis (AC). In one study of 19 patients with actinic cheilitis who failed other therapies, ALA was applied to lip lesions using the Levulan Kerastick.[9] Two to three hours later, lesions were exposed to a PDL (595 nm at 7.5 J/cm² fluence, 10 ms pulse duration, 10 mm spot size, 2–3 passes). Lesions were retreated at monthly intervals (up to three sessions in total) until they cleared clinically. Results are shown in Table 4.4.

In Spain, another group tested topical ALA in combination with an intense-pulsed light device called Epilight (EAC/Sharplan Medical Systems, Needham, MA).[10] In this trial, 20% ALA was applied to 38 AKs on the faces and scalps of 17 patients. The ALA was occluded by plastic film for 4 h, and AKs were then exposed to the IPL (590–1200 nm, 615 nm filter, 40 J/cm² fluence, double-pulse mode of 4.0 ms with 20 ms delay between pulses). Treatments were repeated 1 month later. Clinical assessments were made 1 and 3 months after the second treatment. Results are shown in Table 4.4.

MAL Photodynamic Therapy

Technique of Application

A metabolic precursor of ALA, 16.8% methyl amino-levulinate cream (Metvixia, MAL) is also used as a photosensitizer in PDT for the treatment of AKs. The FDA-approved protocol for MAL PDT differs from the protocol for ALA PDT. Before treatment with MAL PDT, crusts and scale are gently debrided with a sharp curette to facilitate cream absorption and light penetration. A 1-mm thick layer of MAL cream is then applied to AKs with a 5-mm margin of normal skin. The cream is then occluded with a non-absorbent dressing for 2.5–4 h. Physicians should limit the use of MAL cream to 1 g (one half tube) per application session. Physicians need to wear nitrile gloves during the application step because MAL cream penetrates through other types of gloves.

After cream application, patients are advised to avoid exposure of the treated sites to sunlight and bright indoor lighting. Prior to sunlight exposure, patients should protect the treatment sites with a wide-brimmed, opaque hat. Importantly, sunscreens will not protect treated skin from visible light. Patients should also avoid exposure to extreme cold after MAL cream application. MAL cream is then cleansed off AKs using gauze and saline. Finally, AKs are exposed to light with the CureLight Broad Band Model Cure-Light 01 (570–670 nm) with a fluence of 75 J/cm^2. Before treatment, the patient and all attendants in the room are provided with glasses that screen out light between 570 and 670 nm. The treated area should be protected from light exposure for at least 48 h after treatment. Lesions are re-treated in 1 week and reassessed clinically 3 months after the second treatment. Clinical trials results are shown in Table 4.4.

Techniques with Off-Label Light Sources

Small studies have tested the use of other light sources in combination with MAL cream for the treatment of AKs. One group in the UK and Ireland tested the use of a light-emitting diode (AktiliteCL128 lamp; Galderma; Photocure) in combination with 160 mg/g MAL cream (Metvix) for the treatment of 758 AKs

in 119 patients.[12] MAL cream was applied to lesions for 3 h as directed in the FDA label. AKs were then exposed to the LED operating at 630 nm and a fluence of 37 J/cm^2. Non-responding lesions were retreated at week 12. Patients were assessed again for response at week 24. Clinical trial results are shown in Table 4.4.

Photodynamic Therapy for Squamous Cell Carcinoma In Situ, Superficial Basal Cell Carcinoma, and Nodular Basal Cell Carcinoma

Patient Selection

A variety of techniques are available for the treatment of SCCIS, sBCC, and nBCC. Studies have demonstrated superior cosmetic outcomes using PDT. Other studies have demonstrated a clear patient preference for PDT over other invasive treatments. Finally, because PDT treats a field of skin, it is especially effective for patients presenting with multiple skin cancers. For this reason, patients with nevoid basal cell carcinoma syndrome are often referred for PDT at the Roswell Park Cancer Institute.

At the Roswell Park Cancer Institute, we biopsy all lesions suspicious for SCCIS, sBCC, and nBCC prior to performing PDT on these lesions. Patients referred to us for the treatment of nevoid basal cell carcinoma syndrome serve as an exception to this rule, however. These patients often present with hundreds of sometimes pleomorphic basal cell carcinomas. In these special cases, we biopsy approximately 10% of lesions to facilitate a clinical diagnosis of the remaining lesions. Finally, we have pathologists at our institute review slides and confirm all diagnoses made at outside institutions before proceeding with PDT for SCCIS, sBCC, and nBCC.

A variety of factors must be considered before treatment of SCCIS, sBCC, and nBCC with PDT. For example, contraindications to PDT should be considered before initiating therapy (Table 4.4). In addition, if patients require treatment of more than eight SCCIS, sBCCs, and/or nBCCs, anesthesiology is consulted for the administration of monitored anesthesia care (MAC) prior to the treatment. See accompanying illustrative case 4.3.

Illustrative Case 4.3

JE is a 44-year-old male with nevoid basal cell carcinoma syndrome who presented for photodynamic therapy.

JE has been seen for follow-up at 9 months and 10 months following treatment, and on both dates a complete clinical response for all lesions was noted (Fig. 4.13).

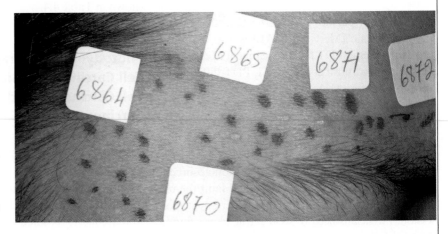

Fig. 4.12 Nodular basal cell carcinomas on the right forehead of a patient with nevoid basal cell carcinoma syndrome, prior to treatment with PDT

JE has a history of more than 100 basal carcinomas treated by a variety of modalities. He also has multiple sclerosis, an untreated meningioma, a left hip chondrosarcoma status post-chemotherapy, two hip replacements in 1992 and 1994, and a decreased ejection fraction (45%) due to chemotherapy. His cardiologist and neurologist have cleared him to undergo monitored anesthesia care (MAC).

Physical examination revealed multiple 2–4 mm pearly, telangiectatic papules—consistent with basal cell carcinomas—on the face (Fig. 4.12).

PDT was performed on 29 basal cell carcinomas using topical ALA and argon and diode lasers under MAC. ALA was applied to lesions for 18 h. Area 6871, described as two "skin-colored papules," was treated with the argon laser with the following parameters: 150 mW/cm^2, 200 J/cm^2, 633 nm, 1,333 s, and treatment field of 1.8 cm. There were no complications.

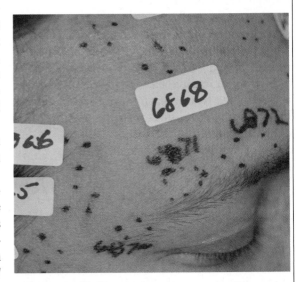

Fig. 4.13 Resolution of nodular basal cell carcinomas after treatment with PDT

Patient Education and Consent

Before patients are treated with PDT, they are thoroughly educated about the procedure. A special education form is provided to patients undergoing MAC (Fig. 4.14). They are also asked to read and sign a consent form.

ALA Photodynamic Therapy

Technique of Application at the Roswell Park Cancer Institute

In the case of nBCC, sBBC, or SCCIS, a circular 0.5-cm margin of normal skin is demarcated around

Roswell Park Cancer Institute

PHOTODYNAMIC THERAPY (PDT) with ALA under MAC Anesthesia

Introduction

Photodynamic Therapy (PDT) using topical aminolevulinic acid (ALA) is a two-step investigational cancer treatment that uses a light-sensitive drug and a visible red light source with proper stability and wave length to destroy cancer / abnormal cells.

On the first day of treatment, blood work EKG and chest x-ray are performed at 7 AM. At 8 AM, we will photograph, measure, and map the lesions. We will apply ALA to the entire lesion and surrounding treatment field, cover it with a clear plastic dressing and a dressing to prevent light penetration. The dressing is to remain dry and in place for 4-6 or 18-24 hours dependent on the parameters of the protocol.

On the second day of treatment, the second application of ALA, if warranted by protocol, is performed at 6-8 AM. Patients receiving conscious sedation are admitted to the day inpatient bed and prepared for the procedure. Patients are transported to either the operating room or the PDT room as warranted by need. Once in the appropriate treatment area, the PDT team removes the dressing, re-checks measurements and sets up for the red light treatment. Anesthesia initiates the conscious sedation and PDT is performed.

After the PDT treatment, the patient is transported to a recovery area to wake up. The patient is then transported back to the day inpatient bed room and is cleared for discharge.

Aminolevulinic Acid (ALA)

After 4-6 or 18-24 hours, the amount of ALA in normal tissues is minimal, but high levels of the drug are in the cancer cells. Visible red light with proper stability and wavelength is applied after the prescribed time. This light activates the ALA and causes destruction of cancer cells.

Benefits

ALA is easy to apply, has a short healing time, has a low infection rate and causes minimal if any scarring

Side Effects

ALA does not get absorbed into the blood stream. This means you will *not* be sensitive to bright lights, or sunlight, except in the area of ALA application. During the treatment it is likely that you will experience moderate pain or discomfort. After treatment some patients have chills or feel faint, but this is rare. These effects last only a short time and are easily managed. However, if you do have chills or feel faint, notify your doctor or nurse immediately.

Photodynamic Therapy (PDT) Red Light Treatment

Your red light treatment will be given either 4-6 hours or 18-24 hours after we apply the ALA to the skin cancer.

Treatment:

Red light with proper stability and wavelength is directed over the area of the affected skin. Treatment is usually done on an outpatient basis in the dermatology PDT clinic area.

Generally, there is moderate pain or discomfort with the light application. We will use conscious sedation to decrease the pain,

The time for the red light treatment will vary depending on the number of lesions and area to be treated. After treatment, the lesions may become swollen, red or sore. There may be considerable discomfort for approximately 6-8 hours. If needed, medication will be ordered to relieve pain or reduce swelling. Ice packs are applied immediately to decrease discomfort and swelling.

There might also be some "weeping" or oozing in the lesion area. Eventually, a scab will form which will heal very much like a brush burn would. Specific care of the area will be explained to you at the time of treatment.

QUESTIONS

If you have any problems with sunburn, fever, chills, pain, infection or anything that is unusual, please contact your nurse or physician immediately.

Nurse: _____

Physician Assistant: _____

Nurse Practitioner: _____

Attending Physician:_____

Fig. 4.14 Instruction sheet given to PDT patients undergoing monitored anesthetic care

the lesion using a marking pen. Next the Levulan Kerastick is prepared in the same manner as described previously for its use for AKs. ALA is applied to the lesion in question and the 0.5-cm margin of normal skin within the circle. The ALA is permitted to dry for 1 min before a second layer is applied. Treated skin is then covered with a transparent dressing, such as Opsite, using Mastisol as the adhesive. Finally, this dressing is covered with black duct tape to protect the treated surface from light. Four- to six-hour and 18–24 h incubation periods lead to similar protoporphyrin IX levels for SCCIS, sBCC, and nBCC. However, recent unpublished data, gathered by the authors, indicates that 4–6 h applications give somewhat better outcomes. Ultimately, the incubation period may be chosen according to patient and physician preference.

After the incubation period, the lesion is rinsed with water and patted dry. The tumor is then injected with 1% lidocaine (with 1 part 8.4% bicarbonate in 10 parts final volume) until analgesia is achieved. The tumor is then exposed to an argon laser (630–635 nm, 200 J/cm^2, 1,333 s, 150 mWatts). After the procedure, treated skin is covered with Neutrogena Ultra Sheer SPF 70 Dry Touch Sunblock. Wound care instructions are given, and a sheet summarizing the instructions is provided to patients (Fig. 4.15). Finally, patients are contacted by a health care professional within a week of treatment to evaluate for side effects (Fig. 4.7).

Patients are seen back in 6 months. If the SCCIS, sBCC, or nBCC has not responded completely at this time, the lesion is re-treated. If the tumor responded completely at 6 months, the patient is seen again with yearly follow-ups.

Off-label use of Levulan Kerastick and BLU-U for treatment of SCCIS is generally performed with the same exposure time and fluence as for treating AKs. We do not treat sBCC, or nBCC with the BLU-U.

MAL Photodynamic Therapy

Technique of Application

Methyl aminolevulinate hydrochloride cream (160 mg/g, 16.0%) sold under the name Metvix is approved for the treatment of SCCIS, sBCC, and nBCC (Table 4.2). According to the Summary of Product Characteristics published in the UK (UK SmPC), the lesion should first be debrided to remove scales and crusts and roughen the surface.[13] A 1-mm thick layer of Metvix cream is then applied with a spatula to the lesion and 5–10 mm of surrounding normal skin. Health care providers should wear nitrile gloves during cream administration to prevent exposure to MAL. In case of SCCIS, the lesion is then covered with an occlusive dressing for 3 h. The dressing is then removed and the lesion is cleansed with saline. The SCCIS lesion is then exposed to red light with a continuous spectrum of 570–670 mm and a total fluence of 75 J/cm^2. According to the UK SmPC, red light with a narrower spectrum providing equivalent activation of porphyrins may be substituted. Directions from the lamp's manual should be followed closely, since factors such as size of the lamp and distance between lamp and skin influence the total fluence delivered. Protective eyewear designed to block red light should be worn by the patient and all attendants in the room during light administration. Treated skin needs protection from light for at least 48 h after treatment.

Lesions of SCCIS are retreated in 1 week. Patients are again evaluated after 3 months, and lesions that have not responded may be retreated at this point. In clinical trials, patients were followed for 24 months to evaluate for recurrences.[14] Ultimately, response to treatment should be verified by a biopsy, and close, long-term follow-up of the lesion is recommended. The UK SmPC notes that lesions larger than 20 mm have a lower response rate than smaller lesions, and SCCIS larger than 40 mm have not been treated. Clinical results are summarized in Table 4.5.

Patients are treated similarly for sBCC and nBCC. In the case of nBCC, any epidermal keratin layer or tumor should be removed before MAL application. After treatment, patients are again evaluated after 3 months, and lesions that have not responded may be re-treated at this point with 2 sessions of PDT 1 week apart. Ultimately, response to treatment should be verified by a biopsy, and close, long-term follow-up of the lesion is recommended. Clinical results are summarized in Table 4.5.

Roswell Park Cancer Institute
Dermatology Clinic / Photodynamic Therapy (PDT)
Care of Site(s) after PDT

Treated areas will be sun sensitive for the next 24-48 hours and require application of sun block during that time period.

Ice packs may be used to help reduce the swelling. Apply the pack to the treated area(s) as soon as possible after treatment. Apply for 10 minutes each hour as tolerated.

If area(s) were treated on your scalp, face or elsewhere on your head, you may experience facial swelling, but not always. To help reduce and/or prevent swelling of the face from PDT treatment:
sleep on several pillows if you can; use ice packs as directed above; use any medications given as directed

The treated site may become red, swollen, sore and drain fluid. Eventually a scab may form which will fall off or be removed by your physician. This process will vary, and may take between 2-6 weeks or longer.

FOR THE FIRST THREE TO SEVEN DAYS:
1. Wash your hands and remove the dressing(s) or band aid(s) if applied.

2. A thin scab is normal. To clean this scab, gently clean with a mixture of equal parts water and peroxide 2 times a day. Pat dry the area, **do not rub vigorously or make bleed**.

3. If you develop an eschar (thick scab), soak the wound with equal amounts of peroxide and water on gauze for 15 minutes 2-3 times a day. Gently cleanse the wound with a Q-tip or gauze. Pat dry the area, **do not rub vigorously or make bleed**.

4. For the first three to seven days, apply a thin layer of antibiotic ointment (Polysporin® or Bactroban® *if prescribed*) to the wound. Do not use Neosporin. After that, keep the areas from drying out with a small amount of Aquaphor® ointment or Vaseline® applied 2 times per day.

5. If facial lesions were treated: gently wash face. Do not use facial makeup until after you are seen at one week visit and given the ok to do so.

6. You may shower.

7. Apply dressing as needed. After 2-3 days, a dressing may be optional.

8. If you develop any of the following listed below:

   ___ bleeding, increase in the amount of drainage, any odor or change in color of drainage

   ___ increased tenderness, redness, swelling or bruising at site

   ___ fever above 100, lasting over 24 hours

       call...   Department of Dermatology   (XXX) XXX-XXXX
                8:00 a.m.-4:00 p.m.   **Monday through Friday (EST)**

   For weekends or evenings, call the operator and explain that you need to speak with a physician from Dermatology for an emergency: **Roswell Park Operator (XXX) XXX-XXXX.**

Fig. 4.15 Wound care instructions given to patients after ALA PDT of superficial squamous cell carcinoma, superficial basal cell carcinoma, or nodular basal cell carcinoma with an argon laser

Table 4.5 Selected clinical outcomes for PDT of non-melanoma skin cancer

Cancer type	Light source (λ in nm)	Photosensitizer	Incubation period	Number of treatments	Complete response rate	Reference
Squamous cell carcinoma in situ	570–670	MAL (Metvix)	3 h	2	60% at 24 months	5
Superficial basal cell carcinoma	570–670	MAL (Metvix)	3 h	Up to 4	78% at 24 months	15
Nodular basal cell carcinoma	570–670	MAL (Metvix)	3 h	Up to 4	76% at 5 years	16

MAL—methyl-aminolevulinate.

Summary

Photodynamic therapy, when performed appropriately for precancerous lesions and superficial cancer, is effective and especially useful in patients with multiple non melanoma skin cancer sites.

Acknowledgements The authors are sincerely grateful to Anne Paquette, RN, BSN, CCRC, and Michelle McCarthy, RPA-C, for their assistance in preparing this manuscript.

References

1. Marcus SL, McIntyre WR. Photodynamic Therapy systems and applications. *Expert Opin Emerg Drugs*. 2002;7:331–334.
2. Tierney EP, Eide MJ, Jacobsen G, Ozog D. Photodynamic therapy for actinic keratoses: survey of patient perceptions of treatment satisfaction and outcomes. *J Cosmet Laser Ther*. 2008;10:81–86.
3. Kaufmann R, Spelman L, Weightman W, Reifenberger J, Szeimies RM, Verhaeghe E, et al. Multicentre intraindividual randomized trial of topical methyl aminolaevulinate-photodynamic therapy vs. cryotherapy for multiple actinic keratoses on the extremities. *Br J Dermatol*. 2008;158:994–999.
4. Surrenti T, De Angelis L, Di Cesare A, Fargnoli MC, Peris K. Efficacy of photodynamic therapy with methyl aminolevulinate in the treatment of superficial and nodular basal cell carcinoma: an open-label trial. *Eur J Dermatol*. 2007;17:412–415.
5. Levulan Kerastick. FDA Label (NDA 020-965). 2003. http://www.fda.gov/cder/foi/label/1999/20965lbl.pdf. Last accessed February 3, 2009.
6. Ehrig T, Cockerell C, Piacquadio D, Dromgoole S. Actinic keratoses and the incidence of occult squamous cell carcinoma: a clinical-histopathologic correlation. *Dermatol Surg*. 2006;32:1261–1265.
7. METVIXIA (methyl aminolevulinate) Cream, 16.8%. FDA Label. 2007.
8. Smith S, Piacquadio D, Morhenn V, Atkin D, Fitzpatrick R. Short incubation PDT versus 5-FU in treating actinic keratoses. *JDD*. 2003;2:629–635.
9. Alexiades-Armenakas M, Geronemus R. Laser-mediated photodynamic therapy of actinic cheilitis. *J Drugs Dermatol*. 2004;3:548–551.
10. Ruiz-Rodriguez R, Sanz-Sanchez T, Cordoba S. Photodynamic Photorejuvenation. *Dermatol Surg*. 2002;28: 742–744.
11. Karrer S, Baumler W, Abels C. Long-Pulse Dye Laser for Photodynamic therapy: Investigations in Vitro and in Vivo. *Lasers Surg Med*. 1999;25:51–59.
12. Morton C, Campbell S, Gurg G. Intraindividual right-left comparison of topical methyl aminolaevulinate-photodynamic therapy and cryotherapy in subjects with actinic keratoses: a multicentre, randomized controlled study. *Br J Dermatol*. 2006;155:1029–1036.
13. United Kingdom Summary of Product Characteristics. 2007. http://www.medicines.org.uk/. Last accessed 1/20/09.
14. Australia Summary of Product Characteristics. 2007. Australian Regulatory Guidelines for OTC Medicines. http://www.tga.gov.au/docs/html/argom.htm. Last accessed 1/20/09.
15. Horn M, Wolf P, Wulf HC, Warloe T, Fritsch C, Rhodes LE, et al. Topical methyl aminolaevulinate photodynamic therapy in patients with basal cell carcinoma prone to complications and poor cosmetic outcome with conventional treatment. *Br J Dermatol*. 2003; 149:1242–1249.
16. Rhodes LE, de Rie MA, Leifsdottir R, Yu RC, Bachmann I, Goulden V, et al. Five-year follow-up of a randomized, prospective trial of topical methyl aminolevulinate photodynamic therapy vs surgery for nodular basal cell carcinoma. *Arch Dermatol*. 2007;143:1131–1136.

Chapter 5
Intralesional and Perilesional Treatment of Skin Cancers

Christopher J. Arpey, Nicole M. Annest, Stephen B. Tucker, Ronald P. Rapini, and Deborah F. MacFarlane

In this chapter, various intralesional and perilesional agents that have been used in the treatment of skin cancers will be presented by practitioners familiar with their use. The four medications reviewed—methotrexate, interferon, 5-fluorouracil, and bleomycin—have been in widespread use for many years in the treatment of cutaneous neoplasms and extracutaneous neoplastic and inflammatory conditions. Therefore, the efficacy, toxicity, delivery, indications, and costs for these agents are well established, and they are widely available. However, the most common routes of administration for such medications are oral, intravenous, and topical. An intralesional and perilesional approach to therapy is less often utilized, leading to less familiarity in clinical practice. It is our hope that a detailed review of these agents delivered in such a manner, along with a variety of clinical examples, will facilitate their use in practice and increase the variety of treatment options available to patients with cutaneous tumors.

I. METHOTREXATE

Methotrexate (MTX) has an appealing mechanism of action for the potential treatment for rapidly growing tumors, as it inhibits DNA synthesis in actively dividing cells. A folic acid analog, methotrexate irreversibly binds to dihydrofolate reductase, thereby blocking the formation of tetrahydrofolate and subsequently preventing the downstream synthesis of the purine nucleotide thymidine.[1]

Although methotrexate has demonstrated activity against a number of cutaneous malignancies including malignant melanoma,[2,3] squamous cell carcinomas,[4,5] and basal cell carcinoma,[6,7] its use in most of these settings has been in combination with other chemotherapeutic agents, and through oral, intravenous, intra-arterial, or intrathecal routes of administration.

Intralesional MTX, however, has gained increasingly widespread recognition for its utility in the treatment of solitary keratoacanthoma (KA),[8] and this first section will emphasize the application. Keratoacanthoma is a cutaneous neoplasm that some consider a less-aggressive subtype of cutaneous squamous cell carcinoma while others claim it is a distinct, typically benign neoplasm that occasionally behaves more aggressively. Its classification and pathophysiology remain enigmatic and have been debated in the literature over many years.[9–14]

Despite difficulties in characterization, classification, and predicting the course of KA in individual patients, this tumor has potential for local tissue destruction, disfigurement, and occasionally may metastasize.[14] Given these realities, in settings where destructive or surgical modalities may be less desirable, intralesional therapy with methotrexate has proven safe and useful in a number of instances.

Other agents, including bleomycin, interferon, 5-fluorouracil, and rarely corticosteroids have been injected into KA tumors.[15–25] The utility of intralesional interferon, 5-fluorouracil, and bleomycin for cutaneous tumors is discussed later in this chapter.

For patients with multiple or syndromic keratoacanthomas,[11,12,26–28] including well-accepted subtypes

D.F. MacFarlane (ed.), *Skin Cancer Management*, DOI 10.1007/978-0-387-88495-0_5,
© Springer Science+Business Media, LLC 2010

such as Witten-Zak, Grzybowski, and Ferguson Smith, intralesional therapy is usually not indicated, and systemic retinoids[29,30] may be more useful in treatment and chemoprevention (see Chapter 21).

Indications and Contraindications

KA typically occurs as a solitary lesion on sun-exposed skin in older patients. These tumors usually develop rapidly over several weeks or a few months, and display distinct histology, with a keratin-filled crater lined by a proliferating, atypical squamous epithelium, often with the rim forming an overhanging appearance—the so-called "buttress." While these tumors may eventually involute spontaneously, some do not, and occasionally may metastasize.[9,10,14]

KA tumors that are most amenable to intralesional MTX are those with a classic clinical course, and where surgery would otherwise be challenging. Typical locations would be close to critical facial structures such as the periorbital region, perioral area, nose, and ears. Another common clinical scenario is if the tumor is not in a critical anatomic location, but of a size where surgery would produce excessive tension on nearby tissue, or require a flap or graft repair. Those who are often excellent candidates for MTX injection include patients who might tolerate surgery poorly because of the duration required to complete an excision, or who have comorbidities such as anticoagulation, diabetes, liver disease, or alcohol or tobacco abuse.

Caveats include patients who are immunosuppressed by medications for autoimmune disease or organ transplantation, or advanced human immunodeficiency virus (HIV) disease. These patients warrant similar concern if watchful waiting for involution is the initial management approach chosen, given their relative lack of tumor immunity. Patients who have difficulty with several weeks of wound care or who are intolerant to a more prolonged clinical course might be better served by one of the other treatment approaches described elsewhere in this text. Since MTX causes tumor necrosis, KA typically become more friable, and

eventually ulcerate before resolution. The appearance of the site, and the care required, are not tolerated well by some patients.

There are many alternatives to injectable methotrexate for solitary KA, including standard excision,[9,10] Mohs excision,[31,32] radiotherapy,[33,34] curettage and electrodesiccation,[35–37] and intralesional 5-fluorouracil (IL-5-FU).[22–25] The recent literature suggests intralesional interferon alfa-2b[38] and topical imiquimod[39] may have utility, but these approaches are less established.

Pre-treatment Considerations

From a global management perspective, it is our most common practice that cases of suspected KA be confirmed histologically prior to any non-excisional therapy, since high-risk, rapidly growing squamous cell carcinomas or other aggressive cutaneous malignancies may be confused with KA. In addition, despite histopathological confirmation of KA, any tumor that does not respond following two MTX injections should be reevaluated and possibly sampled again for microscopic assessment.

Patients who fail to respond demonstrate the importance of clinical judgment in treating patients with suspected KA. Ultimately, the diagnosis of KA is highly dependent on clinicopathologic correlation. The possibility that a suspected KA is truly a squamous cell carcinoma must always be considered, and the failure to respond to intralesional or other non-surgical approaches should prompt alternative evaluation and intervention. Fortunately, successful treatment courses with intralesional MTX for KA last less than 2 months, allowing caregivers to establish an alternative therapeutic path should injectables fail.

Two cases of pancytopenia occurring in patients treated with single 25-mg doses of IL-MTX have been reported.[40,41] These were patients with hemodialysis-dependent renal failure who presumably lacked sufficient renal excretion after systemic absorption of the MTX, leading to transient bone marrow suppression. Other significant adverse effects have not been reported to date in patients without renal disease, but given the potential for subclinical cytopenia, obtaining a baseline and 1-week-post-injection complete blood count (CBC) for all patients is reasonable. In patients with known renal dysfunction, such precautions are strongly suggested.

The use of intralesional MTX for KA should be kept in clinical perspective. Standard excisional surgery is the treatment of choice for many solitary KA, offering both prompt definitive treatment as well as providing a complete specimen for histologic evaluation. Smaller KA, in particular, may resolve after biopsy alone. Surgical intervention, however, may lead to sizable defects in some cases, along with significant functional or cosmetic morbidity.[41,42] Some patients with comorbidities such as cardiovascular disease, poorly controlled diabetes, or chronic liver disease may be poor surgical candidates. In these circumstances, IL-MTX may offer the advantage of being less invasive, quickly administered, and tissue-sparing, as well as being cost-effective. Cosmetic results for KA treated with MTX are typically quite good. Intralesional 5-FU has been demonstrated to be an effective treatment for KA and is a worthy alternative. Intralesional 5-FU may require more frequent injections and may require more local anesthesia; however, these aspects vary with practitioner experience.[42]

Injectable MTX is relatively inexpensive. At our institutions, MTX solution is ordered from the hospital pharmacy at a cost of approximately $2 for a 2-ml vial at a concentration of 25 mg/ml. The brevity of time required to administer the injection also contributes to the overall low therapeutic expense.

Preparing MTX for Injection

Since MTX is a chemotherapeutic agent, most pharmacies require more stringent precautions for mixing than for agents such as corticosteroids or anesthetics. A telephone conversation with a local pharmacy or community hospital pharmacy several days in advance of the planned injection is helpful. The medication should be prepared at the pharmacy, and placed in a Luer-lok 3 ml syringe with a secure cap before delivery. Refrigeration is not required, but the medication should be administered within 24 h of preparation. A concentration of either 12.5 or 25 mg/ml should be chosen—typically the lower concentration for smaller tumors (less than 1 cm), or the higher concentration for larger ones. Depending on clinical response after the first injection, the dose can be maintained if a second injection is required, or altered. If the tumor becomes substantially necrotic and nearly resolves after the first injection, the lower dose should be chosen for the next injection. If the tumor responds minimally, then a higher dose should be chosen for the subsequent injection.

Description of Technique

Our standard practice for injection is as follows: using a 27-gauge needle, 0.3–2.0 cc of MTX in a concentration of either 12.5 mg/ml or 25 mg/ml is injected at each treatment session. We tend to favor the lower concentration for smaller tumors. Small KAs, less than 1 cm, are typically injected in a single central point at the base of the lesion whereas larger KAs are injected in four quadrants as well as at the central lesion base. Very large KA may require more than four injection points, working around the tumor circumferentially and aiming toward the center. The skin is usually just prepped with an alcohol swab and MTX is injected until an endpoint of uniform tumor blanching is achieved. Given the poor cohesion between tumor cells, roughly 50% leakage of the total injected MTX volume typically occurs and can be sponged off with clean gauze. The procedure is well tolerated in most patients without the use of local anesthesia, though use of injected lidocaine or topical anesthesia may be utilized without loss of efficacy. The overall approach to MTX injection for KA is highly analogous to injecting keloids with corticosteroids, though the pressure on the plunger required to inject a KA is less than that needed for the typical keloid. The volume instilled, the depth of injection, and the attempt at uniform distribution through the quadrants and base is quite similar. Patients feel the pain of injection, but as with triamcinolone, the discomfort afterward is minimal.

Treatment Pearls

1. Review all options and expectations with the patient before proceeding with injection.
2. A baseline and post-injection complete blood count, blood urea nitrogen, and creatinine should be considered, especially for patients with underlying chronic medical conditions or advanced age, given the rare reports of cytopenias in patients with renal insufficiency.
3. Local anesthesia is a reasonable option prior to MTX injection, especially for larger KA or anxious patients.
4. Leakage of MTX through the central crust or prior biopsy incisions is expected and should not reduce clinical efficacy.
5. Eye protection and Luer-lok™ syringes are important protective measures prior to injection. Usually, a 30-gauge needle is sufficient; ½ in for smaller KA, and 1 in for larger KA.
6. KA smaller than 1 cm can usually be injected with a single well-placed needle insertion from a peripheral site with the target for the needle tip located at the deeper central portion of the lesion. Larger KA benefit from several injections placed serially around the periphery and directed toward the center. The technique is highly analogous to injecting corticosteroids into hypertrophic scars.
7. Crusting and necrosis are expected 7–10 days after each injection. Gentle debridement of necrotic tissue prior to the next injection assists in delivering the agent to viable residual neoplastic tissue as opposed to injection into the crust.

Post-injection Care

A non-adherent dressing with a small amount of petrolatum centrally is sufficient to protect the recently injected KA. Thereafter patients may cleanse the area daily or twice-daily with dilute acetic acid or dilute hydrogen peroxide before reapplying a dressing. Soaking the surface first with a clean damp cloth or in the shower may help if the crusting is significant.

Expected Course of Treatment and Follow-Up

We recently reported our own experience with injectable MTX for KA over a 15-year period, and combined our data with that published by others over the past several decades.[8] Detailed information on our clinical approach to such patients follows shortly. However, a brief summary of our findings regarding technique, efficacy, and caveats is provided first. The results are also summarized in Table 5.1.

Table 5.1 Injectable methotrexate for keratoacanthoma recent study and review[8]

Total number of patients	38
Mean tumor size	1.9 cm (1.0–4.0 range)
Anatomic location	~75% head and neck
Histopathologic confirmation at baseline	~66%
Methotrexate concentration utilized	12.5 mg/ml in 49% of patients
	25 mg/ml in 51% of patients
Methotrexate mean volume	1.0 ml
Methotrexate cumulative mean dose	36 mg
Mean interval between injections	18 days
Mean number of treatment sessions	2 (range 1–4)
Complete response rate	92% (35/38)
Mean time of follow-up	1.8 years

In our study and review, the average age of the 38 evaluable patients was early 60–70 s, gender distribution was even, and tumors were between 1.0 and 4.0 cm with a mean of 1.9 cm. Nearly 75% were located on the head and neck, with the remainder on trunk and extremities. Histologic confirmation was determined in advance in 2/3 of cases. Patients typically received either 12.5 mg/ml (49% of injections) or 25 mg/ml (51% of injections) concentration of MTX per injection, spaced 2–3 weeks apart. Specifically, the mean interval between injections was 18 days, and the total cumulative average dose for each of the 38 patients was 36 mg of MTX. The mean volume injected was 1.0 ml per treatment session, and the concentration selected appeared to be related more to institutional bias rather than tumor characteristics. The average number of treatment sessions was 2, with a range of 1–4.

Our study revealed a complete response rate of 92% (35 of 38 patients). KA resolution was determined by physical examination and clinical behavior in the vast majority of cases (33/38) while tumor resolution was also determined histologically in 5 of 38 patients. The mean interval of follow-up was 1.8 years. Importantly, 8% (3/38) of KA tumors did not resolve and subsequently required surgical extirpation. Non-respondent lesions were somewhat larger than the 92% of KA that did respond: 2.8 cm versus 1.9 cm, respectively. Two of the non-responders had tumors on the face and the other was a recurrent hand lesion failing prior surgical excision. No significant adverse events occurred in all of the 38 cases examined.

Several case examples follow that illustrate the typical clinical course for patients treated with intralesional MTX for KA.

Illustrative Case 5.1

A 70-year-old Caucasian woman presented with a 1-month history of a rapidly enlarging, mildly pruritic nodule on the right forehead. Her general health was excellent and she was on no medications. Her examination revealed a solitary keratotic 1.5 cm nodule on the right forehead with no lymphadenopathy (Fig. 5.1). Wedge biopsy demonstrated a keratoacanthoma-like squamous cell carcinoma.

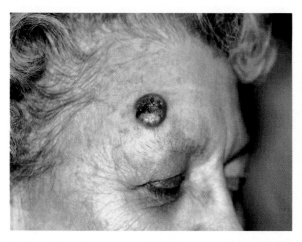

Fig. 5.1 A 70-year-old woman with biopsy-confirmed 1.5-cm keratoacanthoma of the right temple prior to initial intralesional injection of 1.0 ml methotrexate at 25 mg/ml concentration. The tumor developed over 1 month

Three days later she underwent injection of 1 ml of 25-mg/ml concentration MTX. She developed additional crusting over the surface of the nodule, with partial resolution noted 3 weeks later (Fig. 5.2). At that time, she underwent a second injection at the same concentration and volume. One month subsequently, there was minimal residual eschar, and no remaining nodule (Fig. 5.3). She continued to heal well over the next month (Fig. 5.4) with moist occlusive wound care and remained free of recurrence 1 year later, with an excellent esthetic result (Fig. 5.5).

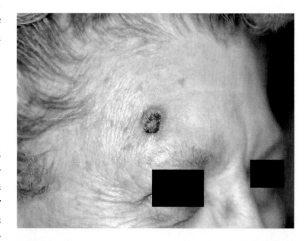

Fig. 5.2 Central and inferior crusting of the keratoacanthoma 3 weeks after initial injection, and prior to the second injection of methotrexate at the same concentration and volume

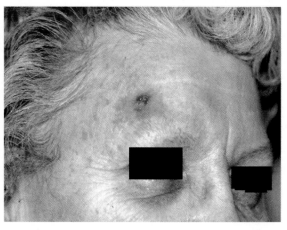

Fig. 5.3 Minimal clinically evident residual keratoacanthoma and eschar 1 month after the second injection

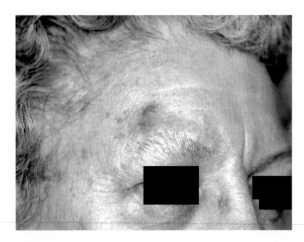

Fig. 5.4 Nearly complete healing 10 weeks after the initial injection of methotrexate

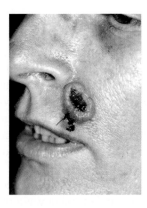

Fig. 5.6 A 48-year-old woman after wedge biopsy confirming well-differentiated squamous cell carcinoma with keratoacanthoma-like features of the *left upper* cutaneous lip, measuring 2.3 × 1.4 cm. The tumor rapidly evolved to this size over 2 months. She underwent initial methotrexate injection at 25 mg/ml concentration and volume of 1.0 ml at this time

Biopsy revealed a well-differentiated squamous cell carcinoma with keratoacanthoma-like features.

After discussing surgical and non-surgical options, she underwent injection of 1 ml MTX at a concentration of 25 mg/ml. At 3 weeks the lesion was approximately 50% of its prior height, though its peripheral dimensions were similar to baseline (Fig. 5.7). The size of the central crater was greatly diminished. The patient underwent a second MTX injection at the same concentration and volume that day. Four weeks subsequently, the overall size of the

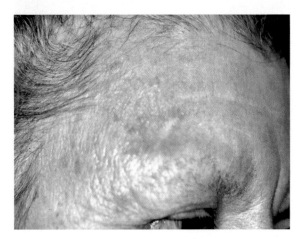

Fig. 5.5 Right temple 1 year after injection with excellent clinical and esthetic results

Illustrative Case 5.2

A 48-year-old Caucasian woman, with no prior medical conditions and on no medications, developed a rapidly growing nodule of the left upper lip and melolabial fold over a 2-month time period. The lesion had failed to respond to a 10-day course of oral antibiotics prescribed by a previous health care provider. On examination, there was a 2.3 × 1.4-cm hyperkeratotic and crusted nodule with a central crater. A suture was in place at the inferior border at the site of a recently performed wedge biopsy (Fig. 5.6). There was no clinical lymphadenopathy.

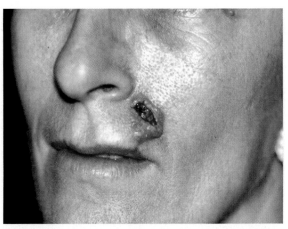

Fig. 5.7 Appearance of the tumor 3 weeks later at the time of the second injection. Note the additional crusting and central necrosis. Peripheral dimensions are similar, though tumor bulk is greatly diminished. She underwent a second injection of methotrexate at the same volume and concentration

lesion was 1.5 × 1.0 cm (Fig. 5.8). A final injection of MTX—once again at 25 mg/ml concentration and 1 ml total volume—was performed. One month later, a small, smooth 4-mm area of tissue remained inferiorly and clinically appeared to be a small scar (Fig. 5.9). This was confirmed by punch biopsy 6 weeks later, which also effectively smoothed the clinical residual. She had no recurrence of disease 2 years later, but did develop one additional small squamous cell carcinoma of the left shoulder in the interim, excised with clear margins and an uneventful post-operative course.

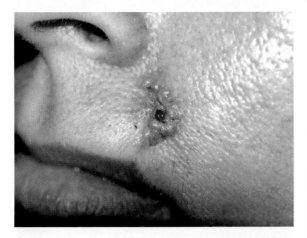

Fig. 5.8 After an additional 3 weeks, the keratoacanthoma continues to involute. She underwent a third and final injection of methotrexate, once again at a volume of 1.0 ml and concentration of 25 mg/ml

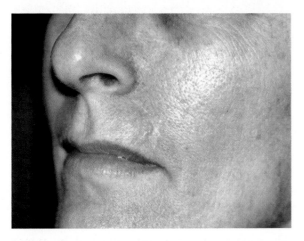

Fig. 5.9 Appearance of the *upper* lip 6 weeks later, showing a small fold of skin at the prior inferior border of the keratoacanthoma. A punch biopsy demonstrated scar and no residual tumor

Illustrative Case 5.3

An 87-year-old Caucasian female with multiple prior basal cell carcinomas developed a rapidly growing nodule on the right temple above the right eyebrow over a 3-month period. She noted occasional tenderness, crusting, and intermittent yellow drainage. The patient also had multiple underlying medical problems, including Parkinson's disease, a prior cerebrovascular accident, hypothyroidism, cervical cancer, and hypertension. Examination revealed a 2.6 × 2.4-cm keratotic plaque on the right temple adjacent to the eyebrow (Fig. 5.10). There was no lymphadenopathy. A wedge biopsy demonstrated squamous cell carcinoma with keratoacanthomatous features.

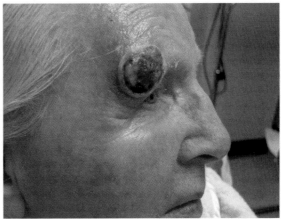

Fig. 5.10 An 87-year-old woman with a 2.6 × 2.4-cm nodule rapidly developing over 3 months on the *right* temple adjacent to the *eyebrow*. A wedge biopsy confirmed squamous cell carcinoma with keratoacanthomatous features

Given her age and multiple comorbidities, she underwent injection of MTX 25 mg/ml concentration and a volume of 1 ml. She received 4 ml of 1% lidocaine with 1:100,000 epinephrine prior to MTX administration (Figs. 5.11, 5.12, and 5.13). Three weeks later, the center had become necrotic (Fig. 5.14) and was removed prior to injection of the base and periphery with an additional 1 ml of MTX at the same concentration (Fig. 5.15). After three additional weeks, healthy granulation tissue was evident at the base, and no additional injections were required

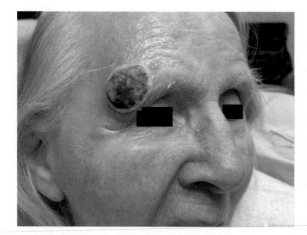

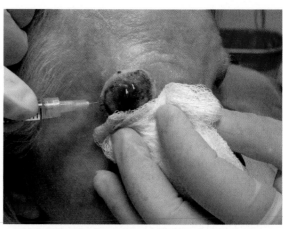

Fig. 5.11 Blanching of the skin surrounding the tumor resulting from administration of 4 ml of 1% lidocaine with 1:100,000 epinephrine prior to intralesional methotrexate injection

Fig. 5.13 Injection of an additional aliquot of 0.2 ml of methotrexate at the lateral aspect of the tumor. The inferior and medial injections followed, but are not depicted in this series

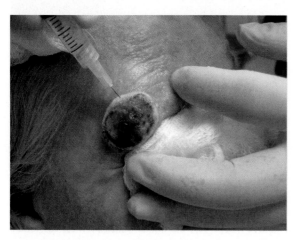

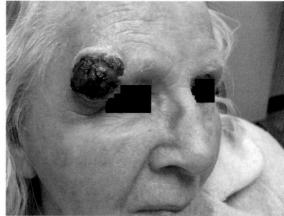

Fig. 5.12 Injection of methotrexate at 25 mg/ml concentration through the superior rim of the tumor with a 30-gauge 1-inch needle directed centrally and parallel to the skin surface. Approximately 0.2 ml was administered, with the remaining volume to be distributed around the periphery, sequentially. The 4 × 4-inch gauze serves both to protect the eye from extravasating methotrexate and to absorb any drug that extrudes through the crust

Fig. 5.14 Crusted and necrotic center of the keratoacanthoma 3 weeks later

II. INTERFERON

Every epithelial carcinoma has been reported to have occasional total regression—stage and tumor burden not withstanding—brought about by immune attack. The immune system routinely kills neoplastic cells, and it is the overwhelming of this function that allows tumors to grow. In an immunocompetent individual, non-melanoma skin cancers are constantly attacked by tumor infiltrating lymphocytes (TIL), and it is through stimulation of these cells that complete regression of skin cancer can occur.[43–47]

(Fig. 5.16). Twice-daily dilute acetic acid soaks followed by the application of white petrolatum, and a non-adherent dressing were employed for the following month, with complete re-epithelialization observed. She had no recurrence of the lesion, or new lesions over the subsequent 3 years (Fig. 5.17).

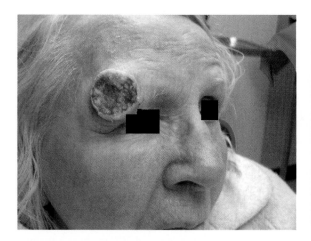

Fig. 5.15 The appearance of the base of the tumor with the crust debrided, and prior to the second methotrexate injection at the same volume and concentration, distributed evenly around the circumference of the residual tumor the same day

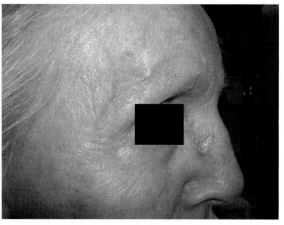

Fig. 5.17 Appearance of the site at 1 year, with excellent healing and no clinical evidence of recurrence. She remains disease-free at 3 years follow-up

be of major concern to the patient. The physician must be comfortable and confident in recommending treatment, and knowledgeable as to the mechanism of action and expected outcome.

The most beneficial treatment for skin cancer is that which eradicates the tumor and produces the least morbidity. Immunomodulatory IFN therapy, which is an alternative to destructive methods, meets these criteria for "most beneficial" with selected tumors.

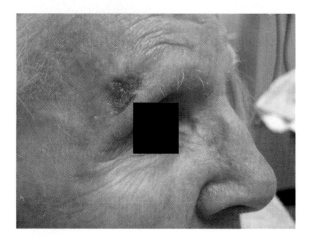

Fig. 5.16 Minimal erosion remaining at the site after an additional 3 weeks. The patient continued moist occlusive wound care without additional methotrexate administration. She completely healed 1 month later

Indications and Contraindications

Essential to the success of perilesional interferon treatment of skin cancer is screening of both the patient and the tumor. The patient should be an individual who understands that immune cells routinely kill cancer cells and one who is comfortable waiting 2–3 months for evaluation of efficacy. Since there are side effects of influenza-like symptoms, even though mild, it is important that this will not

Pre-treatment Considerations: Basal Cell Cancers

The tumors that respond virtually 100% to immunomodulatory treatment are superficial and nodular basal cell carcinomas (BCC).[47] The location where there is a clear cosmetic benefit over destructive/excisional treatment is the trunk. Therefore, a physician who wishes to begin using this therapy should select a superficial or nodular BCC on the trunk. The experience gained will provide confidence and the opportunity to expand the range of tumors treated. Basal cell carcinoma, which is highly differentiated toward adnexal structures (hair follicle, eccrine sweat gland), does not respond to IFN treatment. Periorificial BCC tumors have a somewhat lower response rate, even with typical histology.

Pre-treatment Considerations: Squamous Cell Cancers and Malignant Melanomas

Because of the greater potential for metastatic spread of squamous cell cancer (SCC) and malignant melanoma (MM) great caution in selection of tumors for which injectable interferon (IFN) treatment is "most beneficial" is needed.[48–50] The only SCC suggested for selection are those where the patient has refused surgery (Figs. 5.18 and 5.19), or a superficial or in situ SCC that has failed to respond to previous therapies (Figs. 5.20, 5.21, and 5.22). SCC can invade

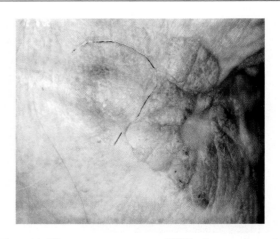

Fig. 5.20 Biopsy-proven verrucous SCC in situ near the medial canthus with lateral extension outlined in ink. Previous treatments over 15 years included multiple cryotherapies, curettages, and curettage with electrodesiccation

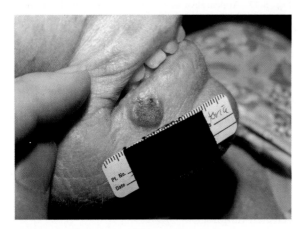

Fig. 5.18 Biopsy-proven large SCC on the lip of an elderly patient who refused surgical treatment

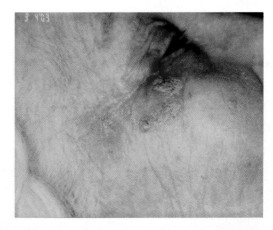

Fig. 5.21 Resolving tumor 1 week after the final IFN injection, typical for SCC but not seen with BCC

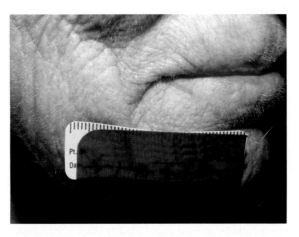

Fig. 5.19 Complete clinical resolution of the SCC on the lip 6 months later with slight delling at the tumor site, and skin markings present

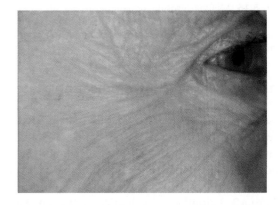

Fig. 5.22 Complete clinical resolution of tumor with intact skin markings. Photo taken 14 months after Fig. 5.21

deeply and be neurotropic—further factors for caution in tumor selection.

Malignant melanoma has great metastatic potential. The only MM suggested for selection are biopsy-proven MM in situ for which surgery is deemed not to be a viable option (Figs. 5.23 and 5.24).[50]

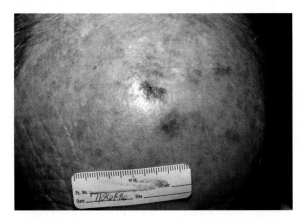

Fig. 5.23 Biopsy-proven recurrent MM in situ 2 years after wide excision

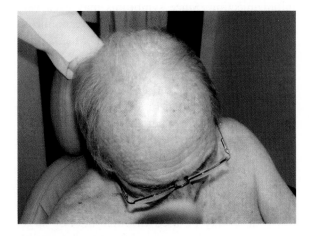

Fig. 5.24 Biopsy-proven and clinically seen complete resolution 7 years after IFN treatment

Obtaining Interferon α2b

Interferon alpha-2b (IFN) is not FDA-approved in the United States but is approved in Europe and Canada. However, approximately one-third of patients may be able to get help from their insurance companies for purchasing IFN. A prescription is given for Intron A, 18 million units, NDC # 0085-1100-01. The manufacturer has labeled this as a "single-use vial," not for intralesional use. However, this is the same solution used in the early trials that showed great efficacy and does not have the risk of reaction to the preservative compounded in vials labeled "for intralesional use."

The diluent that comes in the package is used and additional bacteriostatic saline is further added to bring the concentration to 500,000 U per 0.1 ml (3.6 cc total volume). This vial is immediately and constantly refrigerated except when drawing up the injection. Routine sterile technique is used for multiuse vials. The reconstituted and diluted IFN retains its clinical efficacy when continuously refrigerated for up to 6 months.

The cost to the patient at a nationwide low-cost retail pharmacy is $270. Alternatively, the physician's office may purchase the medication and charge the patient for it. Since approximately 4 million units will be left over after giving all nine injections, the patient may be treated at a slightly reduced medication cost.

Description of Technique (BCC, SCC, MM)

Administering Interferon α2b

The use of 1 cc syringes with plungers that push virtually all fluid into the 30-gauge needle is preferred (Norm-Ject, www.delasco.com). The site is prepared with alcohol and the end of an ice cube is placed on the specific small area where the needle will enter the skin for about 6 s to decrease pain.

Make sure to always:

1. Inject into the dermis, not the subcutis, since the maximum local effect on the immune system depends on intradermal placement.
2. Inject perilesionally, not intralesionally. The solution, if properly placed, will cause swelling and blanching of the surrounding skin as well as

the tumor (Figs. 5.25 and 5.26). Intralesional injection will cause loss of suspended IFN due to leaking of fluid from the less cohesive tumor tissue. It is the immune response in the normal surrounding dermis that attacks the tumor. Some IFN solution may leak out or come out in a spray from hair follicles; adjusting the depth of the needle point or injecting in a different area will correct the loss of medication. Any IFN solution that has leaked onto the skin may be sucked back into the syringe and re-injected.

3. Inject superior to the tumor.
4. Pre- and post-medicate individuals receiving IFN injections. The symptoms that an individual with a cold or flu experiences are due to the body's immune response to the virus, particularly interferon, not the virus itself. These same symptoms can be reproduced by the intradermal injections of interferon and are dose-dependent.

Ibuprofen or acetaminophen—based on patient preference, medical history, and size—is recommended 1 h prior to injection, 3 h after injection (the time of onset of symptoms typically), the evening of the injection, and the following morning. Sensitivity to interferon-induced flu-like side effects varies among individuals. Tachyphylaxis of symptoms occurs if injections are given 2–3 days apart. However, after 5 days without an injection, symptoms are similar to the initial injection. Since symptoms may even vary between injections, the author highly recommends the use of the above regimen for all patients being treated with IFN.

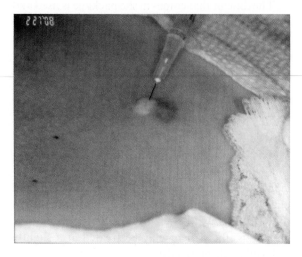

Fig. 5.25 Injection of IFN superior to the tumor with lightening and induration extending into the tumor

The amount of IFN injected depends on the tumor size, the injection sequence, and the sensitivity of the individual to side effects. While the standard dose of IFN per treatment is 1.5×10^6 units (0.3 cc), using a lower dose for the first and second injections—such as 1×10^6 units (0.2 cc)—is recommended. The standard dose of 1.5×10^6 units is given by the third or fourth injection. For a small tumor (e.g., 1×1 cm), the lower dose may be used throughout. For larger tumors, larger doses may be given compatible with patient tolerance. In general, the effective dose range correlates with 1×10^6 units for tumor size 1 cm^2, and increases by 0.5×10^6 units for each additional cm^2. Dilution up to 0.25×10^6 units per 0.1 ml may be made for very large superficial BCC. This flexibility allows for individual variations based on tumor size and sensitivity to side effects.

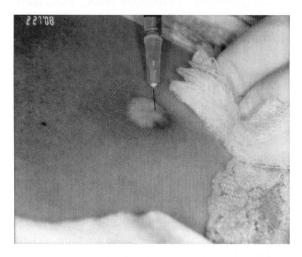

Fig. 5.26 Further extension of IFN into the tumor, complete infiltration of IFN solution with lightening of the area is desired

Treatment Pearls

1. If four or five days have elapsed since the last injection, flu-like symptoms will be stronger, as with the first injection, so the dose may need adjustment.
2. It is the stimulation of the local immune system "over time," not the total dose that produces the desired results. Three large doses given over a week are not as effective as nine small doses given over 3–4 weeks.
3. The dilution of the IFN solution to 0.5×10^6 units per 0.1 cc increases efficacy over more concentrated solutions. When it is more concentrated, the ramifications of losing a small amount of the solution during transferring or injection are greater.
4. Less than 1% of patients treated with this regimen have no response. Another treatment modality is necessary in such cases.
5. Rare individuals will have only a partial response with marked tumor shrinkage. Since the tumor has responded partially, complete response can be obtained if retreatment with another course of IFN is desired by the patient.
6. The location where there is a clear cosmetic benefit of IFN over destructive/excisional treatment is the trunk.
7. The amount of IFN injected depends on the tumor size, the injection sequence, and the sensitivity of the individual to side effects.

Post-injection Care

As with any intradermal injection, local treatment is the placement of petroleum jelly, gauze, and pressure for 2–3 min and/or an adhesive bandage to protect clothing from seepage from the injection site.

Expected Course of Treatment and Follow-Up (BCC, SCC, MM)

Three types of local responses may occur, typically between injections six to nine:

1. The tumor may become red and indurated, sometimes with slight surrounding erythema and rarely with a tender lymph node or folliculitis (Figs. 5.27, 5.28, and 5.29).
2. Slight erythema of the tumor occurs with little induration; and
3. Little to no erythema is observed throughout the course, but slight induration occurs. If local response 1 occurs, 100% tumor resolution has been the rule. However, in greater than 90% of tumors with responses 2 or 3, complete resolution also occurs.

The tumor often stops crusting after injection #6 and less leakage of interferon occurs. Following the ninth injection, the patient is instructed to return for evaluation in 3 months. Little to no regression of BCC is seen during the actual treatment of BCC but occurs weeks later once treatment has finished.

If no response of the tumor is observed (e.g., redness, swelling, induration) surgical removal should be performed. For the other 99% of BCC tumors, the 3-month post-treatment evaluation is sufficient.

SCC often show clinical partial resolution during the 3- to 4-week period of treatment (Figs. 5.20, 5.21, and 5.22). Occasionally, BCC or SCC will develop milia-like cysts, which resolve over the following 3–6 months.[48]

MM resolve in a similar time period to SCC. For pigmented MM, resolution of the pigment, as well as the malignant melanocytes, is expected (Figs. 5.23 and 5.24).

The question of whether there is always a need to biopsy post-treatment is best answered (other than MM which should always be biopsied following treatment) with close evaluation of the treated site. Normal skin lines should return following treatment (Figs. 5.30 and 5.31) in contradistinction to curetted and electrodesiccated lesions (Fig. 5.32). Even with very large and deep tumors, where considerable post-treatment hypopigmentation and/or delling may occur, there is a return of normal skin lines (Figs. 5.33 and 5.34). This allows effective post-treatment clinical follow-up, making biopsy unnecessary.

In the largest double-blind, placebo-controlled study of IFN treatment of BCC, no subclinical tumor was found on excision of the treated site at

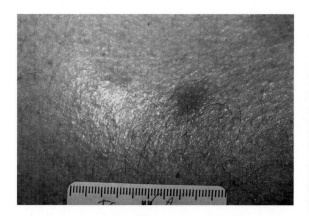

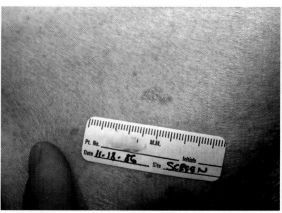

Fig. 5.27 Two superficial BCCs on the chest of a man with numerous truncal BCCs. The man sought treatment for these tumors that would not yield prominent scar formation (see Fig. 5.32)

Fig. 5.30 Superficial BCC on back

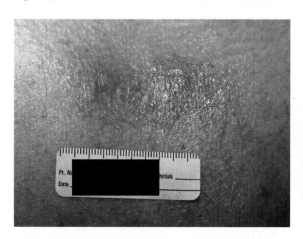

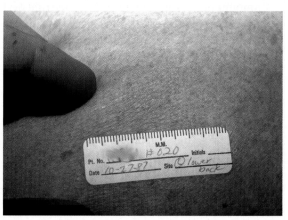

Fig. 5.28 Erythema and induration of the chest BCCs after the seventh IFN injection; typical for a type 1 response to treatment

Fig. 5.31 Complete clinical resolution of superficial BCC with normal skin markings

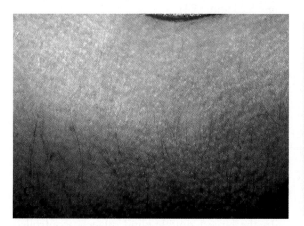

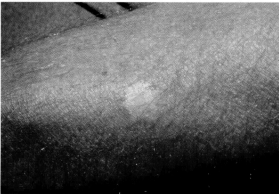

Fig. 5.29 Complete clinical resolution at 6 months post-treatment with slight hypopigmentation and normal skin markings

Fig. 5.32 Electrodesiccation and curettage scar for BCC on the arm of the patient whose chest BCCs are seen in Figs. 5.27, 5.28, and 5.29. Note lack of skin markings after 1 year

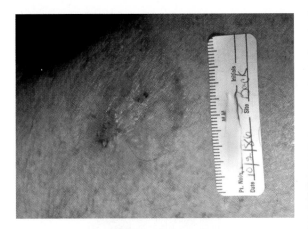

Fig. 5.33 Extensive nodular and superficial BCC on the shoulder prior to IFN treatment, note the hemangioma within the tumor

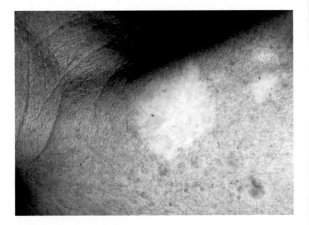

Fig. 5.34 Complete clinical resolution of the tumor photographed 20 years following IFN therapy. Skin markings are present despite the prominent hypopigmentation. The hemangioma was unaffected by IFN therapy as are all benign structures

1-year post-treatment if no tumor was visible by clinical inspection.[51] Long-term follow-up for 10 years or longer has confirmed the extremely low incidence of persistent or recurrent tumor with this immunomodulatory treatment.[47]

III. 5-FLUOROURACIL

5-Fluorouracil (5-FU) is a structural analog of thymidine that interferes with synthesis, resulting in the death of rapidly proliferating malignant cells. It has been used topically for years to treat actinic keratoses, Bowen's disease and superficial basal cell carcinoma (Chapter 2). 5-FU has been used intralesionally in the treatment of keratoacanthomas and nodular basal cell carcinomas (Figs. 5.35, 5.36, 5.37, 5.38, and 5.39).[52]

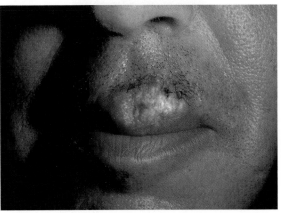

Fig. 5.35 Keratoacanthoma of the lip, pre-treatment

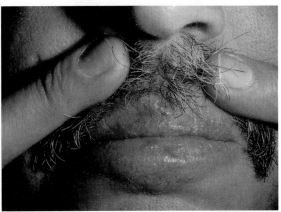

Fig. 5.36 Keratoacanthoma of the lip, 5 months after treatment with intralesional 5-fluorouracil and oral isotretinoin

Keratoacanthomas

Klein was the first to use intralesional 5-FU in 1962 to treat KAs.[22] Since then there have been many reports of KAs treated effectively with intralesional 5-FU.[16,17,24,53–55] In two separate studies, 55 keratoacanthomas located on the face, head,

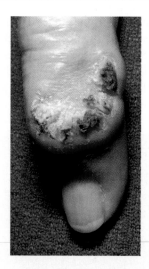

Fig. 5.37 Keratoacanthoma of the finger, pre-treatment

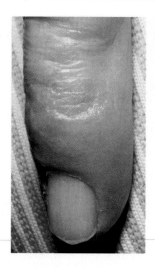

Fig. 5.39 Keratoacanthoma of the finger, 1 year follow-up

Squamous Cell Carcinomas

Intralesional 5-FU has been used to treat SCCs.[56] Twenty-three patients with biopsy-proven SCCs of less than 6 months' duration, located on the face, head, neck, arms, or hands and varying from 0.24 to 7.50 cm were treated with intratumoral 5-FU/epinephrine gel. The patients received weekly injections of 1.0 ml or less of a combination of 30 mg/ml of 5-FU and 0.1 mg/ml of epinephrine gel for 4–6 weeks. Only one patient failed treatment and all had a good to excellent cosmetic result. Morse et al. treated an SCC on the right nasolabial fold with eight weekly injections of 5-FU with doses ranging from 0.8 to 2.4 ml. Histological clearance was achieved and the patient was tumor-free at 5-month follow-up.[18]

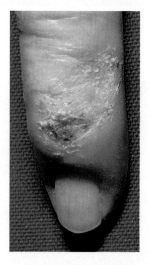

Fig. 5.38 Keratoacanthoma of the finger, 1 month after treatment with weekly intralesional 5-fluorouracil

Basal Cell Carcinomas

and extremities were studied. Following an average of three weekly injections of 0.2–0.6 ml of an aqueous solution of 50 mg/cm^3 5-FU, 53 of the 55 lesions (96%) showed histologic clearing.[53,54] In another case report, Eubanks et al. observed total clearing of all of a patient's 14 KAs treated with doses of IL 5-FU of 0.1–0.2 ml over five to nine weekly injections.[16]

Intralesional injection of 5-FU has been effective in nodular basal cell cancers.[57] At 2-year follow-up, intralesional 5-FU was successful for 3 keratoacanthomas and two of three BCCs. It was found that 5–6 injections were needed to treat the BCCs, a finding in agreement with an earlier study. An average of 8 injections of 5-FU was required to treat the KAs. Odom et al. were able to treat them with 2.8 injections.[53]

Indications

These are similar to MTX, used when a patient refuses surgical intervention, or in cases where a patient's medical condition contraindicates surgery, or in cases where the surgery will result in a large defect.

Contraindications

Hypersensitivity to 5-FU, or difficulty with following the protocol, are contraindications.

Pre-treatment Considerations

These are similar to MTX.

Obtaining and Preparing

Use 5-fluoruracil commercially available for systemic chemotherapy (50 mg/ml). Local anesthesia can be used with it, as an option (1% lidocaine).

Description of Technique

Infiltrate in and around lesion once or twice weekly until neither palpable nor visible. Thorough and complete infiltration of the tumor with 5-FU is essential for efficacy.[58]

Note on Technique

Compared with intralesional methotrexate, intralesional 5-fluorouracil is more painful. The authors have no strong opinion about the relative effectiveness, and we are not aware of a controlled comparison study. It is important to abort the therapy if it clearly is not working, and resort to surgery, radiation therapy, or some other modality. One of the authors (RR) is aware of one case of treatment of a keratoacanthoma of the periorbital area with intralesional 5-fluorouracil that was ineffective, resulting in a lawsuit. The lesion had continued to grow despite the intralesional treatment, and eventually the patient had to have an ocular enucleation.

Post-injection Care

This is similar to intralesional MTX.

Expected Course and Follow-Up

If KAs do not demonstrate necrosis clinically after two to three weekly intralesional 5-FU treatments, alternative treatments should be considered.[58]

Adverse Effects

Kurtis and Rosen reported the development of SCC within a BCC that was treated with intralesional injections of 5-FU.[59] Intralesional injections can result in pain, necrosis, and ulceration. Systemic effects similar to intravenous 5-FU therapy can occur, but generally only when the above doses are exceeded.

IV. BLEOMYCIN

Originally isolated from the fungus *Streptomyces verticillis*, bleomycin is used as an antitumor agent for the treatment of various kinds of malignancy.[60] Other dermatologic uses include the treatment of recalcitrant warts, hypertrophic scars, and keloids. Bleomycin has been shown to block the cell cycle at G2, cleave single- and double-stranded DNA, and degrade cellular RNAs. Bleomycin forms a complex with metal ions such as Fe (II), which is oxidized to Fe (III), resulting in the reduction of oxygen to free radicals which in turn cause cell breaks, leading ultimately to cell death.[61] While systemic bleomycin is FDA-approved for the treatment of SCC of the head and neck, cervix, penis, and skin, Hodgkin's and non-Hodgkin's lymphoma, testicular carcinoma, and malignant pleural effusion, there are no current FDA-approved indications for intralesional bleomycin.[62] The cytotoxic effect of bleomycin is enhanced considerably by coupling it with local anesthetics which increase its cellular uptake.[63] Electrical stimulation also disturbs the cell membrane and enhances bleomycin cytotoxicity in a process known as electrocorporation.[64] While bleomycin alone has not shown desirable outcomes for the treatment of cutaneous malignancies, when combined with electrocorporation, results have been very successful. In electrocorporation, a circular configuration of electrode needles is used to deliver brief, high-intensity, pulsed electrical currents directly into the target tumor.[65] The combined use of electrocorporation and a chemotherapeutic agent is termed electrochemotherapy (ECT).

Squamous Cell Carcinoma/ Keratoacanthoma

Keratoacanthomas have been treated with intralesional bleomycin without ECT. While no controlled, randomized studies have been conducted, in seven cases of KAs treated with intralesional bleomycin alone, a 100% cure rate and no side effects were reported.[19,71] In these cases a 0.5% solution of bleomycin was used, diluted with saline and lidocaine. Using a 27-gauge needle, 0.2–0.4 mg of solution was injected. At most, four courses of treatment were needed at weekly follow-up sessions.

Basal Cell Carcinoma

In a case series of 20 patients with 54 tumors treated with ECT, Glass et al. noted a complete response rate of 94% and a partial response rate of 6%, no reports of non-response or disease progression.[65] No reports on response rates for the different histologic subtypes of BCCs, cost-effectiveness or direct comparison between ECT and conventional treatment. There is one report of ECT and bleomycin used to treat a metastatic BCC with squamous differentiation.[67]

Metastatic Cutaneous Malignant Melanoma

Of the studies performed, treatment protocols varied, with 0.5–1.0U bleomycin per calculated cc of tumor, electrical amplitude between 560 and 15,000 V/cm/s. Complete response rates reported from 72 to 89%, partial response rates (greater than 50% reduction in calculated tumor size-5–10%). Long-term follow-up was not reported.

Indications

Similar to MTX.

Contraindications

Those with Raynaud's phenomenon or peripheral vascular disease should not be treated with bleomycin. It should be avoided in the pregnant or nursing patient.

Pre-treatment Considerations

Same as MTX.

Obtaining and Preparing

A common dilution of bleomycin is to take a vial of 15 international units of powder, and dilute it with 15 ml of normal saline to make a solution of 1 unit per ml. Other authorities have used more dilute preparations.

Description of Technique

One of the authors (RR) generally injects less than 0.6 ml of this solution weekly into a lesion for up to 8 weeks (0.1–0.2 ml for smaller lesions). Care must be taken to inject it specifically into the dermis associated with the lesion, and not into the fat, where larger amounts become easily injected, with very little effect on the malignancy.

Post-injection Care

Similar to MTX.

Expected Course and Follow-Up

One of the authors (RR) used bleomycin in a case of a large verrucous carcinoma of the sole (Fig. 5.40), with the idea that human papillomavirus plays a role in this type of carcinoma. The intralesional

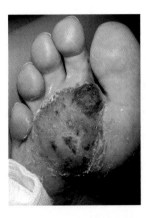

Fig. 5.40 Verrucous carcinoma on sole, pre-treatment

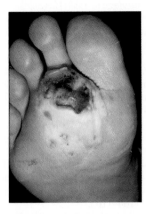

Fig. 5.41 Verrucous carcinoma 1 month after treatment with weekly intralesional bleomycin

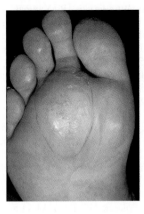

Fig. 5.42 Verrucous carcinoma 3 months after treatment with intralesional bleomycin. The tumor had an excellent response, but did have a partial recurrence later

bleomycin in the illustrated case did very well at eradicating the verrucous carcinoma (Fig. 5.41), but portions of it subsequently recurred (Fig. 5.42).

Adverse Effects

The following reactions occur immediately after injection and include erythema with swelling,[68] pain,[69] and a burning sensation.[70] The pain usually lasts for 72 h and is relieved with acetaminophen. Blackening of the skin and eschar formation have also been observed.[71] Rarely-onychodystrophy,[70] hypopigmentation,[72] atrophic, and hypertrophic scarring.[73] Raynaud's phenomenon, anaphylaxis, and flagellate hyperpigmentation have been reported.[74] If combined with electrical impulses to increase uptake (electrochemotherapy), patients may experience discomfort, local muscle contraction, skin burning, erythema and edema, and muscle fatigue.[75]

References

1. Olsen EA. The pharmacology of methotrexate. *J Am Acad Dermatol.* 1991;25:306–318.
2. Glantz MJ, Jaeckle KA, Chamberlain MC, et al. A randomized controlled trial comparing intrathecal sustained-release cytarabine (DepoCyt) to intrathecal methotrexate in patients with neoplastic meningitis from solid tumors. *Clin Cancer Res.* 1999;5:3394–3402.
3. Nystrom ML, Steele JP, Shamash J, et al. Low-dose continuous chemotherapy for metastatic melanoma: a phase II trial. *Melanoma Res.* 2003;13:197–199.
4. Colevas AD. Chemotherapy options for patients with metastatic or recurrent squamous cell carcinoma of the head and neck. *J Clin Oncol.* 2006;24:2644–2652.
5. Sheen YS, Sheen MC, Sheu HM, et al. Squamous cell carcinoma of the big toe successfully treated by intra-arterial infusion with methotrexate. *Dermatol Surg.* 2003;29:982–983.
6. Coker DD, Elias EG, Viravathana T, et al. Chemotherapy for metastatic basal cell carcinoma. *Arch Dermatol.* 1983;119:44–50.
7. Bason MM, Grant-Kels JM, Govil M. Metastatic basal cell carcinoma: response to chemotherapy. *J Am Acad Dermatol.* 1990;22:905–908.
8. Annest NM, Van Beek MJ, Arpey CJ, et al. Intralesional methotrexate injection for keratoacanthoma tumors: a retrospective study and review of the literature. *J Am Acad Dermatol.* 2007;56:989–993.
9. Beham A, Regauer S, Soyer HP, et al. Keratoacanthoma: a clinically distinct variant of well differentiated

squamous cell carcinoma. *Adv Anat Pathol.* 1998;5(5):269–280.

10. Manstein CH, Frauenhoffer CJ, Besden JE. Keratoacanthoma: is it a real entity? *Ann Plast Surg.* 1998;40(5):469–472.

11. Karaa A, Khachemoune A. Keratoacanthoma: a tumor in search of a classification. *Int J Dermatol.* 2007;46: 671–678.

12. Schwartz RA. Keratoacanthoma: a clinico-pathologic enigma. *Dermatol Surg.* 2004;30:326–333.

13. LeBoit PE. Can we understand keratoacanthoma? *Am J Dermatopathol.* 2002;24:166–168.

14. Hodak E, Jones RE, Ackerman AB. Solitary keratoacanthoma is a squamous cell carcinoma: three examples with metastases. *Am J Dermatopathol.* 1993;15: 332–342.

15. Sanders S, Busam KJ, Halpern AC, et al. Intralesional corticosteroid treatment of multiple eruptive keratoacanthomas: case report and review of a controversial therapy. *Dermatol Surg.* 2002;28:954–958.

16. Eubanks SW, Gentry RH, Patterson JW, et al. Treatment of multiple keratoacanthomas with intralesional fluorouracil. *J Am Acad Dermatol.* 1982;7:126–129.

17. Leonard AL, Hanke CW. Treatment of giant keratoacanthoma with intralesional 5-fluorouracil. *J Drugs Dermatol.* 2006;5:454–456.

18. Morse LG, Kendrick C, Hooper D, et al. Treatment of squamous cell carcinoma with intralesional 5-Fluorouracil. *Dermatol Surg.* 2003;29:1150–1153.

19. Sayama S, Tagami H. Treatment of keratoacanthoma with intralesional bleomycin. *Br J Dermatol.* 1983; 109:449–452.

20. de la Torre C, Losada A, Cruces MJ. Keratoacanthoma centrifugum marginatum: treatment with intralesional bleomycin. *J Am Acad Dermatol.* 1997;37:1010–1011.

21. Andreassi A, Pianigiani E, Taddeucci P, et al. Guess what! Keratoacanthoma treated with intralesional bleomycin. *Eur J Dermatol.* 1999;9:403–405.

22. Klein E, Milgram H, Traenkle HL. Tumors of the skin. II: Keratoacanthoma; local effect of 5-fluorouracil (5-FU). *Skin.* 1962;1:153–156.

23. Bergin DJ, Lapins NA, Deffer TA. Intralesional 5-fluorouracil for keratoacanthoma of the eyelid. *Ophthal Plast Reconstr Surg.* 1986;2(4):201–204.

24. Parker CM, Hanke CW. Large keratoacanthomas in difficult locations treated with intralesional 5-fluorouracil. *J Am Acad Dermatol.* 1986;14:770–777.

25. Thiele JJ, Ziemer M, Fuchs S, et al. Combined 5-fluorouracil and Er:YAG laser treatment in a case of recurrent giant keratoacanthoma of the lower leg. *Dermatol Surg.* 2004;30:1556–1560.

26. Feldman RJ, Maize JC. Multiple keratoacanthomas in a young woman: report of a case emphasizing medical management and a review of the spectrum of multiple keratoacanthomas. *Int J Dermatol.* 2007;46:77–79.

27. Mangas C, Bielsa I, Ribera M, et al. A case of multiple keratoacanthoma centrifugum marginatum. *Dermatol Surg.* 2004;30:803–806.

28. Vergara A, Isaría MJ, Domínguez JD, et al. Multiple and relapsing keratoacanthomas developing at the edge of skin grafts site after surgery and after radiotherapy. *Dermatol Surg.* 2007;33:994–996.

29. Street ML, White Jr JW, Gibson LE. Multiple keratoacanthomas treated with oral retinoids. *J Am Acad Dermatol.* 1990;23:862–866.

30. Benoldi D, Alinovi A. Multiple persistent keratoacanthomas: treatment with oral etretinate. *J Am Acad Dermatol.* 1984;10:1035–1038.

31. Benest L, Kaplan RP, Salit R, et al. Keratoacanthoma centrifugum marginatum of the lower extremity treated with Mohs micrographic surgery. *J Am Acad Dermatol.* 1994;31:501–502.

32. Larson PO. Keratoacanthomas treated with Mohs micrographic surgery (chemosurgery): a review of forty-three cases. *J Am Acad Dermatol.* 1987;16: 1040–1044.

33. Goldschmidt H, Sherwin WK. Radiation therapy of giant aggressive keratoacanthomas. *Arch Dermatol.* 1993;129(9):1162–1165.

34. Caccialanza M, Sopelana N. Radiation therapy of keratoacanthomas: results in 55 patients. *Int J Radiat Oncol Biol Phys.* 1989;16(2):475–477.

35. Reymann F. Treatment of Keratoacanthomas with curettage. *Dermatologica.* 1997;155(2):90–96.

36. Nedwich JA. Evaluation of curettage and electrodesiccation in treatment of keratoacanthoma. *Australas J Dermatol.* 1991;32(3):137–141.

37. Sheridan AT, Dawber RP. Curettage, electrosurgery and skin cancer. *Australas J Dermatol.* 2000;41(1):19–30.

38. Oh CK, Son HS, Lee JB, et al. Intralesional interferon alfa-2b treatment of keratoacanthomas. *J Am Acad Dermatol.* 2004;51(6):1040.

39. Dendorfer M, Oppel T, Wollenberg A, et al. Topical treatment with imiquimod may induce regression of facial keratoacanthoma. *Eur J Dermatol.* 2003;13 (1):80–82.

40. Goebeler M, Lurz C, Kolve-Goebeler ME, et al. Pancytopenia after treatment of keratoacanthoma by single lesional methotrexate infiltration. *Arch Dermatol.* 2001;137(8):1104–1105.

41. Cohen PR, Schulze KE, Nelson BR. Pancytopenia after a single intradermal infiltration of methotrexate. *J Drugs Dermatol.* 2005;4(5):648–651.

42. Melton JL, Nelson BR, Stough DB, et al. Treatment of keratoacanthomas with intralesional methotrexate. *J Am Acad Dermatol.* 1991;25:1017–1023.

43. Dudley ME, Wunderlich JR, Yang JC, et al. Adoptive cell transfer therapy following non-myeloablative but lymphodepleting chemotherapy for the treatment of patients with refractory metastatic melanomas. *Clin Oncol.* 2005;23:2346–2357.

44. Greenway HT, Cornell RC, Tanner DJ, et al. Treatment of basal cell carcinomas with intralesional interferon. *J Am Acad Dermatol.* 1986;15:437–443.

45. Mozzanica N, Cattaneo A, Boneschi L, et al. Immunohistological evaluation of basal cell carcinoma immunoinfiltrate during intralesional treatment with alpha 2 interferon. *Arch Dermatol Res.* 1990;282(5):311–317.

46. Tong Y, Tucker SB. Normal human skin lymphocytic and Langerhans' cell responses to intradermal interferon α2b injections. *Am J Med Sci.* 1993;306:23–27.

47. Tucker SB, Polasek JW, Perri AJ, et al. Long term follow-up of basal cell carcinomas treated with perilesional interferon alfa 2b as monotherapy. *J Am Acad Dermatol.* 2006;54:1033–1038.

48. Tucker SB. Interferon-alpha treatment of basal cell and squamous cell skin tumors. *Cancer Bull*. 1993;45:270–274.

49. Edwards L, Berman B, Rapini RP, et al. Treatment of cutaneous squamous cell carcinomas by intralesional interferon alfa-2b therapy. *Arch Dermatol*. 1992;128: 1486–1489.

50. Carucci JA. Intralesional interferon alfa for treatment of recurrent lentigo maligna of the eyelid in a patient with primary acquired melanosis. *Arch Dermatol*. 2000; 136:1415.

51. Cornell RC, Greenway HT, Tucker SB, et al. Intralesional interferon therapy of basal cell carcinoma. *J Am Acad Dermatol*. 1990;23:694–700.

52. Miller BH, Shavin JS, Cognetta A, et al. Nonsurgical treatment of basal cell carcinomas with intralesional 5-fluoruracil injectable gel. *J Am Acad Dermatol*. 1997;36:72–77.

53. Odom RB, Goette DK. Treatment of keratoacanthomas with intralesional fluorouracil. *Arch Dermatol*. 1978; 114:1779–1983.

54. Goette DK, Odom RB. Successful treatment of keratoacanthoma with intralesional fluorouracil. *J Am Acad Dermatol*. 1980;2:212–216.

55. Kurtis B, Rosen T. Treatment of cutaneous neoplasms by intralesional injections of 5-fluorouracil (5-FU). *J Dermatol Surg Oncol*. 1980;6:122–127.

56. Kraus S, Miller BH, Swinehart JM, et al. Intratumoral chemotherapy with fluorouracil/epinephrine injectable gel: a nonsurgical treatment of cutaneous squamous cell carcinoma. *J Am Acad Dermatol*. 1998;38:438–442.

57. Avant WH, Huff RC. Intradermal 5-flurouracil in the treatment of basal cell carcinoma of the face. *South Med J*. 1976;69:561–563.

58. Hanke CW. Treatment of squamous cell carcinoma with intralesional 5-FU (Comment). *Dermatol Surg*. 2003; 29(11):1153.

59. Kurtis B, Rosen T. Squamous cell carcinoma arising in a basal cell epithelioma treated with 5-fluorouracil. *J Dermatol Surg Oncol*. 1979;5:394–396.

60. Umezawa H, Maeda K, Takeuchi T, et al. New antibiotics, bleomycin A and B. *J Antibiot*. 1966;19: 200–209.

61. Burger RM, Peisach J, Horwitz SB. Activated bleomycin: a transient complex of drug, iron and oxygen that degrades DNA. *J Biol Chem*. 1981;256:1636–1644.

62. Saitta P, Krishnamurthy K, Brown LH. Bleomycin in dermatology: a review of intralesional applications. *Dermatol Surg*. 2008;34:1299–1313.

63. Mizuno S, Ishida A. Selective enhancement of bleomycin cytotoxicity by local anesthetics. *Biochem Biophys Res Commun*. 1982;105:425–431.

64. Belehradek M, Domenge C, Luboinski B, et al. Electrochemotherapy, a new antitumor treatment. *Cancer*. 1993;72:3694–3700.

65. Glass F, Pepine M, Fenske N, et al. Bleomycin-mediated electrochemotherapy of metastatic melanoma. *Arch Dermatol*. 1996;132:1353–1357.

66. Torre C, Losada A, Cruces M. Keratoacanthoma centrifugum marginatum: treatment with intralesional bleomycin. *J Am Acad Dermatol*. 1997;37:1010–1011.

67. Fantini F, Gualdi G, Cimitan A, et al. Metastatic basal cell carcinoma with squamous differentiation. *Arch Dermatol*. 2008;144(9):1186–1188.

68. Omidvari S, Nezakatgoo N, Ahmadloo N, et al. Role of intralesional bleomycin in the treatment of complicated hemangiomas; prospective clinical study. *Dermatol Surg*. 2005;31:499–501.

69. Bunney M. Intralesional bleomycin sulfate in treatment of recalcitrant warts. *Clin Dermatol*. 1985;3:189–194.

70. Miller R. Nail dystrophy following intralesional injections of bleomycin for a periungual wart. *Arch Dermatol*. 1984;120:963–964.

71. Polluck B, Sheehan-Dare R. Pulsed dye laser and intralesional bleomycin for treatment of resistant viral hand warts. *Lasers Surg Med*. 2002;30:135–140.

72. Susser W, Whitaker-White D, Grant-Kies J. Mucocutaneous reactions to chemotherapy. *J Am Acad Dermatol*. 1999;40:367–398.

73. Pienaar C, Graham R, Geldenhuys S, et al. Intralesional bleomycin for the treatment of hemangiomas. *Plastic Reconstruct Surg*. 2006;117:221–226.

74. Smith EA, Harber FE, Leroy EG, et al. Raynaud's phenomenon of a single digit following local intradermal bleomycin sulfate injection. *Arthritis Rheum*. 1985; 28:459–461.

75. Heller R, Jaroszeski M, Reintgen D, et al. Treatment of cutaneous and subcutaneous tumors with electrochemotherapy using intralesional bleomycin. *Cancer*. 1998;83:148–157.

Chapter 6
Electrodesiccation and Curettage

Gloria F. Graham

Curettage alone or in combination with electrodesiccation has been used for the treatment of skin cancer. While the curette was developed in the 1870s,[1] electrodesiccation was first used in 1911 by Clark when a high-voltage, low-current electrode was applied to the skin and resulted in drying of tissue.[2] It was not until later that the combination of curettage and electrodesiccation gained acceptance for low-risk lesions such as superficial and nodular basal cell carcinomas.[3]

Since there is impaired adherence between the tumor cells and the basement membrane and a mucinous stroma around the tumor, the soft tissue can be curetted easily. Other tumors such as warts, actinic keratoses, and keratoacanthomas may respond well to this technique. The differentiation between the healthy fibrous tissue from the softer tumor tissue provides a plane for defining the clinical border of the tumor.[4] Curettage has also been used prior to excision, cryosurgery, and Mohs surgery. Debulking the tumor and better establishing the clinical borders provide a defining step prior to these other procedures. In general terms, electrodesiccation and curettage are used for smaller more superficial lesions and those in less critical locations such as the cheek, temple, forehead, ear, chest, and back. In recent studies, curettage alone has been shown to be effective in over 96% of lesions that adhered to a specific protocol.[5]

Indications/Contraindications

The lower risk sites for this procedure are the neck, trunk, and extremities. Moderate risk sites include sites that are determined by depth and found on the scalp, forehead, around the ear, and the malar areas. Higher risk areas are around the nose, nasolabial folds, eyelids, periorbital areas, lips, chin, and some tumors on the ears.[6] Cure rates of greater than 96% have been found with this technique for lesions 2 cm or less in size. Larger lesions that are not superficial or that are in high-risk sites are best treated by other techniques. Morpheaform basal cell carcinomas (BCCs) are difficult to remove by electrodesiccation and curettage and are best treated by Mohs micrographic surgery, as are infiltrative BCCs, which may be more aggressive and tend to recur more often. Recurrent BCCs extending into scar tissue from previous treatments are infrequently amenable to curettage and electrodesiccation. This technique is contraindicated for most lentigo maligna and for lentigo malignant melanomas, as cancerous cells may extend down the hair follicle and for several millimeters beyond the clinical edge of the tumor.

While this technique is useful in patients on anticoagulants, electrodesiccation should be avoided in patients with pacemakers. Similarly, electrodesiccation should be avoided in those prone to hypertrophic scars and keloids and cryosurgery used instead.

Preoperative Considerations

A history of pacemaker, anticoagulants, or immunosuppressive drugs is important to note.[7] The procedure, anticipated results, and complications should be explained to the patient and informed

D.F. MacFarlane (ed.), *Skin Cancer Management*, DOI 10.1007/978-0-387-88495-0_6,
© Springer Science+Business Media, LLC 2010

consent obtained prior to treatment. The borders of the tumor should be outlined in ink prior to beginning the procedure—include a safety margin of 4–5 mm. The skin should be cleansed with a nonflammable antiseptic solution or dried carefully if alcohol is used to avoid inadvertent fire. Local anesthesia is provided with 1% lidocaine with epinephrine using a 30-gauge needle.

Important considerations prior to making the decision to use electrodesiccation include flammable substances on the skin, oxygen flowing in the room, and elevation of the tumor from superficial nerves and tendons.

If electrodesiccation is used around the anal canal, a moist packing should be provided to prevent the ignition of methane.[8–10]

Description of Technique

Remove the tumor when obtaining a biopsy by shave excision, then perform curettage if the procedures are to follow in sequence. Removal of the bulk of the lesion with the curette is followed by electrodesiccation, which removes persistent tumor cells at the base and rim of the lesion. A curette may be held like a pencil. Curettes vary in size from 1 to 7 mm, but a 3–4-mm diameter is most frequently used. The scooping motion involves holding the curette at a downward angle and vigorously scraping in all directions. After the obvious portion of the tumor is removed, the base and margins may be removed. Holding the curette like a pencil is effective for smaller tumors. With the non-dominant hand, hold the skin around the lesion taut while holding the curette in the dominant hand, between the thumb, index, and middle finger, and resting the remainder of the hand on the skin. Starting at the more distal end of the lesion, firm strokes are carried through the tissue and repeated several times until the entire tumor has been removed. For larger lesions, the curette is held in a position similar to a potato peeler; the thumb stabilizes the movement and holds the skin taut as does the other hand. Curettage is continued until pinpoint bleeding is noted.

If the curette penetrates into subcutaneous fat, curettage should be stopped since the tumor may extend too deeply for removal by this technique.[11]

Electrodesiccation using a Hyfrecator is performed on the base and rim of the lesion for at least 2 mm around the rim of the tumor. For more intense tissue damage, the electrocautery mode using biterminal with low voltage and high amperage is carried out to a 4–6-mm margin and repeated at least three times to ensure that all tumor cells are removed. While electrodesiccation destroys tumor cells, it also aids hemostasis and seals lymphatic vessels.[12] The sequence of steps is illustrated in Figs. 6.1, 6.2, 6.3, 6.4, 6.5 and 6.6.

Variations of this basic technique include curettage alone,[5] electrosurgery followed by curettage,[4] curettage followed by cryosurgery,[13] curettage followed by a course of imiquimod,[14] or curettage and electrodesiccation followed by imiquimod.[15]

One theory proposes that electrosurgery precede curettage. This is believed to cause more tissue destruction and to reduce the need for curettage, but may interfere with the curette's ability to differentiate normal from abnormal skin.[12,16]

Curettage with electrodesiccation cure rates ranges from 95 to 98% depending on size, depth, location, and tumor type.[9] Curettage alone will also be reviewed briefly and in select patients can give a 96% chance of cure.[5]

Spiller reported a cure rate of 99.4% for smaller tumors excluding those on the nose or nasolabial fold.[17] Daily application of imiquimod following curettage was found to be effective in treating primary nodular BCC on the trunk and extremities.[14,15] Ninety-four percent of patients did not have a recurrence at 3 months and had an excellent cosmetic result.[14] Once-daily application of imiquimod for a month following curettage and electrodesiccation resulted in a decrease in the frequency of residual tumor.[15]

Postoperative Care

The area should be cleansed daily with soap and water, hydrogen peroxide, or other cleansers and covered with the twice-daily application of an antibiotic ointment or white petroleum jelly. Leaving the wound open is also associated with excellent

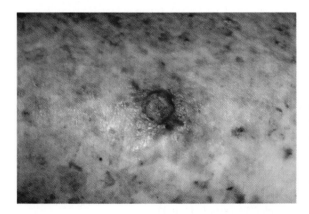

Fig. 6.1 Suspected SCC on the leg of a 46-year-old female with a past history of irradiation and numerous NMSCs

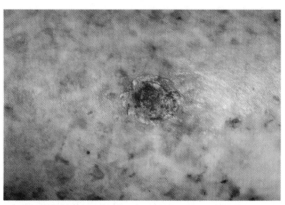

Fig. 6.4 Appearance following curettage

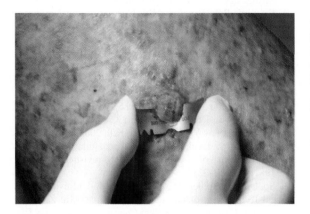

Fig. 6.2 Shave biopsy of suspected SCC

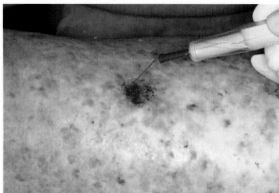

Fig. 6.5 Electrodesiccation to the base and rim of the lesion

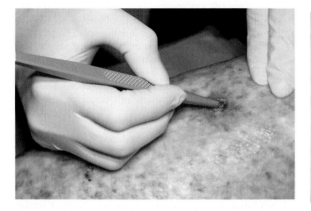

Fig. 6.3 Curettage of lesion base. Note how the curette is held and that the non-dominant hand stabilizes the skin

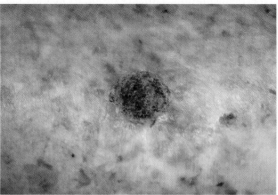

Fig. 6.6 Appearance of the lesion base following ED and C

healing. Pain is minimal, but over-the-counter analgesics may be used if needed. If swelling of a treated lesion occurs on the lower extremities, a compression bandage or support hose may be used. Healing is accomplished within approximately 2–4 weeks with minimal scarring.[8]

Use of Curettage Alone

How effective is curettage alone? Barlow et al. looked at this in a study of 302 low-risk basal cell carcinomas and found a 5-year cure rate of 96%.[5] Curettage alone has been found to be effective for tumors meeting certain strict criteria. The criteria included only primary tumors with nodular or superficial histology, discrete borders, less than 6 mm, not in high-risk areas (nose, nasolabial area, eyelids, medial canthi, ear, or lips), and not more than 2 cm in size. Superficial BCCs of any size were included. Cosmetic results were considered better than when curettage and electrodesiccation were used, as the latter technique has been shown to increase the chance of hypertrophic scarring and hypopigmentation in some locations.[17–19]

Complications

A depressed scar with atrophy or even hypertrophic scarring may result and there may be hypo- or hyperpigmentation. Patients prone to keloids may have a greater tendency to develop one after electrodesiccation than after cryosurgery.

Summary

Curettage and electrodesiccation is an effective, simple, and cost-effective treatment for superficial as well as some nodular basal cell carcinomas in 95–98% of selected cases.[12,16] Curettage alone has also been shown in several studies to clear more than 96% of selected lesions.[17–19]

References

1. Wigglesworth E. The curette in dermal therapeutics. *Boston Med Surg J.* 1876;94:143.
2. Clark WM. Oscillatory desiccation in the treatment of accessible malignant growths and minor surgical conditions. *J Adv Ther.* 1911;29:169–183.
3. Crissey JT. Curettage and electrodesiccation as a method of treatment for epitheliomas of the skin. *J Surg. Oncol.* 1971;3:287–290.
4. Sheridan AT, Dawber RP. Curettage electrosurgery and skin cancer. *Aust J Dermatol.* 2000;41(1):19–30.
5. Barlow JO, Zalla MJ, Kyle A, et al. Treatment of basal cell carcinoma with curettage alone. *J Am Acad Dermatol.* 2006;54(6):1039–1045.
6. Silverman MK, Kopf AW, Grin CM, et al. Recurrence rates of treated basal cell carcinomas. Part 2: Curettage-electrodesiccation. *J Dermatol Surg Oncol.* 1991;17:720–726.
7. Riordan A, Gamache C, Fosko S. Electrosurgery and cardiac devices. *J Am Acad Dermatol.* 1997;37(2 Pt 1):250.
8. Roenigk RK, Roenigk HH. Current surgical management of skin cancer in dermatology. *J Dermatol Surg Oncol.* 1990;16:136–151.
9. Zalla MJ. Basic cutaneous surgery. *Cutis.* 1994;53:172–186.
10. Adam JE. The technique of curettage surgery. *J Am Acad Dermatol.* 1986;15:697–702.
11. Vejjabhinanta V, Singh A, Patel SS, Nouri K. Curettage and electrodesiccation. In: Nouri K, ed. *Skin Cancer.* Vol 44. 1st ed. New York: McGraw-Hill; 2008:536–541.
12. Whelan CS, Deckers PJ. Electrocoagulation for skin cancer: An old oncologic tool revisited. *Cancer.* 1981;47:2280–2287.
13. Spiller WF, Spiller RF. Cryosurgery and adjuvant surgical techniques for cutaneous carcinomas. In: Zacarian SA, ed. *Cryosurgery for Skin Cancer and Cutaneous Disorders.* St. Louis, MO: The C.V. Mosby Co.; 1985:187–198.
14. Wu JK, Oh C, Strutton G, et al. An open-label, pilot study examining the efficacy of curettage followed by imiquimod 5% cream for the treatment of primary nodular basal cell carcinoma. *Aust J Dermatol.* 2006;47(1):46–48.
15. Spencer JM. Pilot study of imiquimoid 5% cream as adjunctive therapy to curettage and electrodesiccation for nodular basal cell carcinoma. *Dermatol Surg.* 2006;32(1):63–69.
16. Williamson GS, Jackson R. Treatment of basal cell carcinoma by electrodesiccation and curettage. *Can Med Assoc J.* 1962;86:855–862.
17. Spiller WF, Spiller RF. Treatment of basal cell epithelioma by curettage and electrodesiccation. *J Am Acad Dermatol.*1984;11:808–814.
18. Kopf AW, Bart RS, Schrager D, et al. Curettage-electrodesiccation treatment of basal cell carcinomas. *Arch Dermatol.* 1977;113:439–443.
19. Silverman MK, Kopf AW. Recurrence rates of treated basal cell carcinomas, part 2: curettage-electrodesiccation. *J Dermatol Surg Oncol.* 1991;17:720–726.

Chapter 7
Cryosurgery

Gloria F. Graham

The history of cryosurgery in dermatology dates back to the 1890s, when White, a New York dermatologist, dipped a cotton-tipped applicator into liquefied air in 1899 and successfully treated warts, keratoses, and skin cancers.[1] Torre[2] and Zacarian[3] both published their findings on the use of freezing for treating skin cancer in the mid-1960s. The Spillers first described its use with curettage and this is a technique that is often used today.[4]

Basic Cryobiology

Heat moves from warm to cold objects, so when a cold applicator (or "heat sink") is applied to a warm target a temperature differential results that drains heat from the tissue. As tissue is frozen, further thermal conduction is facilitated by the formation of what is known as an "ice ball." The size of the applicator as well as physical factors such as the temperature of the cryogen determines the size of the ice ball that can be created and how deep the thermal gradients develop within this ice ball. While the depth of freezing is less important in benign lesions, it is of crucial importance in the treatment of malignances. The rates of temperature fall, of rewarming, and of solute concentration, as well as the length of time the cells are exposed to below-freezing temperatures, are all important parameters.

If a tissue is frozen too slowly, the target tissue primarily produces extracellular ice crystals, whereas rapid cooling can produce intracellular ice, which is most destructive. Intracellular ice can shear the membrane of the cell and concentrate intracellular solutes. Repeating the freeze–thaw cycle produces additional destruction.[3] The inflammatory response releases cytokines and may form useful antibodies to enhance an immune response.[5,6]

Unassisted thawing to room temperature is preferable, but if excessive freezing has occurred in a location, thawing with a warmer object—even one's finger tip—can hasten thawing and lessen destruction. The solutes within tissue become more concentrated as the ice is forming, and this chemical insult adds to the destruction of cells and a greater oxidative insult to the tissue. During recrystallization a phenomenon occurs that is called "grain growth," which produces maximum damage to cells.[6]

Maximum destruction occurs around –50°C and is believed to be the preferred target temperature most used today, but in the 1960s it was felt that –20 to –25°C was satisfactory for cancer cell destruction.[6]

Varying degrees of apoptosis on the outer perimeter of tumors is observed at temperatures of –6 to –46°C.[7] Liquid nitrogen is the preferred cryogen, capable of producing sufficient depth-of-freeze for cancer destruction.[6] Helium is also capable of this, but it is not readily available. Small superficial lesions may be removed with carbon dioxide and Freon gases, but these cryogens are not used in the United States for skin cancer treatment. Nitrogen oxide units available in Europe, and especially in France, have been engineered to develop low enough temperatures for the treatment of malignancies (Table 7.1).

D.F. MacFarlane (ed.), *Skin Cancer Management*, DOI 10.1007/978-0-387-88495-0_7,
© Springer Science+Business Media, LLC 2010

Table 7.1 Cryogens historically used in cutaneous surgery

Agent	Temperature
Solid CO_2	−79.0°C
Liquid N_2O	−88.5°C
Helium	−185°C
Liquid N_2	−195.8°C

Indications

Patients with multiple tumors on the arms, legs, chest, face, and back have been successfully treated by cryosurgery or electrodesiccation, and a combination of the above with shave excision and curettage may prove most effective. In general this involves electrodesiccation and curettage for lesions of minimal to moderate depth and cryosurgery for deeper lesions in the 3–4-mm range. Excision or Mohs surgery is preferred for deeper lesions, especially around the nose, and for more aggressive subtypes such as micronodular, infiltrative, or metatypical basal cell carcinomas (BCCs). Immunosuppressed patients with multiple lesions respond well to both electrodesiccation and cryosurgery. Results vary depending on the tumor type, location, and skin color. It is important to consider the patient's preference once the techniques and potential outcomes have been explained to them.[8] Patients who are keloid formers, have multiple cancers, are on anticoagulants, have a pacemaker, or are otherwise poor risks for more extensive surgery may be ideal candidates for cryosurgery.

Contraindications

Cryosurgery should be avoided in patients with a history of cold anaphylaxis or cold urticaria if severe attacks have occurred. While cold urticaria is often not significant when small lesions are treated, a large tumor treated on the head or neck could produce severe periorbital edema or edema of the skin of the neck, and the patient must be forewarned. Contractures may develop around the eye, nose, and mouth, but in the author's experience these are rare. Relative contraindications include cryoglobulinemia, multiple myeloma, autoimmune diseases including pyodema gangrenosum, Raynaud's disease, areas of vascular compromise, and darkly pigmented skin.[6]

- Patient selection of prime importance
- Excellent technique for keloid formers
- Discuss potential changes in skin: hypopigmentation, alopecia, uncommon numbness, scarring
- Obtain informed consent.

The appropriate selection of patients and tumor sites is vitally important, as hypopigmentation and alopecia can occur. Transient numbness may also occur on the sides of the fingers, neck, or elbow. These potential side effects should be discussed before the patient signs an informed consent. A patient with pigmentary problems such as ephelides, lentigenes, or telangiectasia may be at greater risk for a less-than-satisfactory cosmetic result since the isolated area of pigment loss will be more obvious and this should be discussed with the patient. Inform the patient that more scarring may result when treating a more extensive malignancy for palliation. Mohs surgery or excision may be a preferable option.

Preoperative Considerations

A shave excision for biopsy may be performed prior to or at the time of freezing or electrodesiccation for diagnostic confirmation. The lateral margins may prove helpful in diagnostic considerations, especially in squamous cell carcinoma that is arising from an actinic keratosis. The shave, tumor type, and depth are all important in the final decision-making process. The shave followed by curettage allows an even better determination of depth and, with experience, one can make a reasoned judgment about whether a destructive technique, excision, imiquimod, or Mohs surgery would be the preferred method for definitive treatment. Another consideration in selecting a method is the proximity of a surgeon skilled in Mohs surgery. A long driving distance makes this selection more difficult for some older patients.

Discuss with patients the cure rates and potential side effects from cryosurgery. Since hypopigmentation is the most significant cosmetic change, explain to patients that this leaves the skin more like the color of sun-protected skin. If pigment is removed from photodamaged skin, a more obvious area is appreciated than if the skin is of lighter color. The same is true with telangiectasia in the malar region where freezing may leave a lighter area devoid of the finer superficial vessels. Atrophic scarring may be noted with deeper freezing.[9] Caution patients regarding alopecia on scalp, eyebrow, and temple or other areas of cosmetic significance to the patient.

Equipment

The equipment primarily used in cryosurgery consists of a cotton swab, spray, and probe (Fig. 7.1). A swab with a large cotton reservoir may give a limited increase in depth-of-freeze but is not sufficient for the routine treatment of skin cancer. Since viruses can survive in liquid nitrogen, a change in swab between patients is recommended.

While swab cryosurgery was used from the late 1940s for benign and precancerous tumors, it was never widely used for skin cancer because it reaches a depth of destruction of only 2–3 mm and is considered an inadequate heat sink for skin cancers.[10] Spray and probe freezing with liquid nitrogen are more effective and are used for skin cancers greater than 3–5 mm in depth. The most widely used instruments today are handheld spray and probe units that sit on table tops and are filled from a large Dewar holding liquid nitrogen. A 32-liter tank will last 2–4 weeks with moderate use, and the static holding time for the handheld sprays is 24 h and with moderate use during the day, 24 h.

Technique

With the spray technique, a central spray using intermittent pulses, or spiral pattern starting at the center of a lesion and progressing to the periphery is customary.

A 1-cm lesion is best treated with an A tip or probe that fits the lesion. For larger lesions a paintbrush pattern, passing back and forth over the lesion is used. A 5-mm halo around the tumor is desired for skin cancer and a 2-mm halo for precancerous lesions. Spraying into an insulating cone using a Cryoplate with openings of various diameter (4 mm, 7 mm, 9 mm, 12 mm) provides a deeper, more even depth-of-freeze similar to that obtained with a probe. The average spray time for a skin cancer 3 mm in depth is around *one minute*. Cryoprobe techniques are generally slower than sprays but result in a deeper depth-of-freeze to lateral spread-of-freeze ratio.[10]

- Cryosurgery: Field Therapy
- Three basic techniques are swab, spray, and probe.
- The three spray patterns are central, spiral, and paint brush.

Various sizes and shapes of cotton swabs, probe, and spray tips are available and can vary the shape of the ice ball produced in the target. While cotton swabs are not generally used for treatment of other than the most superficial skin cancers, probes are excellent where there is a well-defined small lesion, one in a difficult-to-reach location, or one on the eyelid where there is a danger of getting liquid nitrogen sprayed into the eye. There are also large probes for the treatment

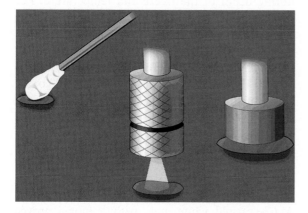

Fig. 7.1 Use of cotton swab, spray tip, and probe are all commonly used techniques in cryosurgery. Reprinted with permission from Graham GF, Barham KL

of large deep tumors and in areas where palliation is the goal. An assortment of spray tips of varying sizes are available.

> A plastic Jaeger retractor may be used to protect the eye as well as a plastic cone, but metal retractors should not be used around the eye when freezing due to possible adherence of the metal to the surrounding tissue.

Monitoring of Freeze Depth

Accurate assessment of freeze depth is critical in cryosurgery. An ice halo may be observed around the frozen tumor. The lateral progression of this halo corresponds to the depth of the freeze. A 6-mm halo on the surface approximates a freezing depth of 6 mm. For most procedures, a single thermocouple needle is used and inserted at the border or under the tumor depending on tumor size (Fig. 7.2). This provides an accurate assessment of depth and quality of freeze and may be obtained from Brymill Cryogenic Systems. Clinical judgment determines the placement of the needles, but if in

doubt the needle can be placed at the dermal subcutaneous border.[11] With experience the need for the thermocouple becomes less.

Basal Cell and Squamous Cell Carcinomas Cure Rates

Cryosurgery offers cure rates in the 96–98%[12–14] range when appropriately selected lesions are treated. Proper selection and attention to detail will produce the highest cure rate.

To obtain cure rates in the range of 96–98%, follow well-established criteria. Outline the border of the lesion with a marking pen so that the progression of the ice ball can be appreciated. When the area becomes white, the boundary of the tumor is no longer visible; so outlining the lesion with a surgical marking pen prior to infiltrating with local anesthetic is crucial. The elevated portion of the tumor is removed by shave or scoop biopsy and submitted for pathology. When cryosurgery is used, many cryosurgeons prefer to curette the base of the lesion prior to freezing.

If a novice at using cryosurgery, use a thermocouple needle implanted under the deepest part of the tumor and freeze using the spray or probe until a 5 mm halo of ice is obtained around the tumor. This will most often require a freeze time of approximately 60 s of intermittent freeze.

Cryosurgery is a field therapy with a target temperature of –50°C, which may be measured by monitoring depth of the freeze and temperature. For superficial basal cell carcinomas on the back, a single freeze is adequate unless the first thaw time is short of the 60 s, in which case a second freeze–thaw cycle should be utilized. Record the halo thaw time (HTT) and the clinical thaw time (CTT) of the entire site. The HTT ranges from 60 to 120 s, the CTT 2½–5 min.

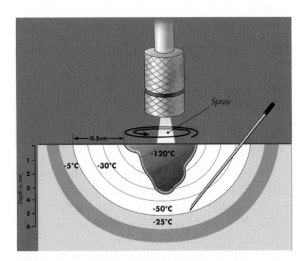

Fig. 7.2 Use of thermocouple needle allows clinician to monitor depth-of-freeze and clinically the extent-of-freeze around lesion by measuring the halo, which should be around 5 mm. Reprinted with permission from Graham GF, Barham KL

Illustrative Case 7.1

A 67-year-old white male with a biopsy-proven basal cell carcinoma in the medial canthus 5 mm is treated by cryosurgery (Fig. 7.3a, b, c).

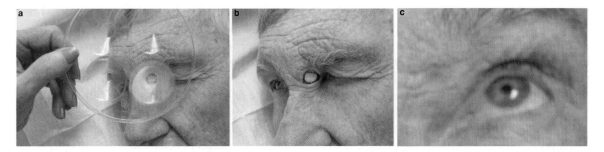

Fig. 7.3 3/19/08. A 67-year-old white male with a biopsy-proven basal cell carcinoma in the medial canthus is treated by cryosurgery. (**a**) A plastic cone is used to protect the eye and confine the spray. (**b**) A 5-mm halo of frozen tissue around the tumor after freezing. Caution patient regarding edema and weeping of the site as well as periorbital edema, which may be observed for 3–5 days postcryosurgery (**c**) At follow up 3 months later, the site is well healed

Times used for Case 7.1:

Cycle 1
Freeze time (FT): 1′ 1″
HTT: 1′ 28″
CTT 3′ 12″

Cycle 2
FT: 1′ 2″
HTT: 1′ 46″
CTT: 3′ 32″

Illustrative Case 7.2

A 69-year-old, white female with a biopsy-proven squamous cell carcinoma (SCC) is treated with shave excision, curettage, and cryosurgery (Fig. 7.4a, b, c, d, e).

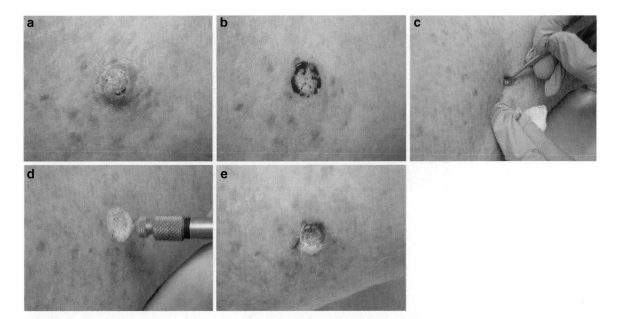

Fig. 7.4 A 69-year-old, white female with a biopsy-proven squamous cell carcinoma (SCC). (**a**) *Right thigh* shows an erythematous nodule with a keratin-filled center. (**b**) After shave excision, *white* base of center of tumor remains. (**c**) With curettage the rest of the friable part of the tumor is removed. (**d**) Area treated by cryosurgery. (**e**) Appearance after 1-min freeze time. Halo thaw time 1 min 33 s, and clinical thaw time 4 min 32 s

Illustrative Case 7.3

A 79-year-old white male, with a biopsy-proven basal cell carcinoma on his right forehead (Fig. 7.5a, b, c, d) is treated with cryosurgery.

Times used:

Cycle 1
1st FT: 1'
HTT: 1' 10''
CTT: 2'

Cycle 2
2nd FT: 1'
HTT: 2' 30''
CTT: 5'

Illustrative Case 7.4

A lesion clinically suspicious for a BCC is noted on the upper back of a 55-year-old muscular male patient (Fig. 7.6a, b, c, d). The area is treated with cryosurgery as the lesion looks superficial and surgery would necessitate a long scar, which would probably spread in this area.

For deeper tumors, most cryosurgeons recommend a double freeze–thaw cycle, with the second cycle following the thawing of the first cycle.[3,8,13,15–18] Local anesthesia may allow longer treatment and thaw times. For a list of diagnoses that can be appropriately treated by cryosurgery see the guidelines of care for cryosurgery (Table 7.2)

Treatment Pearls

- "Fast Freeze, Slow Thaw"
- Repeat freeze–thaw for additional destruction
- Monitoring of depth dose and temperature is important
- Target Temperature –40 to –50°C
- Hypopigmentation expected if freeze over 20–30 s.
- Alopecia may result following 20+ second freeze

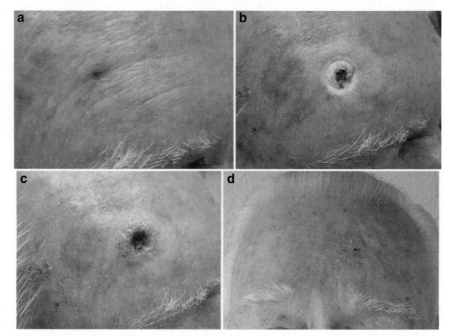

Fig. 7.5 (**a**) A 79-year-old white male, with a biopsy-proven basal cell carcinoma on his right forehead is treated with cryosurgery. (**b**) The tumor is frozen. (**c**) Appearance immediately after cryosurgery. (**d**) At follow-up 2 months later the area has healed well

Fig. 7.6 A lesion clinically suspicious for a BCC on the upper back of a 55-year-old male. (**a**) Appearance prior to cryosurgery. (**b**) Shave biopsy is performed. (**c**) A single freeze is performed as the lesion is superficial and on the back. (**d**) Appearance following cryosurgery with 5-mm rim of freezing obtained

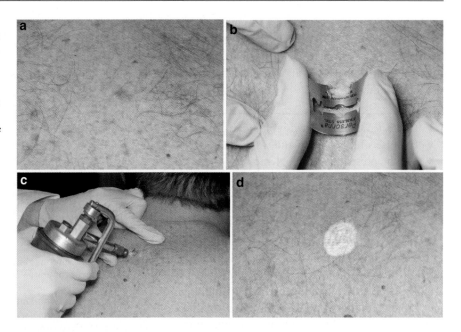

Table 7.2 Lesions that can appropriately be treated with cryosurgery

Precancerous lesions or tumors of uncertain behavior	Malignant lesions
Actinic cheilitis	Basal cell carcinoma
Actinic keratosis	Bowen's disease (carcinoma in situ)
Keratoacanthoma	Kaposi's sarcoma
Lentigo maligna	Squamous cell carcinoma
Bowenoid papulosis	Actinic keratosis with squamous cell carcinoma, adenoid squamous cell carcinoma, de novo squamous cell carcinoma

Reprinted from Drake LA, Ceilley RI, Cornelison RL, et al.[20]

Leukoplakia and Actinic Cheilitis

Freeze with a spray applied in a paint brush manner.

> If the entire lip requires treatment, it is best to treat one half of the lip at each of two sessions, with a freeze time of 10–15 s.[15]

Keratoacanthoma

First biopsy to exclude invasive squamous cell carcinoma by shaving the exophytic portion and then freeze the base for 30–60 s. Holt cleared seven of

eight keratoacanthomas using a 30–60 s freeze time with a 5-mm halo around the lesion.[16]

Postoperative Care

Shortly after the completion of freezing, an erythematous and/or urticarial response may be noted around the lesion. A deep blistering reaction may occur resulting in edema and within 12–24 h, bullae formation followed by weeping of the wound for several days. An eschar forms in approximately 2 weeks. This may be adherent to the underlying tissue for up to 1 month in most locations and on the back or lower leg for 1–3 months. Before complete healing occurs, the eschar must separate and peel away. If delay in healing occurs debridement of the eschar can be performed. Daily cleansing with soap and water may be all that is necessary for most cryosurgical wounds.

- Cryosite acts as its own biologic dressing
- Cleanse site with soap and water daily
- Eschar present for up to 1 month—occasionally on the back and legs it may last 2–3 months
- Debride eschar only if not separating after 4–8 weeks

Patients may resume their daily activities as tolerated, including bathing and swimming. The site acts as its own biological dressing and does not usually need to be bandaged. In fact, bandaging can adhere to the wound, resulting in premature removal of the eschar and a longer healing time.[19]

Patients should be followed carefully for 2 years postoperatively to check for recurrence.

Summary

Cryosurgery is a safe, efficient, and effective procedure for the treatment of many benign, premalignant, and malignant skin lesions. Physicians must be able to distinguish normal reactions to cutaneous freezing from sequelae that require intervention. Physicians who wish to train in cryosurgery are encouraged to do so under the supervision of a person experienced in this technique.

References

1. White AC. Liquid air in medicine and surgery. *Med Rec.* 1899;56:109–112.
2. Torre D. Cradle of cryosurgery. *NY State J Med.* 1967;67:465.
3. Zacarian SA, Adham MI. Cryotherapy of cutaneous malignancy. *Cryobiology.* 1966;2:212.
4. Spiller WF, Spiller RF. Cryosurgery and adjuvant surgical techniques for cutaneous carcinomas. In: Zacarian SA, ed. *Cryosurgery for Skin Cancer and Cutaneous Disorders.* St. Louis, MO: The C.V. Mosby Co.; 1985: 187–198.
5. Baust JG, Gage AA. The molecular basis of cryosurgery. *BJU Int.* 2005;95:1187.
6. Kuflik EG, Gage AA, Lubritz RR, Graham GF. Millenium paper: history of dermatologic cryosurgery. *Dermatol Surg.* 2000;26:715–722.
7. Hanai A, Yang WL, Ravikumar TS. Introduction of apoptosis in human colon carcinoma cells HT29 by sublethal cryoinjury: mediation by cytochrome C release. *Int J Cancer.* 2001;93:26–33.
8. Kuflik EG. Cryosurgery update. *J Am Acad Dermatol.* 1994;31:925–944.
9. Crissey JT. Curettage and electrodesiccation as a method of treatment for epitheliomas of the skin. *J Surg. Oncol.* 1971;3:287–290.
10. Grimmett, R. Liquid nitrogen therapy: histologic observations. *Arch Dermatol.* 1961;83:563–567.
11. Torre D. Cryosurgical instrumentation and depth dose monitoring. In: Breitbart E, Dachow-Siwiec E, eds. *Clinics in Dermatology: Advances in Cryosurgery.* New York, NY: Elsevier Science; 1990:48–60.
12. Graham GF, Clark LC. Statistical analysis in cryosurgery of skin cancer.In: Breitbart E, Dachow-Siwiec E, eds. *Clinics in Dermatology: Advances in Cryosurgery.* Vol 8. New York, NY: Elsevier Science; 1990:101–107.
13. Zacarian SA. Cryosurgery of cutaneous carcinomas: An 18-year study of 3022 patients with 4228 carcinomas. *J Am Acad Dermatol.* 1983;9:947–956.
14. Kuflik EG. Cryosurgery for skin cancer: 30-year experience and cure rates. *Dermatol Surg.* 2004;30:297–300.
15. Graham G. Cryosurgery for benign, premalignant, and malignant lesions. In: Wheeland RG, ed. *Cutaneous Surgery.* 1st ed. Philadelphia: WB Saunders; 1994: 835–867.
16. Holt P. Cryotherapy for skin cancer: results over a 5-year period using liquid nitrogen spray. *Br J Dermatol.* 1988;119:231.
17. Graham G. Cryosurgery. In: Ratz JL, ed. *Textbook of Dermatologic Surgery.* Philadelphia: Lippincott-Raven Publishers; 1998:439–456.
18. Kuflik EG, Gage AA. *Cryosurgical Treatment for Skin Cancer.* New York: Igaku-Shoin; 1990:97–111.
19. Arnott J. *On the Treatment of Cancers by Regulated Application of an Anaesthetic Temperature.* London: Churchill Livingstone; 1855.
20. Drake LA, Ceilley RI, Cornelison RL, et al. Guidelines of care on cryosurgery. *J Am Acad Dermatol.* 1994;31:648–653, with permission from Elsevier.

Chapter 8
Optimizing Surgical Outcomes

Thomas Stasko and Amy Ross

To optimize outcomes associated with cutaneous procedures the surgeon must consider multiple factors. Many of these factors should be addressed prior to the start of surgery and others require attention during or after the procedure. Recognition of these factors can aid in the meticulous planning and attention to detail necessary to obtain the best outcome following surgical treatment of skin cancer.

> It must always be remembered that the primary goal of surgical skin cancer management is complete eradication of the tumor. An outstanding initial cosmetic result is of no avail if the tumor recurs.

There are several approaches to the surgical removal of skin cancer. The approach may differ depending on factors such as tumor type, tumor location, patient health, and health care system limitations. Because of the paramount goal of complete tumor removal, an increasingly common method for removal of skin cancers is Mohs micrographic surgery (MMS). A recent survey indicates up to 40% of all skin cancer treatments in the United States are performed using the MMS technique.[1] The appeal of this approach is its high cure rate and cost-effectiveness.[2,3]

There are situations in which Mohs may not be the most appropriate method of skin cancer removal (see Chapter 11). Tumors that require permanent histological sections for optimum evaluation or tumors that are well demarcated may be best approached with standard surgical excision. It is important to note that until there is pathologic confirmation that a malignant tumor is completely removed, it is inappropriate to repair the resulting defect with a complex flap or graft. If the pathology specimen turns out to be positive for tumor at the margins, closing a wound with a flap or graft may prevent the surgeon from identifying the location of residual tumor in subsequent surgeries.

The dermatologic surgeon must also recognize that there are situations where he or she may not be the most appropriate physician to be treating the patient. The best outcome could be provided by another specialist (see Chapter 20). At some institutions, melanomas greater than 1.0 mm in depth and Merkel cell carcinomas are evaluated by the surgical oncologist for possible inclusion of a sentinel lymph node biopsy at the time of excision. In some circumstances radiation therapy may be the best option for a large tumor in an elderly patient or for an in-transit metastasis. The dermatologic surgeon must be well versed in all aspects of cutaneous oncology to select the proper treatment for the best possible outcome.

Once the dermatologic surgeon has determined that a surgical procedure is the best approach to the treatment of a tumor, there are several steps that will help to optimize the outcome of the procedure. A thorough preoperative assessment and appropriate surgical planning followed by excellent intraoperative technique and vigilant postoperative care are necessary to yield an optimal outcome.

D.F. MacFarlane (ed.), *Skin Cancer Management*, DOI 10.1007/978-0-387-88495-0_8,
© Springer Science+Business Media, LLC 2010

Preoperative Considerations

All patients considered for dermatologic surgery should be questioned regarding pertinent medical history. Commonly this information is first recorded by the patient and then confirmed and elaborated on by a nurse. The physician then utilizes this information to direct their history taking and examination. Figure 8.1a, b show an example of a standard medical information form. This form may be customized to meet the needs of a specific practice population, but should cover the historical factors relevant to all of the considerations listed as follows.

a

Palm Harbor Dermatology
CANCER AND LASER SURGERY CENTER

New Patient History

Patient:_____ Date of Birth: ____/____/_____

Reason for today's visit: _____

Symptoms of today's problem:_____

Skin areas involved: _____ How long has the problem been present: _____

Has there been any previous treatment? **YES NO** If yes, when?_____ Type:_____

Was a biopsy done? **YES NO** If yes, when? _____ By who: _____

Medications you are currently taking:

(including prescriptions, over-the-counter meds, vitamins, and herbals)

Past Medical History:

Yes	No		Yes	No		Yes	No	
☐	☐	AIDS/HIV Infection	☐	☐	Hay Fever	☐	☐	Neurological disorders
☐	☐	Anemia	☐	☐	Healing Problems	☐	☐	Pacemaker
☐	☐	Arthritis	☐	☐	Heart Disease	☐	☐	Pregnant
☐	☐	Artificial Heart Valve	☐	☐	Heart murmur	☐	☐	Psychiatric problems
☐	☐	Artificial Joint	☐	☐	Hepatitis	☐	☐	Respiratory disease
☐	☐	Asthma	☐	☐	High Blood Pressure	☐	☐	Seizures
☐	☐	Bleeding Problems	☐	☐	High Cholesterol	☐	☐	Skin Cancer
☐	☐	Blood Transfusion	☐	☐	Immunosuppression			Type _____
☐	☐	Bruising	☐	☐	Irregular heart beat	☐	☐	Skin Disease
☐	☐	Cancer	☐	☐	Keloid/scarring after surgery			Type _____
☐	☐	Cold sores/fever blister	☐	☐	Kidney disease	☐	☐	Thyroid Disease
☐	☐	Diabetes	☐	☐	Liver disease	☐	☐	Tuberculosis
☐	☐	Eye disease	☐	☐	Lupus	☐	☐	Varicose Veins
			☐	☐	Multiple Sclerosis	☐	☐	Other disorders

Medication allergies: _____

Surgical History: _____

Hospitalizations: _____

Family History of skin cancer: (please circle all that apply)

None   Melanoma   Basal Cell   Squamous Cell   Other _____

Fig. 8.1 Example of a medical information form: (**a**) page one and (**b**) page two

b **New Patient History**   Patient Name: _____
  Social History:
    Occupation _____

    IV drug use **YES NO**

    Smoke **YES NO** packs/day_____

    Alcohol **YES NO** drinks/week_____

    Sunscreen (please circle the one that applies to you) **NO REGULARLY SOMETIMES RARELY**

    At least 1 blistering Sunburn **YES NO**

    Ever used a Tanning Bed **YES NO** Specify _____

  Review of Systems:

Constitutional	**Respiratory**	**Neurology**
Weight change	Cough	Headache
Fatigue	**Endocrinology**	Dizziness
Fever	Excessive sweating	Insomnia
Dermatology	Hot/Cold intolerance	**Gastroenterology**
Rash	**Musculoskeletal**	Nausea
Dry or sensitive skin	Joint stiffness	Vomiting
Suspicious lesions	Leg cramps	Abdominal pain
Itching	Joint pain	Diarrhea
Eyes/Ears/Nose/Throat	Joint swelling	Constipation
Vision changes	Muscle aches	**Female Reproductive**
Hearing impairment	**Psychology**	Sexually active
Nose bleed	Depression	Irregular periods
Sore throat	Sleep disturbances	Normal periods
Cold	Anxiety	Postmenopausal
Cardiology	Suicidal ideation	**Male Reproductive**
Chest pain	**Hematology/Lymp**	Difficulty with erection
Leg swelling	Swollen glands	Diminished sexual drive
Shortness of breath	Easy bruising	**Other:**_____

  Completed by (please circle one): **Patient   Nurse**

  Signed by Patient _____   Date ___/___/___
  Reviewed by _____   Date ___/___/___

Fig. 8.1 (continued)

Bleeding Tendency

Excessive bleeding during or after a surgical procedure may result in a less-than-optimal outcome. Identifying patients at risk for increased bleeding allows the surgeon to take corrective action prior to the procedure when possible and to be prepared to utilize additional tools to minimize any negative effects associated with excessive bleeding.

Exaggerated bleeding is most often related to extrinsic causes (medications and dietary supplements), but may also be related to intrinsic causes such as inherited deficiencies in coagulation factors or problems with platelet production, function, or survival.

Anticoagulant use in today's patient population is high. Table 8.1 lists the commonly prescribed anticoagulants, their mechanism of action, and duration of effect. Many of these anticoagulants are prescribed for use by physicians after cardiac events or stroke; however, increasingly, patients are on low-dose antiplatelet therapy for primary prevention. Historically, many surgeons have been hesitant to operate on patients taking blood thinners;[4] however, recent literature supports the continuation of prescribed medications to prevent potentially deadly consequences.[5,6] There are numerous cases of thromboembolic stroke, pulmonary emboli, cerebral emboli, myocardial infarction, and deep venous thromboses reported after the discontinuation of anticoagulation therapy, with severe consequences in some cases.[7–9]

> The risk of intraoperative and postoperative bleeding must be balanced with the risk of the patient developing a thromboembolic event if anticoagulation is discontinued.

If the patient can safely discontinue aspirin, it should be withheld for 10 days prior to surgery. Clopidogrel and warfarin are most often found

Table 8.1 Prescription blood thinners

Medication	Mechanism of action	Recommendation	Treatment/ Reversal
Aspirin	Irreversibly blocks thromboxane A_2	If for secondary prevention, discontinue 10 days prior to surgery	None
Clopidogrel bisulfate	Irreversible blockade of the adenosine diphosphate (ADP) receptor on platelet cell membranes	Continue, with particular attention to intraoperative hemostasis	Platelet transfusion
Warfarin	Competitively inhibits vitamin K_1-2,-3 epoxide reductase	Continue. Confirm INR <3.0 within 48 h of surgery	Vitamin K, fresh frozen plasma
Heparin	Inhibits factor Xa	Discontinue 6 h prior to surgery	Protamine sulfate
NSAIDs (ibuprofen, naproxen, etc.)	Inhibit cyclooxygenase pathway and prostaglandin synthesis	Discontinue 3 days prior to surgery	None

to be unsafe to discontinue. Unfortunately, in the case of clopidogrel, there is no commonly performed blood test that will inform the surgeon of the degree of anticoagulation present. Reported experience with these patients has been variable, but many surgeons subjectively feel these patients tend to bleed as much as patients anticoagulated with warfarin.

For patients on warfarin, if the physician managing the anticoagulation therapy feels the patient can safely be without therapy for a short period, it is discontinued 48–72 h prior to the procedure and restarted the evening of the procedure, or the following morning. This most commonly occurs in patients on warfarin as prophylaxis because of atrial fibrillation. For patients in whom discontinuation of warfarin therapy is not advisable, such as patients with mechanical heart valves or a recent history of embolic stroke, the authors usually ask that an international normalized ratio (INR) value be checked within 24 h of surgery. In general, the authors will operate on individuals with an INR less than or equal to 3.0. In patients with a long-term history of stable anticoagulation a more remote INR may suffice. Although these patients still require extra precautions during and after surgery and may be subject to more extensive

ecchymosis, cutaneous procedures can usually be successfully performed in these circumstances.

Many patients are on nonprescription supplements that may increase the chance of bleeding, and subsequent complications. There are reports of patients on a variety of supplements developing bleeding complications such as subdural hematomas, hemorrhagic stroke, and vaginal or gingival bleeding unrelated to cutaneous surgery.[10] Some of these supplements and their reported indications for use are listed in Table 8.2. Given that well over 50% of the adult population has reported supplement use in a recent survey,[11] all dermatologic surgery patients should be questioned on the use of these products. Patients should, in general, be advised to discontinue these supplements in preparation for surgery.

One of the most frequently encountered supplements is vitamin E. It is commonly advocated for use in cardiovascular disease prevention, as well as for cancer prevention. It inhibits platelet aggregation and secretion and may cause bleeding.[12] Vitamin E is frequently taken with other supplements, such as garlic, ginseng, and *Ginkgo biloba*, which may also interfere with platelet function. These medications should be discontinued prior to cutaneous surgery.[10]

Ideally, patients with intrinsic clotting problems should be identified preoperatively and managed

Table 8.2 Nutritional supplements to avoid in dermatologic surgery

Supplement	Effect	When to discontinue
Vitamin E	Inhibits platelets	2–3 weeks before
Garlic	Inhibits platelets	At least 7 days before
Ginger (large doses only)	Inhibits platelets	At least 36 h before
Ginkgo biloba	Inhibits platelets	At least 36 h before
Ginseng	Inhibits platelets	At least 7 days before
Ephedra	May react with epinephrine (increases heart rate, blood pressure)	At least 24 h before
Feverfew	Inhibits platelets	2–3 weeks before

in coordination with hematology. The etiology of intrinsic bleeding problems may range from conditions such as hepatic disease to inherited bleeding disorders such as Von Willebrand disease (VWD). An estimated 0.1–1% of the population is affected by VWD,[13,14] making it very likely that a patient with this problem will be encountered in the average practice. Although 20% of patients with VWD have postoperative bleeding as a complication of their disease, there are few standard guidelines for their perioperative management during dermatologic surgery.[15,16] Consultation with the treating hematologist should be completed before there is any decision for surgery, and consideration of pretreatment with 1-desamino-8-arginine vasopressin (DDAVP) or plasma concentrates should be made.

Patients with low platelet counts secondary to idiopathic thrombocytopenic purpura, myeloproliferative disorders, or other extrinsic causes such as chemotherapy, represent a special population. Although there is no data specifically addressing cutaneous surgery in patients with low platelet counts, informed decisions regarding care may be made by reviewing the surgical literature. Thrombocytopenia is strictly defined as a platelet count less than 140,000/µl. The otolaryngology literature suggests surgery with minimal anticipated blood loss may be performed with platelet counts as low as 20,000/µl. However, a platelet count greater than 50,000/µl should be present if more extensive surgery is anticipated. This count should be maintained for 3–4 days following surgery.[17]

Wound Healing

There are three phases of wound healing (Fig. 8.2). Interruption of any of these phases of healing can result in a less-than-optimal outcome. Medications and chronic diseases are the most commonly encountered factors that influence wound healing. Anti-inflammatory medications including glucocorticoids are known to interrupt wound healing and are associated with infection and increased risk of dehiscence.[18] Despite the possibility of impaired wound healing and the need for prolonged wound care, these medications are continued during surgery because the risk of discontinuation is greater than the risk of continuation. Retinoids have been associated with keloidal scarring

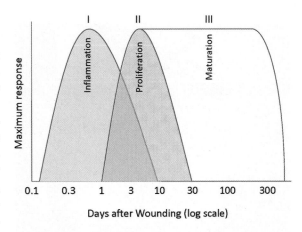

Fig. 8.2 Phases of wound healing

following some procedures. This outcome has not been found to be true following Mohs surgery, and retinoids may be continued through this type of surgery.[19]

Several patient populations historically have increased difficulty with wound healing. Most commonly encountered are patients with diabetes and the frail elderly. Usually there is no reason to defer a needed procedure on these patients, unless they are simply unable to tolerate the surgery. In these patients attention to postoperative care is essential to optimize surgical outcome. For patients unable to care for their own wounds, nursing care should be arranged. In rare cases, hospitalization may be necessary following surgical removal of skin cancer. Most often this is following extensive Mohs surgery prior to repair; however, it may be reasonable to hospitalize frail elderly patients with risk factors for excessive bleeding following a long outpatient procedure. There is published data to suggest dermatologic surgery on patients greater than 80, or even 90 years of age, is safe with few adverse outcomes.[20,21]

History of Hypertrophic Scar or Keloid Formation

Patients with a history of hypertrophic scar or keloid formation should be prepared for a possible similar outcome following skin cancer surgery. This is particularly true of the "V-distribution" (Fig. 8.3) on the trunk (shoulders, central chest,

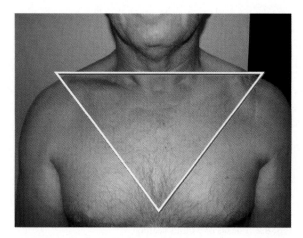

Fig. 8.3 "V" Distribution at risk for keloid formation

upper arms, and upper back) where hypertrophic scarring and keloids tend to occur more often. Close postoperative follow-up and early intervention may allow the surgeon to minimize the adverse outcome of keloid formation following surgery. Strategies to minimize postoperative keloid formation include intralesional steroid injections, as well as pressure devices, and occlusive dressings.[22] Hypertrophic scars may be regarded in a similar manner preoperatively, with the recognition that the problem may be self-limiting and intervention less imperative.

Prophylactic Antibiotics and Antiviral Medication

Prophylactic antibiotics in dermatologic surgery are used for either prevention of endocarditis or prosthesis infection or for prevention of surgical site infection. Almost all the lesions cutaneous surgeons encounter are considered clean or clean-contaminated, and therefore do not require prophylaxis unless the patient has a prosthetic valve, an unrepaired congenital heart abnormality, or a history of endocarditis. It is important to consider the type of wound being manipulated when deciding whether or not antibiotics are appropriate (Table 8.3).

In 2007, the American Heart Association (AHA) revised the recommendations for antibiotic prophylaxis for endocarditis[23] (Table 8.4). The American Academy of Orthopedic Surgeons offers additional guidelines for antibiotic pretreatment for dental and urologic patients with total joint replacements.[24,25] According to these guidelines, patients should receive prophylaxis if their prosthetic joint was implanted less than 2 years prior to the procedure, or if they are considered immunosuppressed or immunocompromised.

In the most recent advisory statement of antibiotic prophylaxis in dermatologic surgery, coverage is recommended for patients with high-risk cardiac conditions and a defined group of patients with prosthetic joints at high risk for hematogenous infection when the surgical site is infected or when the procedure involves breach of the oral mucosa. For the prevention of surgical site infections,

Table 8.3 Wound classification

Type	Class	Characteristics	Risk of infection
I	Clean	Noncontaminated skin Aseptic technique	1–4%
II	Clean–contaminated	Location: gastrointestinal, respiratory, or genitourinary without gross contamination Minor breaks in aseptic technique	5–15%
III	Contaminated	Location: gastrointestinal, respiratory, or genitourinary with gross contamination Major breaks in aseptic technique	6–25%
IV	Dirty and/or infected	Foreign body contamination, wound with acute bacterial infection, ± pus	>25%

Table 8.4 Prophylaxis recommendations

Patients at highest risk for endocarditis[23]
Prosthetic cardiac valve or prosthetic material used in valve repair
Previous infective endocarditis
Congenital heart disease Unrepaired cyanotic CHD, including palliative shunts and conduits For first 6 months following repair of congenital heart defect
Repaired CHD with residual defects at the site or adjacent to the site Cardiac transplantation recipients who develop cardiac valvulopathy
Patients at potential increased risk for hematogenous prosthetic total joint infection[25]
Previous prosthetic joint infection
First 2 years after prosthetic joint replacement
Immunocompromised patients Inflammatory arthropathy (e.g., systemic lupus, rheumatoid arthritis) Drug-induced immunosuppression
Patients with comorbidity Malnourished, HIV, diabetes, malignancy
Antibiotic regimens (administer 30–60 min before procedure[23]**)**
Oral site Amoxicillin 2 g Alternative for penicillin allergy: oral cephalexin 2 g, clindamycin 600 mg, or Azithromycin/Clarithromycin 500 mg
Non oral site Cephalexin 2 g Alternatives as above

antibiotics may be indicated for procedures on the lower extremities or groin, for wedge excisions of the lip and ear, skin flaps on the nose, skin grafts, and for patients with extensive inflammatory skin disease.[26]

Regardless of the recommendations available in current published guidelines, some patients will request prophylaxis. Most often it is because they were once told to take the medication for a "murmur." Even with education, these patients feel very strongly they should take the medication, and often do so with or without the dermatologic surgeon's advice.

Prophylactic antiviral therapy is frequently utilized in patients with a history of frequent flares of herpes labialis (greater than three per year) undergoing facial resurfacing procedures. The risk of reactivation of herpes with resulting spread in incisional surgery near the mouth is probably much less than would be inferred from case reports, and no randomized controlled studies exist to support or refute the use of prophylaxis. Oral acyclovir at a dose of 200 mg five times a day—starting 2–5 days prior to the procedure and continuing for 5 days postoperatively or until the skin has re-epithelialized—may be considered for patients considered at particularly high risk for complications from reactivation and spread; however, a herpes simplex eruption may also be effectively treated by the initiation of antiviral therapy at the first sign of reactivation.[27,28] Alternatively, famciclovir or valacyclovir may be used to reduce dosing frequency.

Allergies

A comprehensive review of allergies is necessary for all first-time patients as well as return patients. Although all medication allergies are important, dermatologic surgeons are most interested in allergies to anesthesia, antibiotics, and pain medications. Patients often report a history of allergy to penicillin, epinephrine, and codeine, which are not true allergies, but adverse reactions. It is important to explore further and determine the nature of the reaction to the medication. Depending on the patient's ability to recall details of the allergic

episode, the physician may use his or her judgment in administering the medication.

True allergies to lidocaine are rare, but do exist. They constitute less than 1% of the total adverse reactions to local anesthesia.[29] Despite this small population of truly allergic individuals, a study detailed that up to 69% of dermatologists report seeing patients presenting with an alleged allergy.[30] These allergies are most often to the ester class of local anesthetics, which is metabolized to para-amino benzoic acid (PABA), a highly allergenic product in some individuals. The commonly used anesthetic lidocaine is an amide, and has a much lower potential to cause an allergic reaction. Patients who have developed a reaction to esters most often may be treated with amide anesthetics without problems (see Chapter 9).

Local anesthesia may be obtained in patients with allergies to amides and ester anesthetics by the injection of bacteriostatic saline. Benzyl alcohol, present as a bacteriostatic agent, acts as a local anesthetic. This relatively painless substitute may be sufficient for a quick punch or superficial shave biopsy; however, its duration is limited to a few minutes and the anesthesia is not profound. It is usually not sufficient for longer, more involved surgical procedures.

Diphenhydramine has been evaluated for its ability to produce local anesthesia. It does produce significant local anesthesia, but the duration is significantly less than that of lidocaine, it is more painful to inject, and necrosis has been reported after local infiltration.[31] Because of the lack of excellent alternatives to lidocaine for involved or extensive procedures, referral to an allergist for evaluation of an uncertain lidocaine allergy may be necessary. General anesthesia may be appropriate for extensive procedures in the lidocaine allergic patient.

Epinephrine, although reported by many patients to cause an allergic reaction, most often causes minor palpitations due to sensitivity to the drug. Diluting epinephrine to up to 1:500,000 limits such reaction in most patients but still provides a reasonable degree of vasoconstriction. For the very sensitive patient, especially those with concomitant cardiac compromise, total avoidance of epinephrine may be necessary.

Patients commonly voice an allergy to penicillin and other antibiotics. On questioning, again, many of these reactions turn out to be adverse reactions, not allergies. Obviously, drugs that have induced allergies or severe adverse reactions should be avoided, if possible, in that individual. Antibiotics are not routinely required in dermatologic surgery; however, if required, the most commonly utilized class of medications is the cephalosporins. Although the risk of cross-reactivity in patients with an allergy to penicillin is low, estimated at 4.4% in a recent review,[32] it is prudent for the physician to avoid this class of antibiotics in patients with documented penicillin allergy.

Implantable Cardiac Devices

Implantable cardiac devices, including pacemakers and defibrillators, are becoming more common in the population of patients with skin cancer. An estimated 4% of Mohs surgery patients have implantable cardiac devices.[33] Electrosurgical instruments used for treatment and hemostasis in dermatologic surgery have the potential to interfere with cardiac devices, and therefore preoperative assessment is crucial in order to ensure that a safe method of hemostasis is employed during the surgery. Electrocautery has been shown to be safe in patients with pacemakers and implanted defibrillators.[34] Handheld disposable electrocautery pens are convenient and often sufficient for hemostasis in this patient population; however, the heat is not adjustable as with tunable, electrically powered thermal cautery units. As a result, the high temperature of disposable units may lead to sectioning of the tissue, increased tissue destruction, and poor hemostasis. Bipolar forceps are also considered safe; however, an electrical current is produced, and cardiac monitoring should be available.

Patient Expectations

Proper informed consent prior to beginning any surgical procedure is essential. Figure 8.4a, b demonstrate a standardized consent form that is reviewed by the nurse, and confirmed by the physician prior to starting any surgical procedure. The review of the procedure by multiple team members and at multiple times helps ensure that the patient is well educated about the procedure and has proper expectations. Documenting preexisting defects with photography is imperative, as many patients do not appreciate asymmetry or recall defects until after their surgery. During the consent process it is important to emphasize the risk of scar formation. Patients rarely seem to understand that the removal of their skin cancer will result in a scar that is likely to be much larger than the primary lesion. A simple explanation of the reasons behind the need for longer or distant excision lines, as well as outlining the excision with a marking pen on the patient prior to surgery, will allow patients to visualize the procedure and prepare for the outcome.

> Often an outcome that the patient perceives as unexpected may have been fully anticipated by the surgeon. Thorough explanations may minimize misunderstandings and prepare patients for the postoperative course.

Intraoperative Considerations

Once potential pitfalls have been addressed preoperatively, it is very important to continue the same diligence while working in the operating suite.

Operating Suite

The organization of the operating suite may play a role in optimizing the surgical outcome. In offices with multiple procedure rooms, the set up will ideally be identical from room to room. This standardization prevents unnecessary wasted time searching for materials or

a

Palm Harbor Dermatology
CANCER AND LASER SURGERY CENTER

INFORMED CONSENT: MOHS MICROGRAPHIC SURGERY& REPAIR

Patient Name: _____   Patient Date of Birth: _____

This form is designed to provide you with the necessary information that you will need to make an informed decision on whether or not you wish to have Mohs Surgery performed. All of the information provided in this form will be or has been reviewed with you by the physician. If you have any questions please do not hesitate to ask us. Do not sign this form until you are instructed to do so.

WHAT ARE THE POTENTIAL COMPLICATIONS AND SIDE EFFECTS OF SKIN SURGERY?

1. **PAIN:** Some mild discomfort is experienced when the area is first anesthetized with the numbing medication. You may experience some mild discomfort during the procedure if the numbing medication has worn off in a particular location. This is easily remedied by immediately giving more anesthetic in that area. After the procedure, some discomfort will be experienced at the surgical site. This is easily controlled with pain medications for a few days.
2. **INFECTION:** Any time that the skin is injured an infection is possible. The rate of infection is very low. Some patients will receive postoperative antibiotics to prevent an infection. If you feel that your wound is infected after surgery please call our office immediately.
3. **BLEEDING:** When you leave our office you will have a pressure bandage applied to your wound. Bleeding is always possible after surgery. Most cases of postoperative bleeding are easily stopped by applying pressure for 20 minutes over the site. If this does not work please call our office immediately.
4. **SWELLING:** After surgery you should expect some swelling where your surgery was performed and around the wound as well.
5. **HEMATOMA:** A hematoma is a collection of blood that forms under the skin. This results from bleeding that occurs after the surgery. A "lump" forms under the skin, which represents the dried blood. If this occurs call our office immediately.
6. **SCAR FORMATION:** Any time that the skin is injured a scar will form. Some scars are more noticeable than others, but a scar is always present. A scar will form after your surgery. Hypertrophic and keloidal scarring are possible. If you have a history of bad scarring please advise us at the time of your visit. The cosmetic appearance following surgery is unpredictable.
7. **WOUND DEHISCENCE:** This means that your wound has broken back open after it has been repaired with sutures. It is very important to take it easy after your surgery so that unnecessary strain is not placed on the wound. This is an uncommon complication.
8. **FAILURE OF FLAP OR SKIN GRAFT:** After your surgery is completed we will need to repair the wound. Some patients are repaired with either a flap or skin graft. A flap is when skin is borrowed from a nearby site to close the defect. A skin graft is when a piece of skin is taken from one site and transplanted to another. A possible complication is the failure of either of these to take at the new site. Smoking is a documented risk for this complication. If you are a smoker it is recommended that you discontinue smoking for one week before and after the procedure.
9. **TEMPORARY OR PERMANENT NERVE DAMAGE:** The primary goal of your surgery is to completely remove the tumor. In order to accomplish this, it is sometimes necessary to damage a nerve. Nerve damage can be temporary or permanent. Recovery usually takes 6 months or more, and rarely can require additional surgery. Nerve damage may be limited to a loss of sensation or may include paralysis.
10. **DISTORTION/ALTERATION OF SURROUNDING ANATOMIC FEATURES:** The repair or healing of surgical wounds may distort the appearance of adjacent structures. Our goal is to completely remove your skin cancer, and then concern ourselves with the function and appearance of surrounding anatomic structures.

Fig. 8.4 Example of a consent form for Mohs surgery: (**a**) page one and (**b**) page two

equipment, particularly while a procedure is ongoing. The most common design of our procedure rooms is depicted in Fig. 8.5. There is certainly significant variation and personal preference associated with room design. There are several good resources available to individuals interested in planning their own office space.[35,36]

Specific equipment details are beyond the scope of this chapter, however, easy access to supplies, clearly marked surgical trays, reliable patient positioning, and excellent lighting are key in optimizing surgical outcomes and ensuring patient safety.

Surgical Site Preparation

Skin Marking

Prior to any intervention, the surgical site is marked with a surgical marking pen. There are numerous pens available, but most are filled with gentian violet. This ink is nontoxic to the skin and can easily be reinforced intraoperatively. Pens are available in sterile form when needed. It is essential to confirm the location of the skin cancer to be removed *with the patient* prior to

b INFORMED CONSENT: MOHS MICROGRAPHIC SURGERY& REPAIR

11. **TUMOR RECURRENCE:** No skin cancer treatment has a guaranteed 100% cure rate. However, Mohs surgery has been shown to have the highest cure rate for the treatment of skin cancer.

The complications of surgery are not limited to the above list.

I acknowledge that I have received and read a copy of the Palm Harbor Dermatology Mohs Micrographic Surgery Brochure. This brochure fully explained to me the procedure and what to expect during and after the procedure. I understand its contents, and all of my questions regarding the procedure have been answered.

I acknowledge that I have read the entire consent form. I understand its contents, and the doctor has adequately informed me of the risks, benefits, advantages, disadvantages, alternatives, and possible complications of skin surgery. I also understand that the postoperative size of the surgical wound after removing the skin cancer, and the method of repair cannot be predicted in advance, and I could require referral for additional closure or revision of the procedure site.

I further request the administration of such analgesia and/or sedative medication as deemed necessary or desirable for the completion of the procedure. I understand that the administration of medication carries risks separate and apart from the risks of the procedure.

I recognize that the results from the practice of medicine and surgery are not absolutely predictable, and I acknowledge that no guarantees or assurances have or can be made concerning the results of such treatment. I further acknowledge that there have specifically been no guarantees as to the cosmetic results from the procedure.

All of my questions and concerns have been answered, and I hereby consent to Mohs surgery and repair if

necessary to be performed by Dr. Ross upon _____ (patient).

I have identified and confirmed the location(s) of my surgical site(s).

I also consent to the taking of photographs before, during, and after the procedure. I understand that these photographs are important to document and follow my progress after surgery. These photographs will belong to Palm Harbor Dermatology, and may be used for educational and scientific purposes. This may include presentation at lectures or publication in medical journals. In such an event, I will not be identified by name. I expect no compensation for any such use of these photographs, and I waive all my rights to any claims for payment or royalties. I also release Dr. Ross from any liability in connection with the use of such photographs.

I agree that any tissue removed during the course of the operation may be examined, documented, preserved and/or disposed of in a manner considered proper for diagnosis, study, and advancement of medical knowledge.

I understand that Palm Harbor Dermatology has recommended that a spouse, relative, or friend accompany me and drive me home following my surgery. If I decide to drive myself home, I understand and assume the risk involved.

Patient's/Guardian's Printed Name _____ Patient's/Guardian's Signature _____

Relationship, if other than patient _____

Date: _____ Time: _____ AM/PM

I confirm that this form has been completely reviewed with the patient. The potential risks, side effects, and complications were all discussed. All of the patient's questions have been answered.

Physician's Signature: _____ Date: _____

Witness Signature: _____ Date: _____

Fig. 8.4 (continued)

marking the surgical site. At our institution, prior to the surgeon marking the skin, the patient is asked to point to the location without direction from the physician. Biopsy sites may heal completely while the patient is awaiting definitive surgery and the patient and the surgeon may have difficulty pinpointing the correct site. There have been several publications suggesting ways to reproducibly document the site of a lesion.[37,38] Digital photographs are an excellent method of documentation. Problems most often arise in patients referred in for a procedure at a time remote from the biopsy.

> If there is any doubt as to the location of the surgical site, the procedure should be delayed until proper identification can be made and all parties are in agreement.

Choice of Antiseptic Solution

Depending on the location of the surgical site, the area is cleansed with either chlorhexidine or iodophore. In most patients, chlorhexidine will be used if the site is not within 2 cm of the orbit, or in the ear.

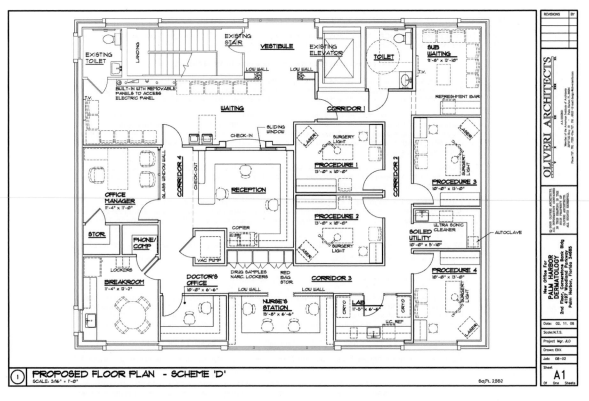

Fig. 8.5 Example of an office design

One of the possibly preventable complications in skin cancer surgery is wound infection. Although the overall infection rate for dermatologic surgery in an outpatient setting is low, at reportedly 0.7–2.45% in several published case series[39–41] surgeons should employ basic standard techniques to ensure minimal risk of infection. These techniques are discussed below; however, the administration of antibiotics should not be considered standard therapy.

Anesthesia

The specifics of anesthesia are covered in Chapter 9; however, a few points are worth emphasizing. The vasoconstrictive effect of epinephrine may take up to 15 min to work. In patients with an increased risk of bleeding, allowing the full 15 min between injection and incision will usually decrease bleeding. The epinephrine in vials of lidocaine is usually at a 1:100,000 dilution. Dilutions as low as 1:500,000 have been shown to provide adequate hemostasis.

Reduction of the amount of epinephrine may be advisable if large quantities of anesthesia are anticipated or will be used in the frail and elderly. To avoid excessive exposure to epinephrine, we routinely use lidocaine with epinephrine 1:300,000.

Another important factor to consider is the use of regional nerve blocks. Although nerve blocks require more time for effect, there are instances in which the use of a nerve block may be beneficial to the patient and the surgeon and help optimize the outcome. For instance, the infiltration of local anesthesia can greatly distort the anatomy of the lip. In this circumstance an infraorbital block for the upper lip, or a mental block for the lower lip, may be beneficial.

There are some instances where tumescent anesthesia may be advantageous. The use of tumescent anesthesia may allow the treatment under local anesthesia of larger tumors or larger surface areas.

In these circumstances conventional anesthesia might be limited over concerns about lidocaine toxicity. In addition, tumescent anesthesia may provide benefits of prolonged duration and decreased bleeding (see Chapter 9).

Staff Preparation

Hand Washing/Surgical Scrubbing

To reduce the risk of postsurgical infections, use of an antimicrobial preparation for hand washing is necessary. There are now numerous waterless surgical scrub products in the market for use as an alternative to traditional cleansers that require rinsing with water after use. We use a solution of chlorhexidine gluconate 1% with 61% by weight ethyl alcohol. This product has been shown to be effective for microbial reduction.[42] There are several other waterless products that have also been found to be effective as antiseptics prior to putting on sterile gloves.[43] These products are strictly alcohol based, and are less costly than the products containing chlorhexidine gluconate. When using products with a significant ethyl alcohol component, care must be taken to assure the preparation has thoroughly dried before there is any exposure to the spark of an electrosurgical instrument or the heat of electrocautery.

Surgical Site Draping

Although most surgeons complete the reconstruction phase of Mohs micrographic surgery (MMS) utilizing sterile technique, there is a difference in sterile technique among surgeons during the taking of Mohs layers. There is evidence indicating that there is no difference in infection rates when stages are taken clean compared to sterile.[44] Utilizing clean technique to take stages can be more cost-effective and efficient compared to the utilization of sterile technique. Nonsterile gloves have also been shown to be generally safe for the practitioner in dermatologic surgery. The rate of perforation of nonsterile examination gloves is published to be 2.3% for routine dermatologic procedures[45] but may increase up to 11.7% for procedures such as MMS.[46] An effective alternative to more costly, but less easily perforated sterile gloves may be to double glove with nonsterile gloves. This has been shown to be an effective method of protection against blood exposure in dermatologic surgery.[47]

Intraoperative Monitoring

Although the American College of Cardiology classifies cutaneous surgery as "low cardiac risk," and recommends no preoperative cardiac evaluation[48] the recording of basic vital signs including blood pressure and heart rate is useful and prudent. Surgery is generally deferred in patients with systolic blood pressures greater than 180 or diastolic blood pressures greater than 100. Except in patients in an exceptionally fragile state or with a high risk of cardiac arrhythmia, intraoperative monitoring is not warranted in low-risk procedures under local anesthesia. All procedure room personnel should have current training in basic life support and physicians should be familiar with more advanced techniques, such as advanced cardiac life support. Every medical office should have a comprehensive emergency plan including immediate access to basic resuscitation equipment such as breathing devices, oxygen, and an automatic external defibrillator, as well as a protocol for activating the local emergency medical response system. Facilities that provide higher risk procedures such as conscious sedation should have more extensive resources and appropriate personnel training.

Tissue Manipulation

After the skin has been incised, it is important to minimize trauma to any tissue that will become part of the closure. A properly utilized skin hook is an excellent way to avoid crush injury to the epidermis, which may result from handling tissue edges with forceps. Figure 8.6 demonstrates the proper handling of skin edges with skin hooks. These instruments, when handled properly by the physician and assistants, are safe and the most effective way to manipulate tissue without

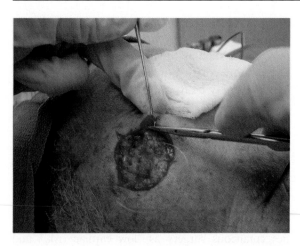

Fig. 8.6 Proper use of the skin hook to allow atraumatic positioning of a subcutaneous suture. Note the careful positioning of the finger behind the hook to stabilize the tissue

significant injury. Crushed skin margins will lead to localized tissue necrosis and detract from the operative result.

> The most effective surgeon is gentle with the patient and the wound.

Optimal closure can often be obtained by undermining the wound edges aggressively with blunt scissors or semi-sharp scissors. Extensive undermining in the proper plane will result in less tension on the sutured wound edges, and ultimately a better cosmetic outcome. Figure 8.7 demonstrates an

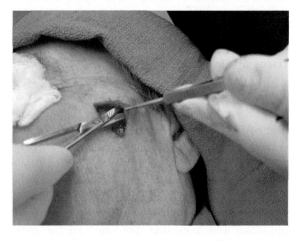

Fig. 8.7 Undermining utilizing scissors and skin hook

appropriate degree and level of undermining for a wound following MMS removal of a nonmelanoma skin cancer. Inadequate undermining may lead to increased tension across the surface of a wound, and suboptimal outcomes.

Hemostasis

Hemostasis must be assured at every stage of the procedure. The approach for obtaining hemostasis should be adjusted to account for the patient's risk factors for bleeding and the operative procedure. In some circumstances, simple prolonged external intraoperative pressure may provide adequate hemostasis. This approach has the benefit of limiting the tissue damage caused by chemical or electrical cauterization.

For wounds that are to be sutured, hemostasis may often be obtained with electrocoagulation or electrodesiccation. It is important to remember that these methods are only effective in a relatively dry surgical field, so attempting to blindly stop bleeding in a pool of blood is futile. Good visualization of the source of bleeding is key in obtaining hemostasis. Although efforts should be employed to minimize postoperative bleeding, the surgeon should resist the temptation to use the electrosurgical device excessively and indiscriminately. Too much char from electrocoagulation or cautery will impede wound healing, especially if applied near the skin edges. Larger vessels may require ligation with suture ties to stop the immediate bleeding and assure continued hemostasis. If this is necessary, an absorbable suture of sufficient gauge such as 4-0 polyglactin 910 suture may be utilized. Ties must be placed securely and encompass as little extra tissue as possible to prevent rebleeding during the immediate postoperative period.

On rare occasions, diffuse bleeding continues despite these measures. This most often occurs in patients on blood thinners, or with coagulopathies. Renewed intraoperative manual pressure for 15–20 min often makes a significant difference in patient bleeding. An open wound may be packed with oxidized cellulose to help control bleeding. If this material is placed in a closed wound, healing may be impaired by the foreign body reaction it induces. A commercially available sponge made of purified porcine skin gelatin (Gelfoam®) may be used in a similar manner with less risk of foreign body reaction. Thrombin is available in several forms to place within the wound bed to control bleeding. Of particular use is thrombin in a gelatin matrix (FloSeal™). Almost any repair can be performed with the material in place. Although expensive, this product is simple to use, and can effectively stop bleeding and prevent potential postoperative complications in patients with a bleeding diathesis.

Alternative, more aggressive approaches in patients with known bleeding disorders, including the use of prophylactic therapy, such as 1-desamino-8-arginine vasopressin (DDAVP) or plasma concentrates, may prevent postoperative bleeding complications. Decisions regarding these prophylactic measures should be made in consultation with a hematologist.

Designing the Closure

There are several fundamental principals to consider in designing an optimal closure. Figure 8.8a, b demonstrate the relaxed skin tension lines on the face of a photo-aged individual. These lines tend to run perpendicular to the underlying muscle, and if possible, the skin closure should be oriented parallel to the relaxed skin tension lines. In some locations, the direction of closure is not clear. In these instances, removing the skin cancer, and undermining around the entire defect may facilitate determining the optimal direction of closure.

> It is important to note that following relaxed skin tension lines on the face should not be done at the expense of crossing cosmetic subunits or placing traction on free margins.

The face is divided into distinct regions (Fig. 8.9). These boundaries represent the cosmetic subunits of the face, and if possible, closures should be designed to be completed within the unit. This will usually result in the least visible and most cosmetically acceptable scar.

Specific techniques regarding excision, flaps, and grafts are covered in other chapters (Chapters 10, 12, and 13); however, it is worth mentioning an important principle:

> The surgeon should always measure twice, and cut once.

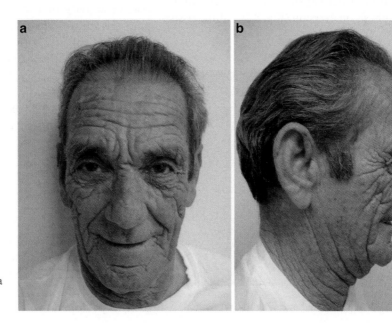

Fig. 8.8 Relaxed skin tension lines on the face of a photo-aged individual: (**a**) front and (**b**) profile

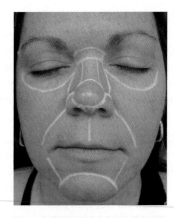

Fig. 8.9 Outline of the cosmetic subunits of the central face

The importance of planning the closure prior to making any additional incisions in the skin should not be underestimated.

Suturing the Wound

Excessive tension on wounds hinders the blood supply, and may result in suboptimal surgical outcomes. As discussed previously, extensive undermining may minimize tension across the entire wound, and precise epidermal apposition with subcutaneous sutures is key to minimizing tension on the epidermis. As scars tend to spread over time, the placement of appropriate deep dermal or subcutaneous sutures and an emphasis on eversion (Fig. 8.10) of the tissue

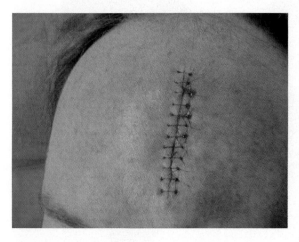

Fig. 8.10 Eversion of a wound under significant tension

will result in a more cosmetically acceptable scar in the long term.

Tension in the wound bed has also been found to influence keloid formation.[49] Extraordinary attention to minimization of wound tension may reduce the risk of postoperative keloid formation.

Postoperative Considerations

After the surgical procedure is complete, the surgical site is cleansed with normal saline, a postoperative photo is obtained, and a dressing is applied.

There are many variations of dressings; however, a key feature of the postoperative dressing is to provide even firm pressure. Figure 8.11a, b, c, d detail a typical postoperative dressing. When the vasoconstrictive effect of epinephrine wears off, patients have a tendency to bleed. A pressure dressing left on for the first 24 h will aid in maintaining hemostasis. Studies have demonstrated a lack of effectiveness in topical antibiotics preventing wound infection.[50] Applying white petrolatum ointment to the wound followed by a nonstick pad, appropriate dry gauze to provide pressure, and tape is sufficient. Patients are instructed to keep the wound covered with ointment and dressing until the time of suture removal. Patients are also advised to avoid heavy lifting, vigorous exercise, or activity that might traumatize the wound until the sutures are removed. Activity should be discussed explicitly with each patient as daily routines vary dramatically. One patient's definition of vigorous activity may be quite different from another's. Postoperative wound care instructions (Fig. 8.12a, b) should be provided in writing as retention of oral instructions after a procedure is quite limited.

Pain Control

All patients should be questioned on their use of, and possible need for, pain medication. It is important to address this issue with patients individually instead of having a standard set of prescriptions for patients postoperatively. Some patients are on pain

Fig. 8.11 (**a**) Wound prior to placement of dressing. (**b**) Wound coated with petrolatum and covered with a nonadherent dressing layer. (**c**) Placement of a layer of dry absorbent gauze. (**d**) Dressing firmly held in place by tape

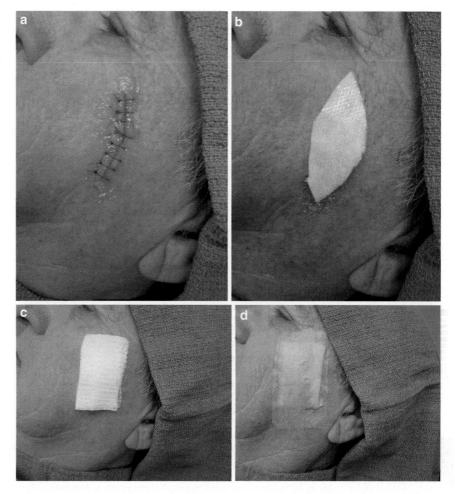

medication preoperatively for an unrelated ailment, while others are completely resistant to taking any narcotic medications. For simple procedures, the patient is advised that acetaminophen will provide adequate pain relief. The patient is always provided with access to a physician if the need for stronger medication develops. This allows evaluation of the patient when necessary in addition to assuring patient comfort. The rest of our patients are told to begin with acetaminophen but are given a prescription for either hydrocodone/acetaminophen or propoxyphene/acetaminophen to take if needed. Except in exceptional circumstances, we always dispense twelve tablets so if there is ever any question from a pharmacy about the legitimacy of the prescription, the staff may be easily alerted to problems.

Antibiotics

Antibiotics following surgery are prescribed very judiciously. As discussed previously, the risk of infection following dermatologic surgery is minimal. We reserve antibiotics for patients with skin grafts, reconstructions with possible compromised vascular supply, patients with a high risk of infection because of underlying disease, or patients who are undergoing excessively long procedures. These patients are most often given cephalexin 500 mg po tid for 7 days, or levofloxacin 750 mg po qd for 7 days if they are allergic to cephalosporins. If the need to provide postoperative antibiotics is anticipated preoperatively, the medication is started preoperatively as it has been demonstrated that having the antibiotic in the tissue at the time of surgery

a

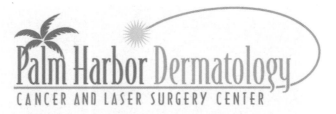

INSTRUCTIONS FOR "CLOSED" (SUTURED) WOUND CARE

MATERIALS

Q-tips, cotton tip applicators
Vaseline
Telfa dressing pads (Non-adherent dressing)
½" or 1" paper tape

PROCEDURE

1. Allow the pressure bandage to remain in place for 24 to 48 hours.
2. Using liquid antibacterial soap and water, gently cleanse the sutures and surgical wound using a Q-tip.
3. Apply a small amount of Vaseline ointment to sutures.

NOTE

1. Keep wound dry for 24 hours
2. Avoid strenuous activity for at least two weeks following surgery.
3. Dressing can be changed as often as necessary; however, dressing change once daily is usually sufficient.

WHAT TO EXPECT FOLLOWING SURGERY

1. Swelling, bruising, and redness around the wound are common. These symptoms typically resolve within several days.

2. Drainage from wound will occur. The drainage may have a yellowish color or foul odor. The drainage and odor will resolve after several days.

3. Significant bleeding is unlikely but may occur. Should you experience significant bleeding it is recommended that you lie down and apply firm, constant pressure to the surgical site for a minimum of 20 minutes. If bleeding continues, repeat the pressure on the surgical wound for an additional 20 minutes. In the event that bleeding persists, please contact our office as early as possible during the day so that we may make arrangements for your evaluation. If you are unable to reach our office or your doctor, please proceed to the nearest emergency room for evaluation and assistance.

4. Discomfort at the surgical site may be experienced for several days following your surgery. One or two **NON-ASPIRIN** pain relievers taken every four hours may be used as needed. **CAUTION: Bufferin, Anacin, Goody Powders, Excedrin, and B.C. Powders <u>all contain aspirin products</u>**.

5. Icepacks may be placed over the wound dressing during the first 24 hours. The icepack is placed over the wound for 15 minutes and may be repeated four times per day. You may also use a bag of frozen peas in substitution for an icepack.

6. Please contact our office or your local physician should you experience excessive bleeding, swelling, redness, fever, or pain.

Further questions can be addressed through our office at 727-786-3810.

Our normal business hours are Monday through Friday 7:30am – 4:30pm.

Fig. 8.12 (**a**) Postoperative wound care instructions for sutured wounds. (**b**) Postoperative wound care instructions for open wounds (see next page)

b

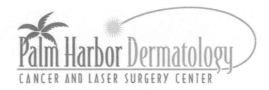

INSTRUCTIONS FOR WOUND CARE (SECOND INTENTION)

MATERIALS
Cotton tip applicator or Q-tips
Vaseline
Telfa surgical dressing pads (non-adherent dressing)
½" or 1" paper tape
Scissors

PROCEDURE

1.   Remove bandage in 24 hours.

2.   Gently cleanse any drainage on or around wound using mild soap and water applied with a Q-tip.

3.   With clean applicator, dry wound.

4.   With clean applicator, spread a thin layer of Vaseline ointment over the wound.

5.   Cut Telfa pad to cover the wound. This is held in place with paper tape. If the Telfa pad adheres to the wound when you remove it at the time of the next dressing change, use more ointment to prevent further sticking. If excessive drainage occurs, cut gauze pad to size and place over Telfa pad.

NOTE

1.   Change the dressing 1-2 times daily for 1-2 weeks and then once daily until the wound is completely healed (some wounds may require 4-6 weeks for complete healing).

2.   Before changing bandages, you may take a shower, wash your hair, shave, etc., then follow the above procedure (the dressing will more than likely get wet, but will act as protection during shower, etc.).

3.   Avoid alcohol, smoking, aspirin, aspirin containing products, and blood thinners as they thin the blood and cause bleeding.

WHAT TO EXPECT

1.   Some swelling, redness and/or bruising around the wound. This usually resolves within a few days.

2.   Some drainage from the wound which may have a foul odor and be yellowish in color. This will resolve in a few days.

3.   Significant bleeding is unlikely, but may occur. Should you experience significant bleeding, it is recommended that you lie down and apply firm, constant pressure to the surgical site for a minimum of twenty minutes. If bleeding continues, repeat the pressure on the surgical wound for an additional twenty minutes. In the event that bleeding persists, please contact our office as early as possible during the day so that we may make arrangements for your evaluation. If you are unable to reach our office or your doctor, please proceed to the nearest emergency room for evaluation and assistance.

4.   Discomfort at the surgical site may be experienced for several days following your surgery. One or two **NON-ASPIRIN** pain relievers taken every 4 hours may be used as needed. CAUTION: Bufferin, Anacin, Goody Powders, Excedrin, and B.C. Powders all contain aspirin products.

5.   Icepacks may be placed over the wound dressing during the first 24 hours. The icepack is placed over the wound for 15 minutes and may be repeated 4 times per day. You may also use a bag of frozen peas in substitution for an icepack.

6.   Please contact our office or your local physician should you experience excessive bleeding, swelling, redness, fever, or pain.

Further questions can be addressed through our office at 727-786-3810.

Our normal business hours are Monday through Friday 7:30am – 4:30pm.

Fig. 8.12 (continued)

provides the most effective prophylaxis.[51] Again, topical antibiotics have not demonstrated effectiveness in this situation.

Timing of Suture Removal

The final consideration prior to sending the patient home is establishing the proper follow-up time. The timing of suture removal is key in optimizing surgical outcomes. "Track marks" may result if sutures are allowed to remain in place for too long. Table 8.5 identifies timing suggestions for suture removal. Timing is dependent upon the location of the wound. Many patients drive for considerable distances to have their skin cancer removed. If a local physician can remove the sutures at the proper time, it may save the patient considerable time and travel

Table 8.5 Timing for suture removal

Location	Number of days postoperative	Other considerations
Face	5–7 days	May use fast absorbing gut, or polyglactin 910 rapide if wound under no tension
Scalp	10–14 days	
Neck	7–10 days	
Trunk and Extremities	14 days	If on acral surface, silk sutures for epidermal closure may minimize tissue tearing

expense. If that is not possible, consideration may be given to using absorbable suture such as fast-absorbing surgical gut, fast-absorbing polyglactin 910, or poliglecaprone 25. Patients should be instructed to call with any problems and be provided with easy access numbers. In general, patients are very appreciative of the effort to minimize the inconvenience associated with a noncomplicated suture removal visit.

Summary

In order to optimize outcomes associated with cutaneous surgery, there are many factors to consider in the perioperative period. Many of the most important factors are addressed preoperatively with careful preparation and planning. With appropriate attention to detail, dermatologic surgery can be performed on a wide range of patient populations, safely, and with excellent results.

References

1. Procedure Survey. Dermasurgery Trends and Statistics. Rolling Meadows, IL: American Society for Dermatologic Surgery; 2005. Available from: http://www.asds.net/TheAmericanSocietyforDermatologicSurgeryReleasesNewProcedureSurveyData.aspx. Last accessed February 3, 2009.
2. Kaplan AL, Weitzul SB, Taylor RS. Longitudinal diminution of tumor size for basal cell carcinoma suggests shifting referral patterns for Mohs surgery. *Dermatol Surg*. 2008;34:15–19.
3. Cook J, Zitelli JA. Mohs micrographic surgery: a cost analysis. *J Am Acad Dermatol*. 1998;39:698–703.
4. Kovich O, Otley CC. Perioperative management of anticoagulants and platelet inhibitors for cutaneous surgery: a survey of current practice. *Dermatol Surg*. 2002;28:513–517.
5. Otley CC. Continuation of medically necessary aspirin and warfarin during cutaneous surgery. *Mayo Clin Proc*. 2003;78:1392–1396.
6. Alcalay J, Alkalay R. Controversies in perioperative management of blood thinners in dermatologic surgery: continue or discontinue? *Dermatol Surg*. 2004;30:1091–1094.
7. Schanbacker CF, Bennett RG. Postoperative stroke after stopping warfarin for cutaneous surgery. *Dermatol Surg*. 2000;26:785–789.
8. Alam M, Goldberg LH. Serious adverse vascular events associated with perioperative interruption of antiplatelet and anticoagulant therapy. *Dermatol Surg*. 2002;28 992–998.
9. Kovich O, Otley CC. Thrombotic complications related to discontinuation of warfarin and aspirin therapy perioperatively for cutaneous operation. *J Am Acad Dermatol*. 2003;48:233–237.
10. Chang LK, Whitaker DC. The impact of herbal medicines on dermatologic surgery. *Dermatol Surg*. 2001;27:759–763.
11. Timbo BB, Ross MP, McCarthy PV, et al. Dietary supplements in a national survey: Prevalence of use and reports of adverse events. *J Am Diet Assoc*. 2006;106:1966–1974.
12. Cox AC, Rao GH, Gerrard JM, White JG. The influence of vitamin E quinone on platelet structure, function, and biochemistry. *Blood*. 1980;55:907–914.
13. Ziv O, Ragni MV. Bleeding manifestations in males with von Willebrand disease. *Haemophilia*. 2004;10:162–168.
14. Werner EJ, Broxson EH, Tucker EL, et al. Prevalence of von Willebrand disease in children: a multiethnic study. *J Pediatr*. 1993;123:893–898.
15. Leonard AL, Hanke CW, Greist A. Perioperative management of von Willebrand disease in dermatologic surgery. *Dermatol Surg*. 2007;33:403–409.

16. Nichols WC, Ginsburg D. Von Willebrand disease. *Medicine (Baltimore)*. 1997;76:1–20.

17. Bailey BJ, Johnson JT, Newlands SD. *Head & Neck Surgery—Otolaryngology*. Philadelphia: Lippincott Williams & Wilkins; 2006:217.

18. Busti AJ, Hooper JS, Amaya CJ, Kazi S. Effects of perioperative anti-inflammatory and immunomodulating therapy on surgical wound healing. *Pharmacotherapy*. 2005;25:1566–1591.

19. Abdelmalek M, Spencer J. Retinoids and wound healing. *Dermatol Surg*. 2006;32:1219–1230.

20. Taniguchi Y, Shimizu Y, Inachi S, Shimizu M. Skin surgery in patients 90 years of age and over. *Int J Dermatol*. 1998;37:547–550.

21. MacFarlane DF, Pustelny BL, Goldberg LH. An assessment of the suitability of Mohs micrographic surgery in patients aged 90 years and older. *Dermatol Surg*. 1998;23:389–392.

22. Berman B, Flores F. The treatment of hypertrophic scars and keloids. *Eur J Dermatol*. 1998;8:591–595.

23. Wilson W, Taubert KA, Gewitz M, et al. Prevention of infective endocarditis guidelines from the American Heart Association. *Circulation*. 2007; 116:1736–1754.

24. Scher K, Elston DM, Hedrick JA, Joseph WS, Maurer T, Murakawa GJ. Treatment options in the management of uncomplicated skin and skin structure infections. *Cutis*. 2005;75:3–23.

25. American Academy of Orthopaedic Surgeons Advisory Statement on Antibiotic Prophylaxis for Dental Patients with Total Joint Replacements. http://www.aaos.org/about/papers/advistmt/1027.asp. Last accessed January 21, 2009.

26. Wright TI, Baddour LM, Berbari EF. Antibiotic prophylaxis in dermatologic surgery: advisory statement 2008. *J Am Acad Dermatol*. 2008;59:464–473.

27. Sheridan RL, Schulz JT, Weber JM, et al. Cutaneous herpetic infections complicating burns. *Burns*. 2000;26: 621–624.

28. Fidler PE, Mackool BT, Schoenfeld DA, et al. Incidence, outcome, and long-term consequences of herpes simplex virus type 1 reactivation presenting as a facial rash in intubated adult burn patients treated with acyclovir. *J Trauma*. 2002;53:86–89.

29. Verrill PJ. Adverse reactions to local anaesthetics and vasoconstrictor drugs. *Practitioner*. 1975;214: 380–387.

30. Amsler E, Flahault A, Mathelier-Fusade P, Aractingi S. Evaluation of re-challenge in patients with suspected lidocaine allergy. *Dermatology*. 2004;208:109–111.

31. Dire DJ. Hogan DE. Double-blinded comparison of diphenhydramine versus lidocaine as a local anesthetic. *Ann Emerg Med*. 1993;22:1419–1422.

32. Romano A, Gueant-Rodriguez RM, Viola M, Pettinato R, Gueant JL. Cross-reactivity and tolerability of cephalosporins in patients with immediate hypersensitivity to penicillins. *Ann Intern Med*. 2004;141:16–22.

33. El-Gamal HM, Dufresne RG, Saddler K. Electrosurgery, pacemakers, and ICDs: a survey of precautions and complications experienced by cutaneous surgeons. *Dermatol Surg*. 2001;27:385–390.

34. Lane JE, O'Brien EM, Kent DE. Optimization of thermocautery in excisional dermatologic surgery. *Dermatol Surg*. 2006;32:669–675.

35. Haines RC Jr, Brooks LR. Office space planning and design for medical practices, Part 1: an overview. *J Med Pract Manage*. 2003;18:244–249.

36. Haines RC Jr, Griffin JK. Office space planning and design for medical practices: Part 3, Implementation, design, and construction. *J Med Pract Manage*. 2003; 19:19–26.

37. Lutz ME. Surgical pearl: curettage before cutaneous surgery to identify an unidentifiable biopsy site. *J Am Acad Dermatol*. 2002;46:591–593.

38. Robbins P, Sarnoff DS. Where's the spot? *J Dermatol Surg Oncol*. 1986;12:1251–1252.

39. Futoryan T, Grande D. Postoperative wound infection rates in dermatologic surgery. *Dermatol Surg*. 1995;21:509–514.

40. Whitaker DC, Grande DJ, Johnson SS. Wound infection rate in dermatologic surgery. *J Dermatol Surg Oncol*. 1988;14:525–528.

41. Carmichael AJ, Flanagan PG, Holt PJA, Duerden BI. The occurrence of bacteraemia with skin surgery. *Br J Dermatol*. 1996;134:120–122.

42. Mulberry G, Snyder AT, Heilman J, Pyrek J, Stahl J. Evaluation of a waterless, scrubless chlorhexidine gluconate/ethanol surgical scrub for antimicrobial efficacy. *Am J Infect Control*. 2001;29:377–382.

43. Gupta C, Czubatyj AM, Briski LE, Malani AK. Comparison of two alcohol-based surgical scrub solutions with an iodine-based scrub brush for presurgical antiseptic effectiveness in a community hospital. *J Hosp Infect*. 2007;65:65–71.

44. Rhinehart BM, Murphy ME, Farley MF, Albertini JG. Sterile versus nonsterile gloves during Mohs micrographic surgery: infection rate is not affected. *Dermatol Surg*. 2006;32:170–176.

45. Kupres K, Rasmussen SE, Albertini JG. Perforation rates for nonsterile examination gloves in routine dermatologic procedures. *Dermatol Surg*. 2002;28:388–389.

46. Gross DJ, Jamison Y, Martin K, Fields M, Dinehart SM. Surgical glove perforation in dermatologic surgery. *J Dermatol Surg Oncol*. 1989;15:1226–1228.

47. Cohen MD, Do JT, Tahery DP, Moy RL. Efficacy of double gloving as a protection against blood exposure in dermatologic surgery. *J Dermatol Surg Oncol*. 1992;18: 873–874.

48. Eagle KA, Brundage BH, Chaitman BR, et al. Guidelines for perioperative cardiovascular evaluation for noncardiac surgery: report of the American college of cardiology/American heart association task force on practice guidelines (committee on perioperative cardiovascular evaluation for noncardiac surgery). *J Am Coll Cardiol*. 1996;27:910–948.

49. Chipev CC, Simon M. Phenotypic differences between dermal fibroblasts from different body sites determine their responses to tension and TGFbeta1. *BMC Dermatol*. 2002;2:13.

50. Smack DP, Harrington AC, Dunn C, et al. Infection and allergy incidence in ambulatory surgery patients using white petrolatum vs. bacitracin ointment: a randomized controlled trial. *JAMA*. 1996;276:972–977.

51. Classen CD, Evans RS, Pestotnik SL, et al. The timing of prophylactic administration of antibiotics and the risk of surgical-wound infection. *N Eng J Med*. 1992;326:281–286.

Chapter 9
Anesthesia

Susannah L. Collier and George J. Hruza

Minimizing a patient's pain is one of the most important components of skin cancer surgery. When done well, it makes the surgical experience much more pleasant for both the surgeon and the patient. There are several variables that can make local anesthesia more effective, safer, and less painful including types of and additives to anesthetics, patient-specific cautions, injection techniques, and other tips for increasing patient comfort.

Local anesthetics work on nerve fibers by blocking the sodium channels. The small, unmyelinated C-fibers, which conduct pain, are blocked quickly; while the larger, unmyelinated fibers, which conduct heat and cold, lag behind. The myelinated A-fibers that conduct pressure are harder to block,

which is why many patients will sense the "pulling and tugging" on the skin, but feel no pain.

There are two basic classes of local anesthetics: amides and esters. It is important to know the difference between the two types, as they differ in the way in which they are metabolized and the frequency with which they may elicit allergic reactions (Table 9.1).

Indications and Contraindications

The primary indication for local anesthesia in outpatient skin cancer surgery is pain management. When combined with epinephrine, a secondary indication is hemostasis. Contraindications for

Table 9.1 Esters vs. Amides[1]

	Ester anesthetics	Amide anesthetics
How to recognize	Generic name contains one "i"	Generic name contains two "i"s
Examples	Procaine (Novocain) Chloroprocaine (Nescaine) Tetracaine (Pontocaine) Benzocaine (Hurricaine, Americaine) Cocaine	Lidocaine (Xylocaine, LMX) Bupivacaine (Marcaine) Prilocaine (in EMLA)[*]
Metabolized and inactivated by	Plasma pseudocholinesterases	Liver
Metabolite	Para-aminobenzoic Acid (PABA)	Prilocaine's metabolite oxidizes hemoglobin to methemoglobin
Metabolite excreted by	Kidney	N/A
Caution in patients with	Pseudocholinesterase deficiency, allergy to PABA, severe renal dysfunction	Severe liver dysfunction, risk of methemoglobinemia[*]

[*] Do not use in infants less than 4 months of age or those with G6PD deficiency. Use with caution in those patients less than 12 months of age and in those who are taking sulfa drugs.

D.F. MacFarlane (ed.), *Skin Cancer Management*, DOI 10.1007/978-0-387-88495-0_9,
© Springer Science+Business Media, LLC 2010

local anesthesia include an allergy to the anesthetic or a preservative in the anesthetic (Table 9.2) and those with specific underlying medical conditions (Table 9.3). The addition of epinephrine is contraindicated in a small subset of patients with certain underlying medical problems (Table 9.4).

Preoperative Considerations

A thorough preoperative evaluation should include asking the patient about anxiety, previous anesthetic reactions, allergies, medications, and underlying medical conditions (Tables 9.2 and 9.3). Knowing these facts prior to the day of surgery will allow the physician to solve potential problems before they arise and will save time on the day of surgery.

Easing anxiety is an important part of anesthesia. Though this seems obvious, it is often overlooked in a busy office. Prior to surgery, you should explain to the patient all the steps that you are taking to reduce their pain. When possible, this is best done several days prior to the procedure, so that the patient is more relaxed when coming to the office. If the patient remains very nervous, one could consider a preoperative oral anxiolytic such as Xanax (alprazolam). The patient could be given a prescription for a 0.25 mg pill, which they would then be asked to fill and bring with them to the office. They would also need to have a driver with them for the ride home. Once the patient is in the room, and the consent has been obtained, the patient can take the pill. Once the patient arrives for surgery, creating a calm environment is important. Playing the patient's favorite type of music on a radio can be a great start. Making sure that the patient is physically comfortable for the procedure by adjusting the head rest of the table/chair or by offering a warm blanket is also helpful. When talking to the patient, using a calm voice and a gentle touch can go a long way toward relaxing the patient.

To save time, anesthetics can be drawn up in batches on the morning of the procedure or the day before. If they are filled in advance, care must be taken to label the syringes with the contents and the date they were filled. In our office, the anesthetics are predrawn the night before. They are stored in clearly labeled boxes in the refrigerator.

The addition of epinephrine to local anesthetics helps not only with hemostasis but also prolongs the duration of anesthesia.

> Waiting 20 min after infiltrating anesthetics with epinephrine dramatically reduces intraoperative bleeding.

Epinephrine is supplied at a concentration of 1:1,000, or premixed with local anesthetics at concentrations of either 1:100,000 or 1:200,000. Because epinephrine is only stable in an acidic environment, when it is premixed with local anesthetics, the pH of the mixture is lowered. This acidity is the main reason why the injection of local anesthetics stings and burns.[12,13] Two ways to avoid this problem include avoiding using premixed solutions (Table 9.5) and adding sodium bicarbonate to the anesthetic at a ratio of 1:10 to bring the anesthetic's pH up to neutral[12,13] (Table 9.6). In both instances,

Table 9.2 Allergens in local anesthesia[2,3,4]

Allergen	Where found	How to avoid
The anesthetic itself	In the anesthetic solution	1. Use an anesthetic of another class 2. Use Benadryl or normal saline for small procedures 3. Consider general anesthesia
PABA[*]	The metabolite of ester anesthetics	Use a preservative-free amide
Sodium Metabisulfite	Preservative in epinephrine	Avoid epinephrine
Methyl Paraben[*]	Preservative found in multi-dose vials of anesthetics	Use a preservative-free amide

[*]PABA and methyl paraben are chemically related. Both should be avoided if an allergy to one is suspected.

Table 9.3 Common anesthetics[1,4,5,6]

Common anesthetics	Class	Onset of action	Duration (without Epinephrine)	Duration (with Epinephrine)	Cautions*
Bupivacaine hydrochloride (Marcaine)	Amide	5–8 min	2–4 h	3–7 h	Stings on injection Use with caution in patients with severe CAD or arrhythmias as circulatory arrest due to bupivacaine may be refractory to treatment
Lidocaine (Xylocaine, LMX, Topicaine)	Amide	< 1 min	0.5–2 h	2–6 h	Stings on injection
Prilocaine hydrochloride (in EMLA, Citanest)	Amide	5–6 min	0.5–2 h		Methemoglobinemia risk** and risk for corneal abrasions if used near the eye
Mepivacaine (Carbocaine)	Amide	1–2 min	1–2 h	2–6 h	Slow neonatal clearance
Procaine (Novocain)	Ester	5 min	1–1.5 h		
Tetracaine (Pontocaine)	Ester	7 min (<1 min for conjunctiva)	2–3 h (<1 h for conjunctiva)		
Benzocaine (Hurricaine, Topex, Cetacaine)	Ester	<1 min for mucosa	< 1 h for mucosa		Frequently causes contact dermatitis Methemoglobinemia risk** if sprays are used in the mouth or throat

* Also refer to Esters vs. Amides table for class-specific precautions.
** Do not use in infants less than 4 months of age or those with G6PD deficiency. Use with caution in those patients less than 12 months of age and in those who are taking sulfa drugs.

Table 9.4 Epinephrine precautions[7,8,9,10,11]

Avoid epinephrine or use dilute with caution in patients	Due to
Taking tricyclic antidepressants	Risk of hypertensive crisis
Taking MAO inhibitors	Risk of hypertensive crisis
Taking adrenergic blockers	Risk of hypertensive crisis
Taking nonselective beta-blockers	Risk of hypertensive crisis and reflex bradycardia
With narrow angle glaucoma (avoid use periorbitally)	Increased intraocular pressure
With severe peripheral vascular disease (avoid use on digits)	Risk of digital ischemia
Who are pregnant	Pregnancy Class C
Allergic to sulfites	Risk of allergic reaction
With severe coronary artery disease	Risk of coronary artery vasospasm
With hyperthyroidism	Risk of hypertensive crisis
With a pheochromocytoma	Risk of hypertensive crisis
With unstable angina or uncontrolled hypertension	Risk of hypertensive crisis and/or myocardial infarction

Table 9.5 Lidocaine and epinephrine[14]

Epinephrine concentrations desired	Plain lidocaine	Epinephrine (1:1000)*
1:100,000	50 ml	0.5 ml
1:200,000	50 ml	0.25 ml
1:500,000	50 ml	0.1 ml

*1:1000 dilution means 1 mg of epinephrine per ml.

Table 9.6 Buffered lidocaine with epinephrine[18]

Lidocaine and Epinephrine 1:100,000	Sodium bicarbonate 8.4%
50 ml	5 ml

fresh solutions should be made frequently in order to keep the epinephrine active.

> Buffering lidocaine and epinephrine with sodium bicarbonate is essential to reduce pain of anesthetic infiltration. Preparing anesthetic syringes ahead of time is very efficient. Keeping the syringes refrigerated maintains clinically useful epinephrine activity for at least 1 week.[15]

Topical Anesthesia

Topical anesthetics can be a useful adjunct to injectable anesthetics for skin cancer surgery. When used on the skin, they can decrease the pain associated with a needle stick. When used topically in the eye, they can decrease the pain of a conjunctival injection and can anesthetize the eye to the irritation caused by anesthetics or blood running into the eye. Finally, they can be used on the oral mucosa prior to an injection for a nerve block.

There are several varieties of topical lidocaine that can be used safely on intact skin. A very common prescription preparation is the mixture of 2.5% lidocaine and 2.5% prilocaine, which is marketed under the trade name EMLA® (AstraZeneca, London, UK). It is applied to intact skin, 1 h prior to surgery, thick (like frosting on a cake), and occluded (plastic wrap from the grocery store works well).[5]

Lidocaine is also available in 4 and 5% creams under the trade name L.M.X.4® or L.M.X.5®,

(Ferndale Laboratories, Ferndale, MI) without a prescription, "behind" the pharmacy counter. For best results, it should be applied in a manner similar to EMLA®. It also should be used on a limited surface area of intact skin. Contact with eyes should also be avoided.

For the eye, two common anesthetic drops are proparacaine and tetracaine. Both are ester anesthetics and should not be used in patients who are allergic to esters. Both eye drops cause some stinging upon instillation, tetracaine more than proparacaine.[16] For each, the topical anesthesia lasts approximately 10 min and can be re-instilled as needed. Neither should be used in a patient with narrow angle glaucoma.

The oral mucosa can be anesthetized quickly and easily, making subsequent injections relatively painless. The oral mucosa should first be dried with a piece of gauze. A topical anesthetic such as lidocaine jelly or viscous lidocaine can then be applied with a cotton-tipped applicator or a second gauze pad. This is held in place for 1–2 min. Care should be taken to ensure the patient avoids swallowing the anesthetic.

> A 5–10% solution of cocaine is very useful for intranasal procedures. The cocaine achieves very effective anesthesia of the nasal mucosa with excellent hemostasis due to cocaine's vasoconstrictive properties. As cocaine is a controlled substance, additional record-keeping rules must be followed.

Complications

There are some risks to topical anesthetic use including toxicity from applying to too large a surface area (something that should rarely be a problem in skin cancer surgery), on mucosal surfaces, or over skin with impaired barrier function. EMLA, specifically, may cause an alkaline burn if it gets in the eye, possibly leading to a corneal abrasion.[5] Prilocaine can cause methemoglobinemia in susceptible patients (Table 9.1). Symptoms of methemoglobinemia can range from cyanosis to seizures.

Infiltrative Anesthesia

Simple infiltrative anesthesia is the most common and simplest approach for skin cancer surgery. It is fast and effective. Though there are many types of anesthetics to choose from (Table 9.3), lidocaine is the most commonly used in skin surgery due to its rapid onset of action and its excellent safety profile. It does sting upon injection, but this discomfort may be reduced by injecting the medicine at a slower rate. Bupivacaine is often used as a secondary agent to extend the length of anesthesia, but is infrequently used alone due to its significant pain on injection and its slow onset of action. A risk to consider when using bupivacaine is its depressive effect on the conduction system of the heart, which can lead to arrhythmias and, while bupivacaine is in the patient's system, these arrhythmias may be unresponsive to cardioversion.[1]

By following a few simple rules, the pain of injection of the anesthetic can be minimized. Several things affect the pain of an injection. The size of the needle, the diameter of the syringe, the direction of the bevel, the laxity of the skin, the rate of injection, and the order of multiple needle sticks are all important. The smaller the needle and the smaller the diameter of the syringe, the less pain there is on injection. A 30-gauge needle on a 1-ml or 3-ml syringe should be used whenever possible. The bevel of the needle should be up and the injection should be made through taught skin. If the skin is loose, one can stretch the skin slightly during injection. The rate of injection should be as slow as possible. Though it seems time consuming for a busy office, slowing the injection down, especially initially, will take less than 30 s. The dramatic increase in patient comfort is always worth the extra time. Finally, one should use one needle stick whenever possible, but if multiple injections are required, one should always re-enter the skin through an area that is already numb.

Certain areas of the body are more sensitive to pain than others. These places include the nose, the lips, and the digits. In these locations, distraction techniques can be a great benefit. Many surgeons will pinch the skin at or near the injection site just prior to the needle stick, while others will apply ice to the injection site for a minute or so prior to injection.

> Using an ice cold air blower (e.g., Zimmer Cryo Cold Air Device) on the skin prior to injection reduces pain of injection. The cold air needs to be kept away from the injection needle as it will freeze the anesthetic in the needle and prevent further injection.

Rubbing the skin can also be effective (the gate theory of pain). Even better is the use of a simple vibrating apparatus, which can be placed near the injection site just prior to and during the injection. Having the patient hold the machine can help involve the patient in the procedure and gives them a sense of control.

Field Blocks

A field block involves injecting a ring of local anesthetic around the surgical site. Advantages to this technique include lack of distortion of the surgical site and less volume of anesthetic required to anesthetize a large area. The anesthetic should be injected into both the superficial and deep planes to be maximally effective.[17] Sites conducive to this include the scalp, the nose, the ear, the trunk, and the extremities. The only disadvantage is the lack of hemostasis at the central surgical site; therefore, if this is a concern, additional anesthetic mixed with epinephrine could be injected centrally once the ring block has been placed.[18]

Tumescent Anesthesia

Tumescent anesthesia is the infiltration of large amounts of dilute lidocaine (0.05–0.1%) and epinephrine (1:1,000,000) into the subcutaneous fat (Table 9.7). It is used most commonly for liposuction, ambulatory phlebectomy, and hair transplantation, but it can also be used for skin cancer surgery. It produces swelling and firmness (tumescence) of the targeted area[19] and can be used to aid in dissection by separating tissue planes and leaving vital structures out of harm's way. Other advantages include prolonged anesthesia and decreased intraoperative bleeding.[20] Because dilute lidocaine is absorbed slower in the subcutaneous fat, doses as high as 35–50 mg/kg have been found to be safe.[18]

Table 9.7 Tumescent anesthesia formula[*18]

Ingredient	Quantity (ml)
Lidocaine 1%	50–100
Epinephrine 1:1000	1
Sodium bicarbonate 8.4%[**]	10
Normal saline 0.9%	900–950

[*]Final concentration: 0.05–0.1% lidocaine and 1:1,000,000 epinephrine.
[**] If solution is freshly prepared, do not include sodium bicarbonate.

The tumescent solution is infiltrated with the help of one of several pumps or large 30-ml syringes, with the injection carried out through long 18–20-gauge 3.5-inch spinal needles or specially designed multiport cannulas. The infiltration rate is started slowly with small needles, and gradually increased by the use of spinal needles and, finally, infiltration cannulas. The deep subcutaneous plane is infiltrated first, followed by the superficial fat compartment. The solution is injected until firm tumescence of the tissue has been achieved. Anesthesia and epinephrine-induced hemostasis develop within 20 min and last for several hours.[18]

Regional Nerve Blocks

Peripheral nerve blocks are a great way to anesthetize large areas with few injections, and are achieved by anesthetizing around a nerve root to produce anesthesia in the distribution of that nerve.[17] Other benefits include a reduced volume of anesthetic is used and distortion of the operative site is avoided. Nerve blocks are especially helpful when working on the lips or the nail units, where local injections are notoriously painful. Using a 30-gauge needle to make an intradermal wheal prior to performing the block can make the procedure less painful. The primary disadvantage of a nerve block is the lack of epinephrine placed in the operative field, which would have otherwise provided hemostasis. Most of the anesthetics used on the skin can be used for a nerve block. Though epinephrine is not used for hemostasis, it can prolong the duration of anesthesia and is safe to use for facial nerve blocks. Epinephrine's use in digital blocks is more controversial.[21]

Nerve blocks should be performed at least 10–20 min prior to surgery, as it may take that long for the block to take effect. If local hemostasis is required, a local anesthetic containing epinephrine may be used in addition. With the nerve block in place, the local anesthetic can be injected quickly and easily, as the patient is already numb.

Facial Nerve Blocks

Facial nerve blocks can be performed at six points on the face. Each point lies above a sensory nerve: the supraorbital nerve superiorly, the infraorbital nerve centrally, and the mental nerve inferiorly. The locations of these injection points and the regions of the face they supply can be seen in Fig. 9.1. At each point, the insertion of the needle should be in the mid-pupillary line, perpendicular to the skin, and deep enough to be just superficial to the periosteum. The needle should not enter the foramen or touch the nerve. If the patient complains of paresthesias during injection, the needle should be withdrawn, as it is likely to be touching the nerve. Usually 1–2 ml of anesthetic is sufficient for each site.[18]

An alternative approach to the infraorbital and mental nerves is intra-orally. Though it may seem

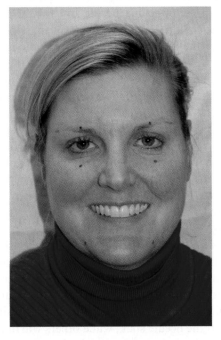

Fig. 9.1 Injection points for facial nerve blocks: supraorbital superiorly, infraorbital centrally, and mental inferiorly

counterintuitive, this approach is much less painful for the patient and there is less swelling and bruising. The needle is inserted at the mid-pupillary line, the landmark for which is the space between the first and second premolars (bicuspids), at the junction of the attached and nonattached mucosa (the labial sulcus) (Fig. 9.2). The needle should be kept just superficial to the periosteum.[18] The prior application of topical anesthesia will decrease the initial pain of the block.

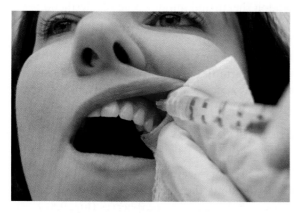

Fig. 9.2 The intraoral injection site for an infraoral nerve block: the needle is inserted between the first and second premolars at the labial sulcus

Digital Nerve Block

Digital nerve blocks are helpful when working on or around the nail. Each digit is innervated by four nerve branches: a ventral pair and a dorsal pair. A simple way to perform the block is with two injections, on either side of the digit (Fig. 9.3). The needle

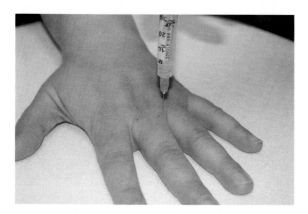

Fig. 9.3 The injection sites for a digital nerve block

is inserted on the dorsal aspect of the digit, lateral and just distal to the MCP joint. The needle is inserted perpendicular to the digit and just lateral to the bone until the skin on the ventral side of the digit begins to protrude. One-half ml of epinephrine-free anesthetic should be injected slowly. Next, withdraw the needle a few millimeters and inject another 1/2 ml of anesthetic toward the dorsal side. Repeat these steps on the other side of the digit. If, at any point, the patient complains of paresthesias, the needle should be withdrawn, as it is likely touching a nerve.[22] For further details of digital blocks see Chapter 14.

Hand Nerve Blocks

The hand is innervated by the radial, median, and ulnar nerves (Fig. 9.4). Depending on where the skin cancer is located, one, two, or all three of the nerves can be blocked.

To block the radial nerve, locate the injection site, at the dorsal wrist, by measuring three-finger breadths proximal to the distal wrist crease or anatomic snuff box, just beside the cephalic vein (Fig. 9.5). Inject 2–5 ml of local anesthetic in a "bleb" just above the tough superficial fascia. Then massage the bleb across the path of the nerve first one way, then the other.[23]

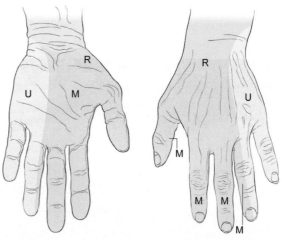

Fig. 9.4 Nerves in the hand. R—radial nerve, U—ulnar nerve, M—median nerve (Illustration by Alice Y. Chen)

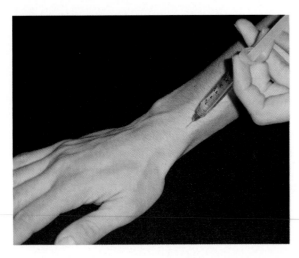

Fig. 9.5 The injection site for the radial nerve block

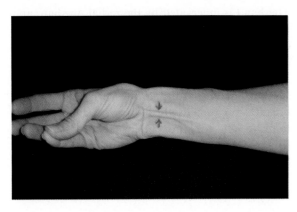

Fig. 9.6 The palmaris longus tendon is easily seen by apposing the thumb and fifth finger with the wrist slightly flexed

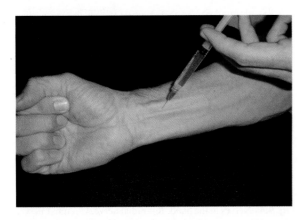

Fig. 9.7 The injection site for blocking the median nerve

The median nerve enters the carpal tunnel at the distal wrist crease where it should not be blocked (neuritis may result). The ideal injection site is just under the tendon of the palmaris longus (PL), three-finger breadths from the distal wrist crease.[23] The PL can be easily seen by apposing the thumb and fifth finger with the wrist slightly flexed[18] (Fig. 9.6). The needle should enter the skin in the groove between the PL and the flexor carpi radialis (Fig. 9.7). Advance the needle slowly to avoid the tendon sheath and inject 3–5 ml of anesthetic.[23]

The ulnar nerve is most easily blocked at the elbow where it travels between the olecranon process and the epicondyle of the humerus. With the patient's arm flexed, the needle is inserted between the bones and 3–5 ml of anesthesia is injected.[18]

Foot Nerve Blocks

The five sensory nerves of the foot are the posterior tibial, the sural, the superficial peroneal, the saphenous, and the deep peroneal nerves (Fig. 9.8).

The posterior tibial and sural nerves are easiest to block with the patient in the prone position. The posterior tibial artery is palpated between the medial malleolus and the Achilles tendon. A 1.5-inch

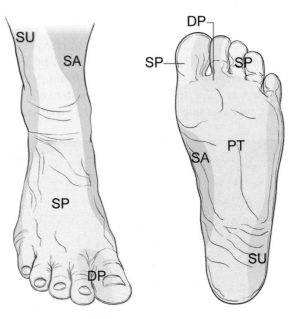

Fig. 9.8 Nerves of the foot. SP—superficial peroneal, DP—deep peroneal, SU—sural, SA—saphenous, PT—posterior tibial (Illustration by Alice Y. Chen)

needle is directed anterior and lateral to the arterial pulse until the bone is touched. The needle is pulled back slightly and 3–5 ml of anesthetic is injected. The sural nerve is blocked by injecting into the groove between the lateral malleolus and the Achilles tendon, in an identical fashion to the tibial nerve injection.[18]

The saphenous and superficial peroneal nerves are easiest to block with the patient supine. Here anesthetic is infiltrated subcutaneously from malleolus to malleolus on the dorsal surface of the foot.[18]

The deep peroneal nerve is easiest to block, locally, between the first and second toes.[18]

Penile Nerve Block

The easiest way to anesthetize the penis is to do a ring block of the shaft. By injecting a ring of epinephrine-free anesthetic in the subcutaneous plane around the base of the penis, most of the penis will be anesthetized. If the surgery is to involve the periurethral region of the glans or the frenulum, additional local anesthetic will be required.[18]

Postoperative Analgesia

Most surgery involving the skin tends not to cause a great deal of postoperative discomfort. Mild pain, usually resulting from swelling, can be relieved with acetaminophen and an ice pack. There are a few exceptions. A large defect on a tight scalp or forehead that is closed primarily can give the patient a headache for a few days. Also, surgery involving the cartilage of the ear or the nail can result in more significant postoperative pain. In these instances, patients may appreciate a prescription for acetaminophen in combination with oxycodone (Percocet, for example). The strengths of oxycodone include 2.5, 5, 7.5, and 10 mg. It is imperative that the patient be warned not to drive or operate heavy machinery while taking oxycodone as it could make them drowsy.

> Exposed ear cartilage often develops a chondritis that is best managed with oral anti-inflammatory drugs taken around the clock for 1–3 weeks.

Unusual Situations and Complications

Common side effects of local anesthesia include local bruising and edema (especially periorbitally), the vasovagal response, and temporary motor paralysis.

Edema from local anesthesia (and the trauma of the surgery itself) can be dramatic. When working on the lower half of the forehead or near the eyelids, patients should be forewarned about the risk of periorbital swelling. Having someone drive the patient home is recommended, as the swelling can interfere with vision. To minimize swelling, the patient should ice the periorbital area for 24–48 h and sleep on a few pillows or in a recliner for the first few postoperative nights.

Vasovagal reactions present with diaphoresis and dizziness and can lead to syncope (Table 9.8). Calming the patient prior to injection can help, but is not always successful. For this reason, it is important to always anesthetize patients while they are lying down. If the patient complains of these symptoms, placing them in the Trendelenburg position with a cool, moist cloth over their forehead will make them feel better quickly.

Patients expect to feel "numb" after surgery, but once the anesthesia wears off they expect to feel normal. Occasionally, there is a temporary paralysis of the local muscle group that may last beyond when the "skin numbness" resolves. This problem should resolve in a matter of hours. Warning the patients of this can alleviate patient anxiety.

More serious complications of local anesthetics, though rare, can happen. These include allergy and epinephrine effect, overdose, and necrosis.

Allergy to anesthetics is rare. True hypersensitivity accounts for less than one percent of adverse reactions seen with injectable local anesthetics.[14] Nonetheless, a true allergic reaction could be life-threatening. For this reason, it is important to take a detailed history of previous reactions and then try to determine the cause.

Symptoms of hypersensitivity include urticaria/hives or other generalized rash, bronchospasm, angioedema, or anaphylaxis (Table 9.8). If any of these symptoms are elicited in the history, one should try to identify exactly to what the patient is allergic. Patients can be allergic to the anesthetic itself, a metabolite of the anesthetic, or a preservative used in either the anesthetic or the epinephrine.

Table 9.8 Differential diagnosis of local anesthetic systemic reactions[18]

Diagnosis	Pulse rate	Blood pressure	Signs & symptoms	Emergency management
Vasovagal reaction	Low	Low	Excess parasympathetic tone; diaphoresis, hyperventilation, nausea	Trendelenburg, cold compress, reassurance, oxygen
Epinephrine reaction	High	High	Excess α(alpha)- and β(beta)-adrenergic receptor stimulation; palpitations	Reassurance (usually resolves within minutes), phentolamine, propranolol
Anaphylactic reaction	High	Low	Peripheral vasodilation with reactive tachycardia; stridor, bronchospasm, urticaria, angioedema	Epinephrine 1:1000 0.3 ml sc, antihistamines, fluids, oxygen, airway maintenance
Lidocaine overdose: 1–6 μg (micrograms)/ml	Normal	Normal	Circumoral and digital paresthesias, restlessness, drowsiness, euphoria, lightheadedness	Observation
Lidocaine overdose: 6–9 μg/ml	Normal	Normal	Nausea, vomiting, muscle twitching, tremors, blurred vision, tinnitus, confusion, excitement, psychosis	Diazepam, airway maintenance
Lidocaine overdose: 9–12 μg/ml	Low	Low	Seizures, cardiopulmonary depression	Respiratory support
Lidocaine overdose: >12 μg/ml	None	None	Coma, cardiopulmonary arrest	Cardiopulmonary resuscitation and life support

Anesthetics in the ester class are the most problematic due to the para-aminobenzoic acid (PABA) metabolite. Using a preservative-free anesthetic from the amide class is the solution. It should be preservative free because these preservatives can be chemically similar to PABA.

Finally, epinephrine contains sodium metabisulfite as a preservative. Patients with sulfite allergies (different from "sulfa" allergies) may need epinephrine-free anesthesia.

In the rare case that a patient is allergic to both classes of anesthetics, one could use injectable diphenhydramine (Benadryl) or normal saline for small procedures. For larger procedures, general anesthesia in a hospital setting is the most suitable option.

If there is any question regarding the source of allergy, a referral to an allergist is beneficial for you and for the patient. If the allergy occurs in your office, and is limited, it can be safely managed with antihistamines and prednisone. However, if the allergy is more severe (i.e., bronchospasm or anaphylaxis), immediate emergency management is required. It is always a good idea to have antihistamines, injectable epinephrine, oxygen, and an automatic external defibrillator in the office so that quick action can be taken.

Common side effects of epinephrine include palpitations, anxiety, tremor, tachycardia, and hypertension. These side effects are usually transient. Potentially life-threatening side effects of epinephrine—such as cardiac arrhythmias, digital ischemia, and cerebral hemorrhage—are rarely encountered at the doses used for skin surgery (Table 9.8). However, patients who are especially susceptible to these side effects, due to underlying medical conditions or certain medications, should be given dilute epinephrine or none at all (Tables 9.4 and 9.9).

Table 9.9 Dilute epinephrine[18]

Epinephrine concentrations desired	Plain lidocaine	Lidocaine with epinephrine 1:100,000*
1:200,000	5 ml	5 ml
1:500,000	4 ml	1 ml

*50 ml contains 500 mg of lidocaine and 0.5 mg of epinephrine.

Table 9.10 Maximum doses of anesthetics[14]

Anesthetic	Maximum total adult dose per procedure[*]	Volume of maximum adult dose if wt > 145 lb/65 kg	Volume of max dose if wt is 120 lb/ 54 kg	Volume of max dose if wt is 100 lb/ 45 kg	Volume of max dose if wt is 80 lb/ 36 kg
Lidocaine 1%: 10 mg/ml 2%: 20 mg/ml	4.5 mg/kg Max:300 mg	30 ml (1%) 15 ml (2%)	24 ml (1%) 12 ml (2%)	20 ml (1%) 10 ml (2%)	16 ml (1%) 8 ml (2%)
Lidocaine with epinephrine 1:100,000 or 1:200,000	7 mg/kg Max: 500 mg	50 ml (1%) 25 ml (2%)	38 ml (1%) 19 ml (2%)	31 ml (1%) 15 ml (2%)	25 ml (1%) 12 ml (2%)
Bupivacaine (Marcaine) 0.25%: 2.5 mg/ml	2.5 mg/kg Max: 175 mg	70 ml	61 ml	45 ml	36 ml
Bupivacaine with epinephrine[**]	Max: 225 mg	90 ml			
Mepivacaine 1%: 10 mg/ml	Max: 400 mg	40 ml			

[*]Maximum doses should be decreased in patients with severe liver disease or severe congestive heart failure due to decreased metabolism by the liver.

[**]Buffering bupivacaine with epinephrine is not advisable as the anesthetic may precipitate out of solution.

Overdose from local anesthetics is rarely encountered in noncomplicated skin cancer surgery. If a high volume of anesthesia is needed, or if the patient is of an especially small build, one should be aware of the recommended limits based on weight (Table 9.10). When overdose occurs, it affects the central nervous system first and is heralded by perioral tingling, numbness of the tongue, metallic taste, or lightheadedness (Table 9.8). If these symptoms occur, an emergency response team should be notified, as the treatment requires oxygen, fluids, inotropes, and close cardiovascular monitoring. If unrecognized, this could progress to seizures (central nervous system [CNS] stimulation) followed then by respiratory arrest (CNS depression). Anesthetic overdose can also depress the cardiovascular system. Usually this happens after the CNS symptoms appear, but can present earlier if the anesthetic is inadvertently injected intravascularly. Initially, bradycardia occurs and can quickly progress to a fatal arrhythmia leading to cardiovascular collapse.

Necrosis of the skin is rare. When it occurs, it is due to local vasoconstriction caused by the addition of epinephrine to the anesthetic. This becomes problematic on the digits of patients with peripheral vascular disease. In these patients, avoiding epinephrine may be prudent.

Summary

Local anesthesia is a critical part of skin cancer surgery. It is often the fear of pain that makes the patient most concerned. When local anesthesia is done well, it will provide the patient with a safe, painless, and anxiety-free experience. This, in turn, will allow the surgeon to concentrate on the bigger job at hand.

References

1. McLure HA, Rubin AP. Review of local anaesthetic agents. *Minerva Anestesiol.* 2005;71:59–74.
2. Eggleston ST, Lush LW. Understanding allergic reactions to local anesthetics. *Ann Pharmacother.* 1996;30:851–857.
3. Malamed SF. *Handbook of Local Anesthesia.* 4th ed. St. Louis: Mosby; 1997.
4. Jackson D, Chen AH, Bennett CR. Identifying true lidocaine allergy. *J Am Dental Assoc.* 1994;125:1362–1366.
5. Friedman PM, Mafong EA, Friedman ES, Geronemus RG. Topical anesthetics update: EMLA and beyond. *Dermatol Surg.* 2001;27:1019–1026.

6. Cohen MJ, Schecter WP. Perioperative pain control: A strategy for management. *Surg Clin North Am.* 2005;85: 1243–1257.

7. Perusse R, Coulet JP, Turcotte JY. Contraindications to vasoconstrictors in dentistry: Part III pharmacological interactions. *Oral Surg Oral Med Oral Pathol.* 1992;74: 687–691.

8. Yagiela JA. Adverse drug interactions in dental practice: interactions associated with vasoconstrictors. Part V. *J Am Dent Assoc.* 1999;130:701–709.

9. Yagiela JA, Neidle EA, Dowd FJ, eds. *Pharmacology and Therapeutics for Dentistry.* 4th ed. St. Louis: Mosby; 1998.

10. Budenz AW. Local anesthetics and medically complex patients. *J Calif Dent Assoc.* 2000;28:611–619.

11. Dzubow LM. The interaction between propanolol and epinephrine as observed in patients undergoing Mohs surgery. *JAAD.* 1986;15:71–75.

12. Stewart JH, Chinn SE, Cole GW, et al. Neutralized lidocaine with epinephrine for local anesthesia-II. *J Dermatol Surg Oncol.* 1990;16:842–845.

13. Stewart JH, Cole GW, Klein JA. Neutralized lidocaine with epinephrine for local anesthesia. *J Dermatol Surg Oncol.* 1989;15(10):1081–1083.

14. Local anesthetic agents, infiltrative administration. http://www.emedicine.com/proc/topic149178.htm. Accessed January 19, 2009.

15. Larson PO, Ragi G, Swandby M, Darcey B, Polzin G, Carey P. Stability of buffered lidocaine and epinephrine used for local anesthesia. *J Dermatol Surg Oncol.* 1991;17: 411–414.

16. Bartfield JM, Holmes TJ, Raccio-Robak N. A comparison of proparacaine and tetracaine eye anesthetics. *Acad Emerg Med.* 1994;1:364–367.

17. Local anesthesia and regional nerve block anesthesia. http://www.emedicine.com/derm/topic824.htm. Accessed January 19, 2009.

18. Hruza GJ. Anesthesia.In: Bolognia JL, Jorizzo JL, Rapini RP, eds. *Dermatology.* 1st ed. St. Louis: Mosby; 2008:2233–2242.

19. Klein JA. Tumescent technique for regional anesthesia permits lidocaine doses of 35 mg/kg for liposuction. *J Dermatol Surg Oncol.* 1990;16: 248–263.

20. Ramirez OM, Galdino G. Does tumescent infiltration have a deleterious effect on undermined skin flaps? *Plast Reconstr Surg.* 1999;104:2269–2272.

21. Thomson CJ, Lalonde DH, Denkler KA, et al. A critical look at the evidence for and against elective epinephrine use in the finger. *Plast Reconstr Surg.* 2007;119: 260–266.

22. Digital nerve block. http://www.nda.ox.ac.uk/wfsa/html/u02/u02_007.htm. Accessed January 19, 2009.

23. Regional blocks at the wrist. http://www.nda.ox.ac.uk/wfsa/html/u12/u1204_01.htm. Accessed January 19, 2009.

Chapter 10
Excision Techniques, Staples, and Sutures

Mollie A. MacCormack

Excisions are one of the most commonly performed dermatologic procedures. It is estimated that more than 650,000 excisions are performed each year in the United States, with dermatologists accounting for about 58% of this number.[1] Excisions are performed for a variety of reasons including diagnosis, the therapeutic removal of malignant and benign growths, as well as simply for improved appearance. While the vast majority of excisions are straightforward in nature, close attention to a few basic tenets will enhance both the efficiency of the procedure as well as overall cosmesis. This chapter will review the basic materials required for a successful excision as well as the most common excision and closure techniques.

Patient Preparation

Patient preparation is of great importance in assuring a successful outcome to any surgical procedure. Early identification of any potential complicating factors can greatly reduce the incidence of adverse events (Table 10.1). Preoperative evaluation should begin with the assessment of patient comorbidities that may prevent them from providing informed consent, lessen their ability to tolerate the procedure, place them at increased risk of infection, or interfere with appropriate wound healing. All women of childbearing age should be asked about potential pregnancy. A complete list of medications is required, with close attention paid to those medications that may affect the ability to obtain hemostasis (antiplatelet therapy, anticoagulants) or potentially complicate wound healing (systemic corticosteroids or isotretinoin use within the last 6–12 months). It should be noted that many food items and herbal supplements can also alter platelet function.[2–4] While in the past it was common practice to discontinue those medications that can make hemostasis more difficult, a number of studies have shown that the actual negative impact of such medications is quite small, while the potential ramifications of discontinuation on overall health (stroke, myocardial infarction, pulmonary embolus, etc.) are devastating.[5–9] For this reason, while patients may be advised to discontinue herbal supplements, nonsteroidal anti-inflammatory drugs (NSAIDs), or aspirin taken for primary prevention, it is strongly recommended that they be maintained on all medically necessary anticoagulation.

Any existing drug allergies should be recorded and avoided. Patients should be evaluated for any electrical devices such as pacemakers, internal cardiac defibrillators, and nerve stimulators that may receive interference from electrocautery. In addition, needle/surgical phobias or simply patient anxiety are not uncommon in the surgical setting and should be addressed. Often a complete explanation of the procedure is all that is required to put such a patient at rest.

> Simple nonpharmacologic interventions such as a peaceful office setting, soothing music, the use of drapes to minimize visualization of surgical instruments and the surgical field, as well as distracting conversation are often quite beneficial.

D.F. MacFarlane (ed.), *Skin Cancer Management*, DOI 10.1007/978-0-387-88495-0_10,
© Springer Science+Business Media, LLC 2010

Table 10.1 Preoperative patient evaluation

Medical Comorbidities	Anxiety
	Arthritis/Severe musculoskeletal disease
	Artificial heart valves or recent prostheses
	Cardiovascular disease/heart valve anomalies
	Clotting disorders
	Dementia
	Diabetes
	History of endocarditis
	History of poor wound healing/ keloid formation
	Hypertension
	Malnutrition
	Peripheral vascular disease
	Pregnancy
Medications/ Herbal supplements	Anticoagulants
	Antiplatelet agents
	Accutane use within the past 6–12 months
	Corticosteroids
	Herbal supplements
	Immunosuppressants
Drug allergies	
Electrical devices	Pacemakers
	Implantable cardiac defibrillators
	Brain stimulators
Social Environment	Patient ability to care for wound/ obtain assistance in wound care

In the extreme case, premedication with low-dose anxiolytics such as lorazepam given orally 1 h prior to the procedure can be helpful (after first ensuring that the patient will not be driving).

Antibiotic Prophylaxis

The vast majority of dermatologic excisions do not require pre- or postoperative antibiotics. Updated guidelines for endocarditis prophylaxis were published by the American Heart Association in 2007. Based upon these recommendations, routine prophylaxis is rarely required and is deemed appropriate only for procedures (including biopsies and suture removal) involving perforation of the respiratory tract/oral mucosa or performed in actively infected tissue in a small subgroup of patients at highest risk of adverse outcome.[10] For

those patients who require prophylaxis, antibiotic choice should be directed toward the eradication of viridans group streptococci for procedures involving perforation of oral/respiratory mucosa and staphylococci and B-hemolytic streptococci if the procedure involves infected skin. Should methicillin-resistant *Staphylococcus aureus* (MRSA) be suspected, clindamycin or vancomycin would be the drug of choice.

While no official guidelines exist addressing the issue of cutaneous surgery and prophylaxis of artificial joints, a joint advisory statement from the American Dental Association and the American Academy of Orthopedic Surgeons recommended against the use of prophylaxis for routine dental work in patients with artificial joints more than 2 years old—procedures that carry a significantly higher risk of inducing bacteremia than clean cutaneous incisions.[11] Tooth brushing alone induces bacteremia rates of 25%,[12,13] while the rate of bacteremia induced by cutaneous surgery is less than 3%.[14,15] The guidelines are less clear for patients whose artificial joints are less than 2 years old, as these joints are noted to be more susceptible to infection.[11] At the current time, there is no evidence to suggest that prophylaxis is required for the vast majority of prosthetic joint recipients with clean cutaneous wounds. However, given the higher risk of bacteremia associated with procedures involving mucosal surfaces, adopting the endocarditis prophylaxis guidelines is often recommended for patients with clean-contaminated wounds.[16] As treatment guidelines for patients who have received their transplants within the past 2 years are unclear, many practitioners have also adopted the endocarditis recommendations for this patient subset.[17] Please see Chapter 8 for further discussion.

Site Preparation and Anesthesia

Preoperative Antisepsis

The ideal cutaneous antiseptic would provide complete, long-lasting sterilization of the operative field with no tissue toxicity. A number of choices are available for antiseptic preparation of the cutaneous surface (Table 10.2). The most commonly

Table 10.2 Antiseptic solutions

Antiseptic agent	Advantages	Disadvantages
Povidone-iodine	Broad spectrum, including fungi	Quickly neutralized by blood, serum proteins, or sputum; irritant; potential systemic toxicity with large body surface area
Chlorhexidine gluconate	Prolonged effect	Keratitis and otitis
Hexachlorophene		Neurotoxicity in infants
Isopropyl alcohol	Inexpensive	Flammable, must allow it to dry

used are 10% povidone-iodine, 4% chlorhexidine gluconate, 70% isopropyl alcohol, and 2% chlorhexidine gluconate combined with 70% isopropyl alcohol. Povidone-iodine has broad-spectrum activity against bacteria and some viruses; however, it is easily inactivated as it is only effective when dry. Chlorhexidine is slower in onset, however, its overall effect is of longer duration and it has been demonstrated to be superior to povidone-iodine in decreasing bacterial load.[18] Comparative studies suggest that the 70% isopropyl alcohol and 2% chlorhexidine gluconate combination, as well as a combined isopropyl alcohol/ povidone-iodine scrub, provide the best immediate and persistent antimicrobial effect.[19–21] While generally well tolerated, caution must be taken when using cutaneous antiseptics. Prolonged, direct contact with chlorhexidine can lead to keratitis and ototoxicity, while iodine preparations are often irritating to the skin and can be toxic in newborns.

Anesthesia

Most cutaneous excisions can be performed under local anesthesia. The most commonly used anesthetic is 0.5–1% lidocaine due to its rapid onset of action and intermediate duration of effect. The addition of epinephrine not only provides increased hemostasis but also extends efficacy. Maximum recommended dose is 4.5 mg/kg for the plain formulation and 7 mg/ kg for lidocaine plus epinephrine.[22] While it was once thought that only plain lidocaine could be used in anatomic areas such as the nose, ear, or penis, this is not the case and there are no

absolute anatomic contraindications to epinephrine use.[23–25] The use of epinephrine should be avoided in patients taking propanolol, a nonselective beta blocker, as it could potentially lead to malignant hypertension.[26] True allergy to anesthetics is rare. It is important to obtain a complete history of reported allergic reactions because what many patients interpret as an allergic response is actually a vasovagal episode or symptoms due to epinephrine effect (palpitations, shaking, sweating, light-headedness). In the uncommon case of actual allergy, the offending agent is often the preservative present in multi-dose vials or a sodium metabolite found in epinephrine-containing products.[27] Should a true lidocaine allergy exist, an ester anesthetic such as procaine can be substituted.

The discomfort associated with anesthesia injection is multi-factorial, in part due to tissue distension and in part due to the acidity of the anesthetic (especially in epinephrine-containing formulations). Simply buffering the anesthetic with sodium bicarbonate in a 9:1 formulation, initiating the injection in the more distensible subcutaneous tissue, and decreasing the speed of infiltration can increase patient comfort substantially.[28] An in-depth review of cutaneous anesthesia is provided in Chapter 9.

Excision Margins

Surgical margins vary based on such factors as tumor type, intent of procedure (diagnostic versus therapeutic), and tumor size/depth. For basal cell carcinomas less than 2 cm in diameter located in low-risk anatomic areas (trunk,

Table 10.3 Recommended surgical margins for melanoma excision[3,7]

Melanoma depth	Clinical margin
In situ	5 mm (larger may be required for lentigo maligna)
<1.01–2 mm	1 cm (consider sentinel node)
2.01–4 mm	1–2 cm (consider sentinel node)
>4 mm	2 cm

extremities), a margin of 4 mm provides a 98% initial cure rate.[29] Larger basal cell carcinomas, as well as tumors with more aggressive histologic growth patterns—such as morpheaform and micronodular tumors—have been shown to have a much greater degree of subclinical extension, and thus should be excised with either greater margins or treated with Mohs micrographic surgery.[29–31] Recurrence rates for primarily excised basal cell carcinomas range from approximately 5–10% at 5 years.[32,33] Well-differentiated squamous cell carcinomas less than 2 cm in diameter and located in low-risk anatomic areas excised with a 4-mm margin have a 95% initial clearance rate; however, moderately/poorly differentiated tumors or tumors greater than 2 cm in diameter require a 6-mm margin.[34] Recurrence is about 8% at 5 years.[35] For tumors in high-risk locations (H-zone of the face, genitalia, hand/feet, ears) or very large tumors, Mohs micrographic surgery may be a better treatment option due to its higher cure rate.[36]

Recommendations for the surgical treatment of melanoma have been made by the National Comprehensive Cancer Network and are outlined in Table 10.3[37] and further discussed in Chapter 15.

Specimen Handling

Handling of tissue specimens should be performed in accordance with the overseeing institution's policies. Most specimens should be immediately placed in formalin to await transport to the lab. To avoid confusion, it is highly recommended that appropriately labeled containers be prepared prior to the start of the procedure and that all specimens are transported directly from patient to jar.

Hemostasis

Obtaining good wound hemostasis is essential for appropriate field visualization as well as avoidance of adverse postoperative events. For very small procedures, simple pressure and suturing may be all that is needed. However, in general, most excisions proceed more smoothly with the use of an external device such as a heat cautery unit, hyfrecator, or electrocautery. Heat cautery can be provided either via disposable handheld units or by a free-standing unit with sterilizable tips and is a good choice for patients with pacemakers, implantable cardiac defibrillators, brain stimulators, or other internal electronic devices as there is no current that could cause potential interference. Hyfrecators work via the emission of monoterminal, high-voltage, low-amperage current, while electrocautery units use high-amperage, lower voltage AC electricity to achieve effect (Table 10.4). Most electrocautery units have "cut" and "coagulation" settings. The "cut" current is a continuous, lower voltage current producing high levels of heat that rapidly vaporizes tissue, while the "coagulation" current is a pulsed, higher voltage current that produces heat more slowly, leading to blood coagulation

Table 10.4 Electrosurgical devices

Device	Circuit	Tissue contact	Voltage	Amperage
Electrofulguration	Monoterminal	No	High	Low
Electrodesiccation	Monoterminal	Yes	High	Low
Electrocoagulation	Biterminal	Yes	Low	High
Electrosection	Biterminal	Yes	Low	High
Electrocautery	None	Yes	Low	High

and more diffuse tissue damage.[38] Monopolar electrocautery units require the use of a ground and entail passage of electrical current through the patient; whereas in bipolar electrocautery units the current should pass only through the tissue placed between the forceps probe, making it a safer choice for patients with internal electrical devices.[39,40]

To obtain hemostasis the wound should first be blotted with gauze or similar material so that active sites of bleeding can be identified. The offending blood vessels can then be treated directly or grasped with a forceps to which the cautery tip is then placed. The desired endpoint is a bloodless field, yet it is important to remember that excessive cautery can delay wound healing and increase risk of infection. On occasion, some vessels are too large to be treated with electrocautery and need to be tied off with suture. As cautery is by its very nature a destructive process, excessive cautery and treatment of the skin edge should be avoided.

Suture Materials

Sutures are classified into two major categories: absorbable and nonabsorbable. Traditionally, absorbable sutures are used for deep closure and nonabsorbable sutures are used for epidermal repair; however, many exceptions to this rule apply. For example, in situations where suture removal is inconvenient, absorbable suture such as 6.0 fast absorbing gut is often used for epidermal closure. The choice of suture material is largely a matter of physician preference; the major characteristics of the most commonly used suture materials are outlined in Table 10.5.[41] As a general rule, the smallest suture providing adequate tensile strength is preferred. Wounds closed under significant tension will benefit from suture that maintains its tensile strength, whereas in low-tension wounds sited in rapidly healing areas this is much less of a concern. Overly tight epidermal sutures, as well as failure to remove epidermal sutures in a timely fashion, may lead to the formation of suture marks resulting from epidermal ingrowth/scarring along the suture line. As a general rule of thumb, facial sutures should come out within 5–7 days, while sutures on the trunk and extremities should be removed between days 10 and 14.

Staples

Staples provide a rapid, secure means of wound closure. While sutures typically allow for more precise alignment of wound edges, in certain areas such as the scalp, staples can provide an equivalent or even slightly improved overall cosmetic outcome.[42,43]

> Staples may provide an alternative for potentially contaminated wounds where delayed primary closure is not elected.[44]

A variety of disposable stapler sizes are available. To place a staple, the stapler tip is firmly placed perpendicular to the wound edge and the handle depressed. Staplers typically provide excellent wound edge eversion; however, if additional eversion is required an assistant can manually evert the wound edge using two-toothed Adson forceps prior to staple discharge. Specialized staple removers enable easy extraction.

Skin Adhesive

Although typically more expensive than suture material, skin adhesive (2-Octyl cyanoacrylate) can be an acceptable choice for closure in low-tension wounds. When used in conjunction with appropriately placed subcutaneous sutures, cosmetic outcome has been shown to be excellent in low-tension repairs.[45–49] However, in areas of high mobility or tension, epidermal sutures may be a better choice.[50]

> For proper application of skin adhesive, the wound should first be completely reapproximated with subcutaneous sutures. The skin surface is cleaned, the ampoule crushed, the wound edges manually everted with forceps, and the adhesive is applied extending at least 1/2 cm beyond the wound edge, gradually building up to 3 or 4 layers.

As skin adhesive forms its own dressing, minimal postoperative care is required. Patients should be instructed to avoid washing the area too vigorously, as this can result in rapid breakdown of the adhesive.

Table 10.5 Suture materials[4,1]

	Suture	Filament type	Tensile strength	Inflammatory response	Absorption	Notes
Absorbable						
	Surgical gut (Plain)	Mono	7–10 days	+ +	70 days	Collagen from sheep/beef intestine
	Surgical gut (Fast absorbing)	Mono	5–7 days	+ +		Treated with heat to speed absorption
						Good for low-tension facial closures, full thickness skin grafts
	Surgical gut (Chromic)	Mono	10–14 days	+ +	90 days	Chromium salts slow absorption and decrease reactivity
	Polyglactin 910 (Vicryl)	Braided Multi	65–75% at 14 days 20–50% at 21 days 10% at 35 days	–	Minimal for 45 days, complete by 70 days	Rapid absorption once tensile strength is lost
	Poliglecaprone 25 (Monocryl)	Mono	50–60% at 7 days 20–30% at 14 days 0% at 21 days	–	120 days	Very pliable, good for subcuticular closure
	Polydioxanone (PDS II)	Mono	70% at 14 days 50% at 28 days 25% at 42 days	+	6 months	Lower initial tensile strength, but longer retention providing extended wound support
Non absorbable						
	Silk	Braided Multi	0% by 1 year	+ + +	+/– 2 years	Handles well, high reactivity Good for mucosal areas (soft)
	Nylon (Ethilon)	Mono	81% at 1 year	–	Slowly hydrolyzed	Good elasticity, high memory
	Polypropylene (Prolene)	Mono	2 years	–	–	Does not stick to tissue, good for subcuticular or other "pullout" closures

Skin Tape

Various types of skin tapes are available, typically composed of nonocclusive, microporous material. While simple tapes such as Steri-Strip® closures (3 M, St. Paul, MN) are more often used to provide additional support to an already closed wound, more complex products such as ClozeX® tape (Clozex Medical LLC, Wellesley, MA), an adhesive film with multiple interlocking filaments that allow for wound edge approximation, have been shown to have good effect.[51] To obtain best adhesive results, the skin should be degreased with alcohol or acetone and Mastisol® (Ferndale Laboratories, Ferndale, MI) or tincture of benzoin applied prior to application.

Closure Techniques

Second Intention

After an excision has been performed it can be left to heal on its own (second intention healing), which, while slow, can be an appropriate choice for defects in areas where primary closure is prohibited due to lack of tissue mobility and/or concerns regarding graft take. In certain instances—for example, concavities such as the medial canthus, nasal alar crease or conchal bowl, as well as for many mucosal surfaces—second intention healing can be the closure of choice providing excellent cosmesis[52] (Figs. 10.1 and 10.2). As second intention wounds contract as

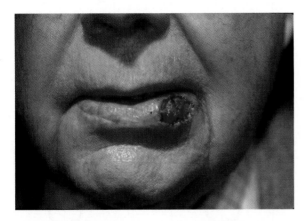

Fig. 10.1 Wound resulting from surgical removal of squamous cell carcinoma. Photograph courtesy of Suzanne Olbricht, M.D.

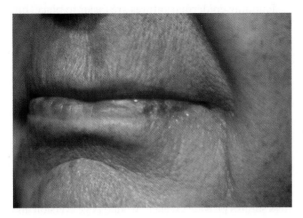

Fig. 10.2 Healed wound by second intention, 4 weeks after initial surgery. Photograph courtesy of Suzanne Olbricht, M.D.

they heal, this type of healing should be undertaken with caution in areas adjacent to free margins such as the eyelid, nasal alar rim, and lip, as unwanted tissue distortion may result.

Layered Closures

The vast majority of excisions are closed primarily and there are a number of techniques available to achieve closure. The simplest closure consists of purely epidermal sutures, a type of repair appropriate only for areas with negligible tension. Should wound tension be present, a layered closure is a more appropriate choice. Deep dermal sutures function to close dead space, approximate wound edges, and provide wound eversion, while epidermal sutures act to further refine edge alignment. When placing dermal sutures, use of the "buried vertical mattress technique" as described by Zitelli and Moy provides an excellent result due to prolonged dermal support and edge eversion.[53] While similar to a traditional dermal suture, this technique is characterized by a few key differences. To begin, the needle should enter the base of the skin flap through the subcutaneous fat, head up toward the superficial dermis and then dive back down to exit the ipsilateral skin edge at the level of the deep dermis, the opposite pattern is repeated on the contralateral side and a buried knot is placed. When drawn together, the central portion of the wound is raised up forming a tightly opposed, well-everted wound (Fig. 10.3a). Some practitioners have found this technique so effective that they forgo additional epidermal sutures.[54,55] In the rare situation where significant eversion is not desired, the dermal suture can be placed in the dermis without the lateral upward arch.

A myriad of techniques exist for epidermal closure. Simple interrupted sutures provide good strength and excellent wound edge alignment, but are considered time consuming by some (Fig. 10.3b). To be properly placed, the needle should enter the skin at 90 degrees within 1–2 mm of the wound edge, the needle should move smoothly through the dermis and subcutaneous fat to the contralateral side following the curve of the needle and exiting the skin in a similar manner. The two ends of suture are typically tied using an instrument tie. To perform this

Fig. 10.3 Various suture techniques for epidermal closure (Illustration by Alice Y. Chen)

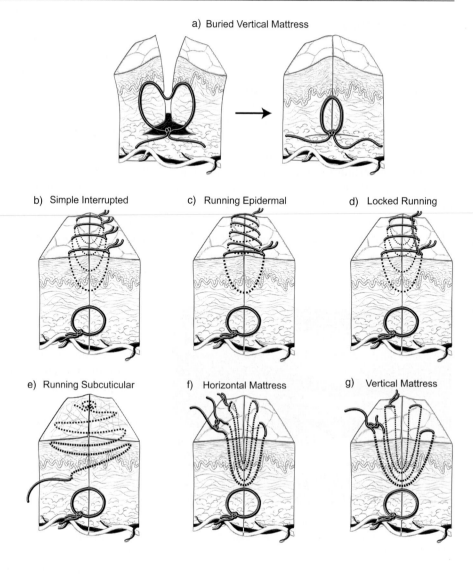

procedure, a double loop (to help prevent knot slippage) should be made around the needle driver tip utilizing the needle end of the suture. The needle driver then grasps the short (free) end of the suture and the two sides are pulled tight. The procedure is then repeated from the opposite direction to create the next knot; however, after the first knot is placed, only a single loop around the needle driver is required. Depending on the type of suture used, between 3 and 6 knots should be placed to avoid untying (more for monofilament as opposed to braided suture). Knots should be tight, but care must be taken to avoid strangulating the skin. One trick is to leave some laxity in the first 1 or 2 knots to accommodate potential swelling.

Running epidermal sutures are faster to place, but sacrifice some precision, run a greater risk of being pulled too tight leading to tissue strangulation, and are more vulnerable should the suture break (Fig. 10.3c). Locked running sutures are similar, allow for slightly more precision in edge alignment, but carry an even higher risk of vascular compromise (Fig. 10.3d). Running subcuticular sutures are faster to place than simple interrupted sutures, and with good technique can provide good wound edge alignment (Fig. 10.3e). Furthermore, if placed with buried knots and absorbable suture the need for suture removal is eliminated. Vertical mattress sutures provide excellent wound edge eversion and are useful in areas, such as the helical rim, where a depressed scar would be quite visible; however, if not removed promptly they carry a high risk of leaving suture marks (Fig. 10.3g). Horizontal mattress sutures are useful for closing areas under high tension, although if there is difficulty in edge approximation, an alternative repair may be a better choice (Fig. 10.3f). High tension not only increases risk of vascular compromise, tissue injury, and poor healing, but also significantly increases risk of scar spread. Even for low-tension wounds, when tying sutures it is important to use the minimal amount of tension necessary to obtain edge approximation.

Description of Procedure

Elliptical Excision

The majority of excisions are elliptical or fusiform in design, in large part due to ease of closure. By designing an excision with a length/width ratio of approximately 3:1 or with apical angles of no more than 30° (on a flat plane), the likelihood of standing cone deformities or "dog ears" is markedly reduced, resulting in a cosmetically elegant flat scar.

> When performing excisions on convex areas, the desired apical angle is often less than 30°, while on a concave surface, apical angles greater than 30° are often well tolerated.

Cosmesis can be further enhanced by orienting the long axis of the excision parallel to existing skin tension lines and/or the intersection of two cosmetic units. When planning an excision, the borders of the tumor should first be marked, the appropriate margins delineated, and the incision line drawn, taking care to place the long axis in the most desirable orientation, as described previously (Figs. 10.4 and 10.5).

Once anesthesia has been obtained, the procedure may begin. The scalpel handle should be held firmly between the first and second fingers, similar to a pencil, with the opposing hand used to provide skin traction.

> In general a #15 blade is used; however, in areas of very thick skin, such as the back, a #10 blade may be more effective.

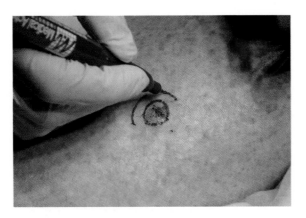

Fig. 10.4 Elliptical excision, marking margins

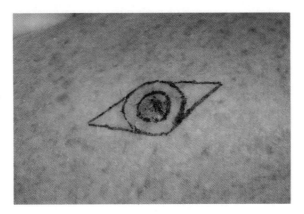

Fig 10.5 Elliptical excision, planned incision line

Starting at one end of the excision site, the skin should be scored in a single pass. This is then repeated on the opposing side, with care being taken to cleanly incise the tips. Utilizing firm pressure, the skin should then be incised completely down to subcutaneous tissue using the minimal number of passes possible (one to two strokes) (Figs. 10.6 and 10.7).

At all times it is important to hold the blade perpendicular to the skin surface to allow for good edge approximation later during closure. For most tumors, excision to the mid to deep subcutaneous fat is adequate; however, when excising melanoma the excision should extend down to fascia. After the excision edges are freed, the specimen is grasped with forceps and separated from the wound base by scalpel blade, scissors, or electrosection. To help maintain an even base, it is helpful to draw the

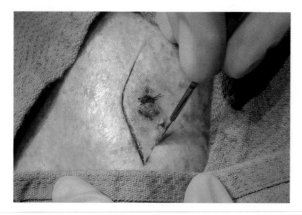

Fig. 10.6 Elliptical excision, initial incision

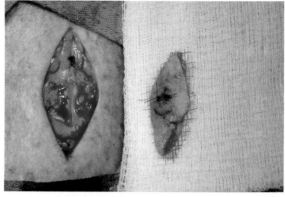

Fig. 10.9 Elliptical excision, specimen removed

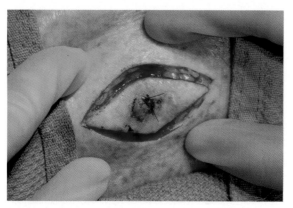

Fig. 10.7 Elliptical excision, incision completed

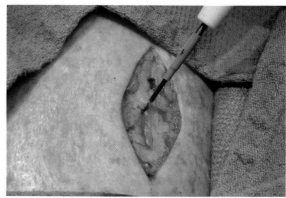

Fig. 10.10 Elliptical excision, obtaining hemostasis

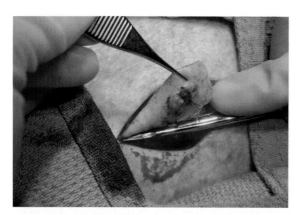

Fig. 10.8 Elliptical excision, separation from subcutaneous tissue

specimen over the blade or scissors while cutting (Fig. 10.8). Once freed (Fig. 10.9), the specimen should immediately be placed in a correctly labeled container.

Hemostasis should be obtained, if needed, utilizing the techniques described previously to provide a clear operative field (Fig. 10.10). If the wound is very small, one can then progress immediately to closure. However, in most cases, wounds will benefit from undermining as it increases tissue mobility, decreases tension, and facilitates edge eversion. The large plate-like scar resulting from wide undermining may even help in the resolution of tissue redundancies/dog ear deformities.[56] It is important when undermining to always be aware of the surrounding anatomy in order to avoid unwanted injury to adjacent nerves, vessels, or other structures.

Undermining can be performed via either blunt dissection or sharp dissection. In blunt dissection, the wound edge is stabilized in a nontraumatic manner, such as with a skin hook. A pair of surgical scissors is inserted with closed blade into the wound, parallel to the skin surface. The blades are then opened, gently separating the subcutaneous tissue. Blunt dissection is a good option for areas where nerve or vessel injury is a concern as these structures are often pushed aside rather than severed. However, blunt dissection can also lead to an uneven dissection plane and is frequently slower than sharp dissection. In sharp dissection, either the scalpel blade or one blade of an open pair of scissors is inserted into the wound—again parallel to the skin surface—and the tissue separated either by cutting, pushing the scissors through the skin in a planing motion, or blade closure (Fig. 10.11). Sharp undermining tends to be faster and allows for more control over the dissection plane. The depth of undermining varies by anatomic site. In general, undermining should be performed at the level of the wound base in the mid to deep subcutaneous fat or just above the fascial layer, however, exceptions apply (Table 10.6).[57] There are no hard and fast rules governing the extent of undermining; each wound must be considered individually with the goal of creating a tension-free repair.

Once the wound has been completely undermined it should be reassessed for hemostasis. When all active bleeding has been controlled the wound is ready for sutures. Dermal sutures are placed first, preferably utilizing the buried vertical mattress technique as described previously. It is often helpful to start at the tips (areas of lower tension), gradually moving in toward the center (area of highest tension). Once the dermal sutures are completed, the

Table 10.6 Recommended undermining planes

Scalp	Subgaleal
Forehead : small	Subcutaneous fat
: large	Subgaleal
Temple	Subcutaneous fat (Need to stay above superficial temporal fascia to avoid temporal branch CN VII)
Nose	Sub-nasalis
Cheek	Subcutaneous fat
Jaw/Neck	Superficial subcutaneous fat (Avoid marginal mandibular nerve, CN XI)
Trunk/Extremities	Deep subcutaneous fat/fascia
Dorsal Hands/ Feet	Subdermal

wound should appear as a slightly raised ridge with the skin edges nicely opposed. The dermal sutures are followed by epidermal sutures, again utilizing one of the aforementioned techniques (Figs. 10.12, 10.13, 10.14, 10.15 and 10.16).

A common variation of the classic elliptical excision gently curves the ends of the incision resulting in an S-shaped repair. S-plasty closure has the advantage of decreasing wound tension and may often result in a more esthetically pleasing scar; however, the resulting scar is often longer than that created by a traditional elliptical procedure.

Purse-String Repair

An alternative to the elliptical excision is the purse-string closure. On occasion, high skin tension prevents immediate closure following elliptical excision, or the long linear scar that would result from elliptical excision is undesirable. In such cases a disc excision with purse-string closure may be a more acceptable alternative. To perform a disc excision one begins by marking the desired surgical margin around the excision site. The lesion is then excised in a circular or disc-like manner leaving a round defect. The wound is gently undermined, hemostasis is obtained, and the wound is ready for closure. Various techniques exist for placing a purse-string suture. The original publication in the dermatologic

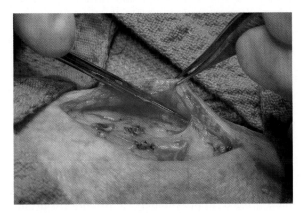

Fig. 10.11 Elliptical excision, tissue undermining

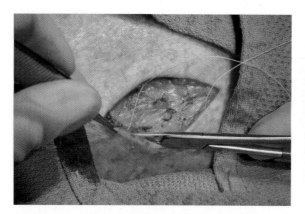

Fig. 10.12 Elliptical excision, initial dermal suture

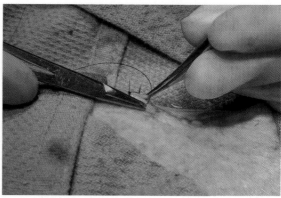

Fig. 10.15 Elliptical excision, epidermal sutures

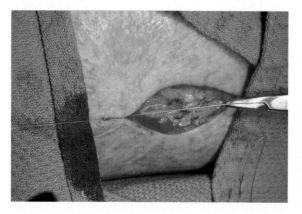

Fig. 10.13 Elliptical excision, initial dermal suture tied

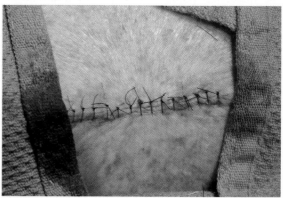

Fig. 10.16 Elliptical excision, final wound

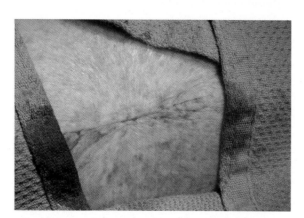

Fig. 10.14 Elliptical excision, dermal sutures completed

The author's preference for purse-string closure is to use an absorbable suture, such as Vicryl, placed horizontally in the mid to deep dermis. As the suture is drawn together and tied, the wound becomes puckered, much like the top of a draw-string purse. Once the wound has been maximally reapproximated, simple interrupted epidermal sutures can be placed to further speed healing.

literature described using a nonabsorbable 3-0 or 4-0 polypropylene subcuticular suture with an epidermal knot at 12 o'clock and escape loops placed at 3, 6, and 9 o'clock.[58]

On occasion, it is impossible to close the wound completely and the central area is closed with a skin graft or is left to heal by second intention. Another excellent alternative is to place a purse-string suture utilizing a nonabsorbable suture, such as polypropylene, using vertically oriented bites placed approximately 5–10 mm from the wound edge. The skin edges can then be further

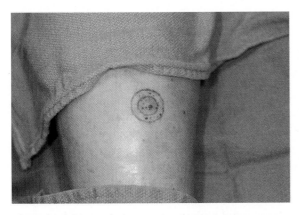

Fig. 10.17 Purse-string closure, margin marked

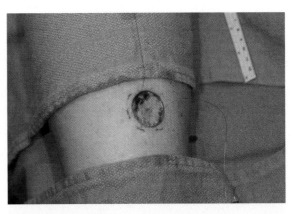

Fig. 10.20 Purse-string closure, purse-string suture of 4.0 Prolene placed

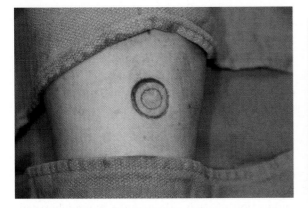

Fig. 10.18 Purse-string closure, margin incised

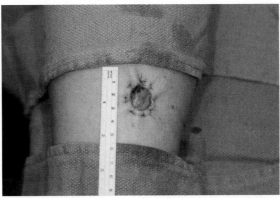

Fig. 10.21 Purse-string closure, purse-string suture tied

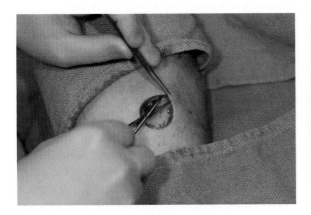

Fig. 10.19 Purse-string closure, undermining

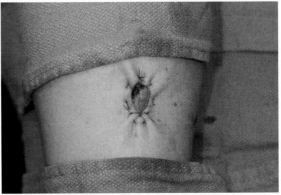

Fig. 10.22 Purse-string closure, further edge approximation

reapproximated using buried vertical mattress sutures and simple interrupted epidermal sutures[59,60] (Figs. 10.17–10.24). All nonabsorbable sutures should be removed at 5–7 days for facial wounds and 10–14 days for nonfacial repairs. The wound will continue to display moderate pleating at

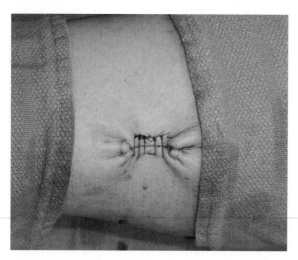

Fig. 10.23 Purse-string closure, final repair

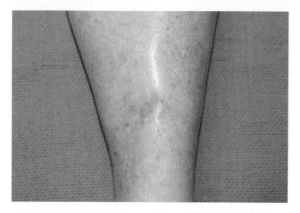

Fig. 10.24 Purse-string closure, 4-month outcome

the time of suture removal; however, as long as the wound is in an area of moderate tension these skin folds almost always resolve.

Standing Cones (Dog Ears)

On occasion, after elliptical excision the wound continues to exhibit vertical elevations at the tips or "dog ears." Many factors can contribute to the formation of tissue redundancies including initial apical angles greater than 30°, inadequate undermining, failure to maintain a 90-degree incision

angle, or unequal side lengths. When an excision borders a free margin, such as the lip or ala, such tissue redundancy presents not as a vertical elevation, but rather as a pushing distortion of that margin. Small dog ears, especially in areas of high tension/tissue mobility, such as the dorsal hand, will often resolve on their own. Larger redundancies, however, are often best resolved at the time of the initial procedure. One of the easiest means of resolution is simply by wound extension. While holding the redundancy steady, an incision can be made through the center of the standing cone to its base. After careful undermining, the two resulting triangular halves can be laid across the initial incision line and neatly trimmed (Figs. 10.25–10.30). As one becomes more proficient in dog ear management, it becomes clear that by utilizing the same principles the tissue redundancy can be removed from almost any direction. The same technique can be applied when performing immediate linear closure following disc excision. In fact, this method of surgical removal has been demonstrated to result in overall shorter scar lengths than those seen with preplanned ellipses.[61]

If a difference in wound edge lengths is appreciated prior to closure it can often be dealt with via "the rule of halves." The first suture is placed in the midportion of each side and the wound bisected. The process is repeated—continuing to divide the unsutured areas in half until the wound is closed—ultimately resulting in a curvilinear repair.

An excellent review of dog ear management has been published by Weisburg, Nehal, and Zide.[62]

Postprocedure Care

Wound dressings serve a number of functions. Not only do they act to keep the wound clean and protected from unwanted exposure, they also act to provide pressure, limiting postoperative bleeding complications and can help support and stabilize the wound. While small procedures require little more than daily cleansing followed by application of ointment (such as petrolatum or topical antibiotic) covered by gauze, larger procedures often benefit from a more substantial dressing. Many patients prefer a "leave-on"

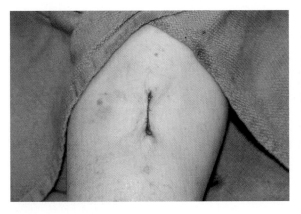

Fig. 10.25 Cutaneous redundancy

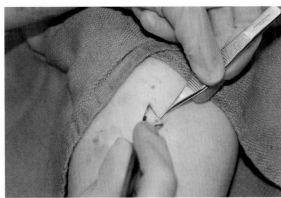

Fig. 10.28 Cutaneous redundancy, second incision

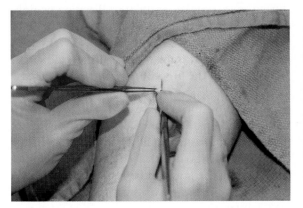

Fig. 10.26 Cutaneous redundancy, initial incision

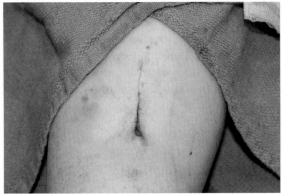

Fig. 10.29 Cutaneous redundancy, dog ear removed

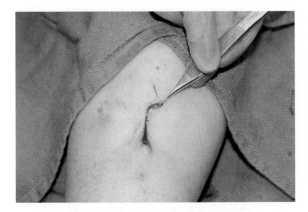

Fig. 10.27 Cutaneous redundancy, tissue overlap

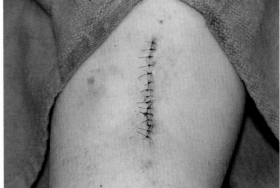

Fig. 10.30 Cutaneous redundancy, final wound

bandage that requires no wound care on the part of the patient. One such example is to begin by applying a thin layer of ointment over the wound edge. Steri-Strips held in place with liquid adhesive are then placed perpendicular to the wound to further enhance edge support. The next layer is an absorptive material such as a hydrocolloid (i.e., Cutinova-Hydro®, Smith &

Nephew, London, UK) trimmed to fit the excision line, which is in turn covered by a breathable, waterproof film (i.e., Tegaderm®, 3 M) allowing the patient to shower. On top of all of this is a pressure dressing composed of gauze and tape, which is removed by the patient at 24–48 h.

Fig. 10.32 Postoperative wound infection

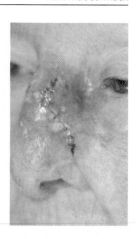

Complications

When properly performed, surgical excisions have a very low complication rate. All patients should be informed preprocedure that some sort of scarring is inevitable and localized cutaneous numbness is not uncommon due to transaction of sensory nerves. With time, typically within 1 year, sensation often returns to normal, and scar cosmesis can be enhanced via proper planning and orientation. Appropriate knowledge of surgical anatomy can prevent inadvertent injury to surrounding vessels and nerves as well as tissue distortion. Allergic reactions to topical antibiotics, dressing materials, or adhesive tape (Fig. 10.31) are not uncommon and can be easily addressed by removal of the offending agent and application of a mild topical steroid. Wound infection occurs in less than 2% of cases and is often heralded by an increase in pain[63,64] (Fig. 10.32). Risk can be minimized by use of good sterile technique and appropriate wound care. Should infection occur, the wound should be cultured, drained if necessary, and the patient started on a suitable antibiotic. Bleeding complications occur in about 3% of cases, but careful attention to intraoperative hemostasis as well as use of a good pressure dressing for the first 24–48 h following the procedure can help to decrease this risk[64] (Fig. 10.33). Wound dehiscence can occur as a result of excessive wound tension, hematoma formation, or infection. In such cases the underlying issue should be addressed and the wound then allowed to heal by second intention. Once healed, the scar can be revised, if necessary. For further discussion on surgical complications see Chapter 12.

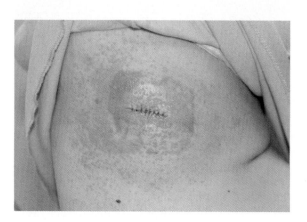

Fig. 10.31 Allergic contact dermatitis to adhesive

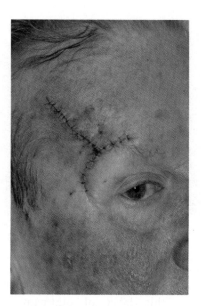

Fig. 10.33 Postoperative hematoma

Summary

Excision remains one of the most frequently performed dermatologic procedures. As time goes on, advances such as improved topical anesthetics or the use of confocal microscopy to help better delineate tumor margins may improve patient comfort and treatment efficacy. However, for the foreseeable future cutaneous excisions will remain one of the mainstays of surgical dermatology.

References

1. Shaffer CL, Feldman SR, Fleischer AB Jr et al. The cutaneous surgery experience of multiple specialties in the Medicare population. *J Am Acad Dermatol.* 2005;52 (6):1045–1048.
2. Chang LK, Whitaker DC. The impact of herbal medicines on dermatologic surgery. *Dermatol Surg.* 2001;27 (8):759–763.
3. Ang-Lee MK, Moss J, Yuan CS. Herbal medicines and perioperative care. *JAMA.* 2001;286(2):208–216.
4. Heller J, Gabbay JS, Ghadjar K, et al. Top-10 list of herbal and supplemental medicines used by cosmetic patients: what the plastic surgeon needs to know. *Plast Reconstr Surg.* 2006;117(2):436–445; discussion 446–437.
5. Lewis KG, Dufresne RG Jr. A meta-analysis of complications attributed to anticoagulation among patients following cutaneous surgery. *Dermatol Surg.* 2008;34 (2):160–164; discussion 4–5.
6. Khalifeh MR, Redett RJ. The management of patients on anticoagulants prior to cutaneous surgery: case report of a thromboembolic complication, review of the literature, and evidence-based recommendations. *Plast Reconstr Surg.* 2006;118(5):110e–117e.
7. Syed S, Adams BB, Liao W, et al. A prospective assessment of bleeding and international normalized ratio in warfarin-anticoagulated patients having cutaneous surgery. *J Am Acad Dermatol.* 2004;51(6):955–957.
8. Alam M, Goldberg LH. Serious adverse vascular events associated with perioperative interruption of antiplatelet and anticoagulant therapy. *Dermatol Surg.* 2002;28(11): 992–998; discussion 8.
9. Otley CC, Fewkes JL, Frank W, et al. Complications of cutaneous surgery in patients who are taking warfarin, aspirin, or nonsteroidal anti-inflammatory drugs. *Arch Dermatol.* 1996;132(2):161–166.
10. Wilson W, Taubert KA, Gewitz M, et al. Prevention of infective endocarditis: guidelines from the American Heart Association: a guideline from the American Heart Association Rheumatic Fever, Endocarditis, afsnd Kawasaki Disease Committee, Council on Cardiovascular Disease in the Young, and the Council on Clinical Cardiology, Council on Cardiovascular Surgery and Anesthesia, and the Quality of Care and Outcomes Research Interdisciplinary Working Group. *Circulation.* 2007;116(15):1736–1754.
11. Antibiotic prophylaxis for dental patients with total joint replacements. *J Am Dent Assoc.* 2003;134(7):895–899.
12. Roberts GJ, Gardner P, Simmons NA. Optimum sampling time for detection of dental bacteraemia in children. *Int J Cardiol.* 1992;35(3):311–315.
13. Sakamoto H, Karakida K, Otsuru M, et al. Antibiotic prevention of infective endocarditis due to oral procedures: myth, magic, or science? *J Infect Chemother.* 2007; 13(4):189–195.
14. Carmichael AJ, Flanagan PG, Holt PJ, et al. The occurrence of bacteraemia with skin surgery. *Br J Dermatol.* 1996;134(1):120–122.
15. Sabetta JB, Zitelli JA. The incidence of bacteremia during skin surgery. *Arch Dermatol.* 1987;123(2):213–215.
16. Babcock MD, Grekin RC. Antibiotic use in dermatologic surgery. *Dermatol Clin.* 2003;21(2):337–348.
17. Hurst EA, Grekin RC, Yu SS, et al. Infectious complications and antibiotic use in dermatologic surgery. *Semin Cutan Med Surg.* 2007;26(1):47–53.
18. Garland JS, Buck RK, Maloney P, et al. Comparison of 10% povidone-iodine and 0.5% chlorhexidine gluconate for the prevention of peripheral intravenous catheter colonization in neonates: a prospective trial. *Pediatr Infect Dis J.* 1995;14(6):510–516.
19. Hibbard JS. Analyses comparing the antimicrobial activity and safety of current antiseptic agents: a review. *J Infus Nurs.* 2005;28(3):194–207.
20. Nishimura C. Comparison of the antimicrobial efficacy of povidone-iodine, povidone-iodine-ethanol and chlorhexidine gluconate-ethanol surgical scrubs. *Dermatology.* 2006;212(Suppl 1):21–25.
21. Hibbard JS, Mulberry GK, Brady AR. A clinical study comparing the skin antisepsis and safety of ChloraPrep, 70% isopropyl alcohol, and 2% aqueous chlorhexidine. *J Infus Nurs.* 2002;25(4):244–249.
22. MICROMEDEX® Healthcare Series. In: POISINDEX® Managements: Thomson Micromedex; 2008. http://www.micromedex.com/products/poisindex/
23. Lalonde D, Bell M, Benoit P, et al. A multicenter prospective study of 3,110 consecutive cases of elective epinephrine use in the fingers and hand: the Dalhousie Project clinical phase. *J Hand Surg [Am].* 2005;30(5): 1061–1067.
24. Denkler K. A comprehensive review of epinephrine in the finger: to do or not to do. *Plast Reconstr Surg.* 2001;108(1):114–124.
25. Thomson CJ, Lalonde DH, Denkler KA, et al. A critical look at the evidence for and against elective epinephrine use in the finger. *Plast Reconstr Surg.* 2007;119(1):260–266.
26. Dzubow LM. Optimizing local anesthesia. The heat is on. *Dermatol Surg.* 1996;22(8):681.
27. Golembiewski J. Local anesthetics. J Perianesth Nurs 2007;22(4):285–288.
28. Burns CA, Ferris G, Feng C, et al. Decreasing the pain of local anesthesia: a prospective, double-blind comparison of buffered, premixed 1% lidocaine with epinephrine versus 1% lidocaine freshly mixed with epinephrine. *J Am Acad Dermatol.* 2006;54(1):128–131.
29. Wolf DJ, Zitelli JA. Surgical margins for basal cell carcinoma. *Arch Dermatol.* 1987;123(3):340–344.

30. Breuninger H, Dietz K. Prediction of subclinical tumor infiltration in basal cell carcinoma. *J Dermatol Surg Oncol.* 1991;17(7):574–578.

31. Salasche SJ, Amonette RA. Morpheaform basal-cell epitheliomas: a study of subclinical extensions in a series of 51 cases. *J Dermatol Surg Oncol.* 1981;7(5):387–394.

32. Silverman MK, Kopf AW, Bart RS, et al. Recurrence rates of treated basal cell carcinomas. Part 3: surgical excision. *J Dermatol Surg Oncol.* 1992;18(6):471–476.

33. Rowe DE, Carroll RJ, Day CL Jr. Long-term recurrence rates in previously untreated (primary) basal cell carcinoma: implications for patient follow-up. *J Dermatol Surg Oncol.* 1989;15(3):315–328.

34. Brodland DG, Zitelli JA. Surgical margins for excision of primary cutaneous squamous cell carcinoma. *J Am Acad Dermatol.* 1992;27(2 Pt 1):241–248.

35. Alam M, Ratner D. Cutaneous squamous-cell carcinoma. *N Engl J Med* 2001;344(13):975–983.

36. Leibovitch I, Huilgol SC, Selva D, et al. Cutaneous squamous cell carcinoma treated with Mohs micrographic surgery in Australia I. Experience over 10 years. *J Am Acad Dermatol.* 2005;53(2):253–260.

37. National Comprehensive Cancer Network (NCCN) clinical practice guidelines in oncology: melanoma. In: v.1. 2008 ed. http://www.nccn.org%3F/. Accessed January 19, 2009.

38. Pollack SV. Electrosurgery of the Skin. New York: Churchill Livingstone; 1991.

39. Martinelli PT, Schulze KE, Nelson BR. Mohs micrographic surgery in a patient with a deep brain stimulator: a review of the literature on implantable electrical devices. *Dermatol Surg.* 2004;30(7):1021–1030.

40. Yu SS, Tope WD, Grekin RC. Cardiac devices and electromagnetic interference revisited: new radiofrequency technologies and implications for dermatologic surgery. *Dermatol Surg.* 2005;31(8 Pt 1):932–940.

41. Ethicon Wound Closure Manual, Somerville, NJ, Ethicon 2007. http://www.jnjgateway.com/public/NLDUT/Wound_Closure_Manual1.pdf. Last accessed October 29, 2008.

42. Kanegaye JT, Vance CW, Chan L, et al. Comparison of skin stapling devices and standard sutures for pediatric scalp lacerations: a randomized study of cost and time benefits. *J Pediatr.* 1997;130(5):808–813.

43. Khan AN, Dayan PS, Miller S, et al. Cosmetic outcome of scalp wound closure with staples in the pediatric emergency department: a prospective, randomized trial. *Pediatr Emerg Care.* 2002;18(3):171–173.

44. Stillman RM, Marino CA, Seligman SJ. Skin staples in potentially contaminated wounds. *Arch Surg.* 1984;119 (7):821–822.

45. Sniezek PJ, Walling HW, DeBloom JR 3rd, et al. A randomized controlled trial of high-viscosity 2-octyl cyanoacrylate tissue adhesive versus sutures in repairing facial wounds following Mohs micrographic surgery. *Dermatol Surg.* 2007;33(8):966–971.

46. Quinn J, Wells G, Sutcliffe T, et al. A randomized trial comparing octylcyanoacrylate tissue adhesive and sutures in the management of lacerations. *JAMA.* 1997;277(19):1527–1530.

47. Holger JS, Wandersee SC, Hale DB. Cosmetic outcomes of facial lacerations repaired with tissue-adhesive, absorbable, and nonabsorbable sutures. *Am J Emerg Med.* 2004;22(4):254–257.

48. Toriumi DM, O'Grady K, Desai D, et al. Use of octyl-2-cyanoacrylate for skin closure in facial plastic surgery. *Plast Reconstr Surg.* 1998;102(6):2209–2219.

49. Coulthard P, Worthington H, Esposito M, et al. Tissue adhesives for closure of surgical incisions. *Cochrane Database Syst Rev.* 2004;2:CD004287.

50. Bernard L, Doyle J, Friedlander SF, et al. A prospective comparison of octyl cyanoacrylate tissue adhesive (dermabond) and suture for the closure of excisional wounds in children and adolescents. *Arch Dermatol.* 2001;137 (9):1177–1180.

51. Kuo F, Lee D, Rogers GS. Prospective, randomized, blinded study of a new wound closure film versus cutaneous suture for surgical wound closure. *Dermatol Surg.* 2006;32(5):676–681.

52. Leonard AL, Hanke CW. Second intention healing for intermediate and large postsurgical defects of the lip. *J Am Acad Dermatol.* 2007;57(5):832–835.

53. Zitelli JA, Moy RL. Buried vertical mattress suture. *J Dermatol Surg Oncol* 1989;15(1):17–19.

54. Sadick NS, D'Amelio DL, Weinstein C. The modified buried vertical mattress suture: a new technique of buried absorbable wound closure associated with excellent cosmesis for wounds under tension. *J Dermatol Surg Oncol.* 1994;20(11):735–739.

55. Hohenleutner U, Egner N, Hohenleutner S, et al. Intradermal buried vertical mattress suture as sole skin closure: evaluation of 149 cases. *Acta Derm Venereol.* 2000;80(5):344–347.

56. Zitelli JA. TIPS for a better ellipse. *J Am Acad Dermatol.* 1990;22(1):101–103.

57. Boyer JD, Zitelli JA, Brodland DG. Undermining in cutaneous surgery. *Dermatol Surg.* 2001;27(1): 75–78.

58. Brady JG, Grande DJ, Katz AE. The purse-string suture in facial reconstruction. *J Dermatol Surg Oncol.* 1992;18(9):812–816.

59. Hoffman A, Lander J, Lee PK. Modification of the purse-string closure for large defects of the extremities. *Dermatol Surg.* 2008;34(2):243–245.

60. Weisberg NK, Greenbaum SS. Revisiting the purse-string closure: some new methods and modifications. *Dermatol Surg.* 2003;29(6):672–676.

61. Hudson-Peacock MJ, Lawrence CM. Comparison of wound closure by means of dog ear repair and elliptical excision. *J Am Acad Dermatol.* 1995;32(4): 627–630.

62. Weisberg NK, Nehal KS, Zide BM. Dog-ears: a review. *Dermatol Surg.* 2000;26(4):363–370.

63. Rogues AM, Lasheras A, Amici JM, et al. Infection control practices and infectious complications in dermatological surgery. *J Hosp Infect.* 2007;65(3): 258–263.

64. Amici JM, Rogues AM, Lasheras A, et al. A prospective study of the incidence of complications associated with dermatological surgery. *Br J Dermatol.* 2005;153(5):967–971.

Chapter 11
Mohs Surgery

Desiree Ratner and Jennifer L. MacGregor

Mohs surgery is named after Dr. Frederic Mohs, who pioneered a technique for removing cancers termed "chemosurgery" and first published his technique in 1941.[1] Dr. Mohs' initial method involved applying a zinc chloride paste directly to the patient's tumor to chemically fix the tissue, after which the patient was allowed to return home. On the following day, the patient came back to the office. The tumor was then removed in precise, serial layers that were horizontally oriented and systematically mapped. This allowed all peripheral and deep margins of the specimen—essentially the interface between the patient and his or her tumor—to be examined under the microscope. If any part of the tumor remained, these steps were repeated until all peripheral and deep margins were clear. The goal of "chemosurgery" was to remove the tumor in its entirety, while preserving the surrounding normal skin. In this original technique, necrotic wounds created by zinc chloride paste were allowed to heal by second intention, as they were unsuitable for surgical reconstruction.

The Mohs surgery technique has been refined to allow the removal of fresh tumor without prior fixation, followed by the mapping of this fresh tissue, and the examination of horizontally oriented frozen sections by the surgeon. The fresh-frozen tissue technique allows for serial tissue layers to be removed from those specific areas that have residual tumor on microscopic examination, without otherwise enlarging the defect. When margins are deemed clear microscopically, the defect may be repaired in the office under local anesthesia, or by another surgical specialist in their operative suite. At times,

secondary intention healing is still employed and may also produce a good cosmetic result. Zinc chloride paste, which causes tissue necrosis, is no longer used, so that the wound edges are fresh and optimal for wound healing either by primary reconstruction or by secondary wound contraction. Today, the Mohs micrographic surgical procedure is recognized as the most precise method of removing skin cancers and is performed by dermatologists who complete additional fellowship training in Mohs micrographic surgery, otherwise known as "Mohs surgery." This training includes comprehensive experience in all aspects of cutaneous oncology, the Mohs technique of tumor removal with precise tissue mapping and orientation, laboratory processing with horizontally oriented frozen sections, pathologic examination of the tissue, and esthetic surgical repair of the resulting wounds. Figure 11.1 compares tumor removal and tissue orientation in standard excision versus excision with Mohs surgery.

Indications for Mohs Surgery

Standard modalities for removing skin cancers such as basal (BCC) and squamous cell carcinomas (SCC) include: excisional surgery, electrodesiccation and curettage, topical chemotherapy, cryosurgery, and radiation. These techniques are appropriate for the majority of nonmelanoma skin cancers. The Mohs technique is more time-consuming and expensive, and requires specialized

D.F. MacFarlane (ed.), *Skin Cancer Management*, DOI 10.1007/978-0-387-88495-0_11,
© Springer Science+Business Media, LLC 2010

Fig. 11.1 Comparison of techniques: A standard excision specimen is fixed and sectioned vertically to assess a representative sampling of the tissue margin. This technique is also termed "breadloafing." The Mohs technique orients the entire margin in a horizontal fashion so that 100% of the peripheral and deep tissue margins can be examined microscopically by the surgeon

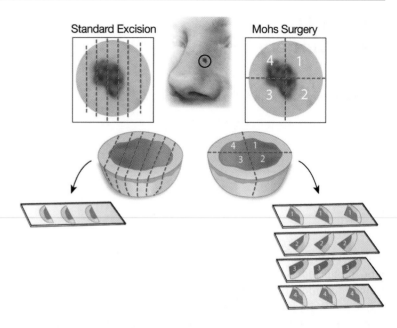

training and expertise. It is therefore reserved for the removal of certain types of skin cancers in sensitive locations or those at high risk for recurrence or metastasis.[2] The specific indications for Mohs micrographic surgery are listed in Table 11.1. The Mohs surgical technique is most commonly used to treat BCC and SCC on high-risk areas of the head and neck, locations where tissue conservation is essential; and subclinical extension beyond the visible margins of the tumor is common. If the tumor border is poorly defined clinically or if the tumor is recurrent after previous surgery, Mohs surgery can identify and remove infiltrating cancer cells with a high degree of accuracy. Those tumors with aggressive histologic subtypes are also treated with Mohs surgery. Finally, patients who are immunosuppressed or those who have received cutaneous irradiation develop aggressive tumors that tend to recur and/or metastasize with greater frequency and should be treated with Mohs surgery. Mohs surgeons also treat other types of skin tumors characterized by locally infiltrative or aggressive growth patterns, including: sebaceous carcinoma, microcystic adnexal carcinoma (MAC), dermatofibrosarcoma protuberans (DFSP), and atypical fibroxanthoma. A more comprehensive list of the types of tumors managed with Mohs surgery is included in Table 11.2.

Table 11.1 Indications for Mohs surgery[2]

High-risk nonmelanoma skin cancer (BCC and SCC)
Large size (>2 cm)
Ill-defined clinical borders
Rapid growth or aggressive clinical behavior
Aggressive or mixed histology
BCC—morpheaform, micronodular, infiltrating SCC—high-grade, deeply penetrating, perineural invasion
High-risk location
Periorbital, perinasal, auricular or preauricular, perioral
Areas where tissue preservation is important
Hands, feet, eyelids, lip, nose, genitalia, etc.
Recurrent
History of incomplete removal
Tumor arising in irradiated skin
Tumor arising in prior scar, burn, or other dermatoses (discoid lupus, lichen sclerosis, etc.)
Patient factors
Immunosuppression
Certain genodermatoses (xeroderma pigmentosum, nevoid BCC syndrome, others)

Cure Rates Following Mohs Surgery

Standard excision or superficial ablative techniques are appropriate treatments for most nonmelanoma skin cancers; however, for high-risk tumors such as

Table 11.2 Types of tumors treated with Mohs surgery[2]

Types of tumors treated with Mohs surgery
Basal cell carcinoma (BCC)
Squamous cell carcinoma (SCC)
Verrucous carcinoma
Erythroplasia of Querat
Extramammary Paget's disease
Keratoacanthomas (aggressive, recurrent, deep, or mutilating)
Lentigo maligna melanoma*
Dermatofibrosarcoma protuberans
Atypical fibroxanthoma
Malignant fibrous histiocytoma
Leiomyosarcoma
Adenocystic carcinoma of the skin
Sebaceous carcinoma
Oral and central facial paranasal sinus neoplasms
Merkel cell carcinoma
Microcystic adnexal carcinoma
Apocrine carcinoma of the skin
Aggressive locally recurrent benign tumors

*Adequate excision is the primary goal of therapy; however, Mohs surgery may be a part of the overall treatment plan for certain patients with melanoma.

those outlined in Table 11.1, Mohs surgery offers superior cure rates. Table 11.3 summarizes the estimated 5-year recurrence rates following Mohs surgery for both primary and recurrent BCC and SCC. It should be noted that there are no prospective, randomized trials comparing standard excision to Mohs surgery, and the majority of patients reported in early published studies were not treated by fellowship-trained Mohs surgeons. Available data regarding recurrence rates following Mohs excision of high-risk lesions is more than 10 years old, making direct comparison of these results with those of tumors treated with standard excision of limited value.

Table 11.3 Recurrence rates following Mohs surgery

	Mohs (%)	Excision (%)
Basal Cell Carcinoma[3,4]		
Primary tumor	1.0–1.4	10.1–17.4
Recurrent tumor	4.0–5.0	10.9–23.2
Squamous Cell Carcinoma[6–12]		
Primary tumor	2.6–6.7	10.9
Recurrent tumor	5.9–10.0	23.3

Basal Cell Carcinoma

Recurrence rates following standard excision of BCC have been best documented by Rowe et al.[3] who reported a 5-year recurrence rate of 10.1% for excision of primary BCC versus 17.4% for recurrent tumors. When the Mohs surgical technique was used, recurrence rates decreased to 1% for primary and 5.6% for recurrent BCC. Recurrence rates may be higher in patients with large tumors (>2 cm), tumors with infiltrative histology, or a mid-facial location (e.g., nose).[3] Interestingly, in an Australian database of 3,370 patients[4] and a similar study of 620 patients in the Netherlands[5] treated with Mohs surgery for BCC, similar 5-year recurrence rates were found. In the Australian study, however, no significant differences relating to tumor size, histology, or location were found.[4]

Squamous Cell Carcinoma

Traditionally, cutaneous SCC was treated with standard excision, with a 5-year recurrence rate of 10.9% for primary tumors and 23.3% for recurrent tumors. Reports of recurrence rates following Mohs for high-risk SCC on the head/neck,[6–12] however, range from 2.6 to 10.0%, with the greatest number of recurrences occurring in tumors with a high-risk location (e.g., lip),[12] prior recurrence, or perineural invasion. A more recent report from the Australian database reported similar recurrence rates.[7] It is likely, however, that immunosuppressed patients or those with hematologic malignancies are at risk for recurrence at much higher rates than those in previous studies. Mehrany et al. reported that patients with chronic lymphocytic leukemia were seven times more likely to develop recurrent SCC following Mohs surgery than controls.[13] Further studies are also needed to assess recurrence rates for SCC following Mohs surgery in the growing population of organ transplant recipients.

Preoperative Considerations

Prior to surgery, patients should have a full skin examination, including a biopsy of their tumor to confirm the diagnosis. A previous history of cutaneous malignancies and their treatments should be reviewed. In addition, a full medical and surgical history should be taken with particular attention to cardiac, pulmonary, renal, hepatic, and infectious diseases. A complete medication list, including supplements and alcohol/drug/smoking history, is essential. Decisions regarding the management of blood thinners and the need for antibiotic prophylaxis should be made in consultation with the primary care physician and/or cardiologist. Patients with implanted cardiac devices, such as pacemakers or defibrillators, can usually undergo Mohs surgery safely with the use of bipolar or heat cautery.

There is no current standard of care regarding the management of anticoagulant and anti-platelet therapy for Mohs surgery, and practice differs between physicians.[14,15] The risks of discontinuing medically necessary blood thinners may outweigh the risk of postoperative bleeding.[15] Warfarin and anti-platelet agents are generally continued during Mohs surgery if they are prescribed to treat or prevent cerebral, cardiovascular, and vascular thrombosis in high-risk patients. The international normalized ratio (INR) value should be checked prior to the procedure and determined to be within the therapeutic range (2–3.5). Patients with levels above this range are at the greatest risk for excessive bleeding and their medications should be adjusted prior to the procedure by their primary physician. Little data exist regarding the management of clopidogrel for cutaneous surgery. Aspirin or nonsteroidal inflammatory medications taken as primary prevention can be discontinued 10 days prior to the procedure, although the continuation of treatment should not adversely affect the surgical outcome if adequate hemostasis is achieved intraoperatively.[16] Patients at risk for unsatisfactory outcomes due to postoperative bleeding or hematoma include those on warfarin, older age (>67 years), or with flaps, grafts, or surgical sites on the ear.[16]

Decisions regarding antibiotic prophylaxis for the prevention of endocarditis and prosthesis infection in high-risk patients are usually individualized, and consultation with the patient's general, cardiac, or orthopedic physician prior to Mohs surgery may be required. According to the latest American Heart Association (AHA) recommendations regarding antibiotic prophylaxis for the prevention of endocarditis in the highest risk individuals, prophylaxis is reasonable for procedures involving oral sites, respiratory tract, or infected skin structures.[17] Procedures involving intact surgically scrubbed skin do not require antibiotics for the purpose of preventing endocarditis in high-risk individuals. For patients with joint prostheses, the American Academy of Orthopaedic Surgeons (AAOS) recommends antibiotic prophylaxis for high-risk patients undergoing procedures involving oral sites.[18] In concordance with this, the most recent advisory statement for antibiotic prophylaxis in dermatologic surgery recommends such prophylaxis for Mohs surgery in patients at risk for infective endocarditis or total joint prosthesis infection when the surgery involves perforation of oral mucosa, an infected site or a noninfected site that is at high risk of surgical site infection. Since Mohs surgical cases are heterogeneous—some, for instance, may breach the nasal mucosa or may extend over many hours—each patient's clinical scenario should be considered individually and decisions regarding antibiotic prophylaxis should be made after taking into account all relevant factors.[19]

Prior to surgery, patients should be educated about the procedure necessary to treat their particular type of tumor, the reconstruction that will follow, and potential risks of surgery, including acute complications, as well as later esthetic or functional problems, which may vary depending upon the size and location of the tumor. Occasionally, additional laboratory testing or imaging will be required. For large or complex tumors invading deeper facial structures—particularly around the eyes, ears, or central face—ophthalmology, otolaryngology, plastic surgery, and/or neurosurgery may also be called upon to evaluate the patient. If multidisciplinary care is required, the procedure may be coordinated with the Mohs surgeon resecting the tumor until margins are microscopically confirmed to be clear, after which another specialist repairs the defect. Patient instructions regarding the possible need for limited activity in the postoperative period, recommendations regarding smoking cessation and alcohol avoidance, and the list of supplies required for wound care should be given. Written instructions are often provided to patients so as to minimize later confusion with respect to preoperative recommendations and postoperative care.

Guide to the Mohs Surgery Procedure

Mohs surgery is usually performed in an outpatient surgical facility under local anesthesia. On the day of surgery, the site should be confirmed with the patient and the original biopsy report reviewed to confirm location and diagnosis. The tumor is measured, photographed, and marked; and the local area is infiltrated with local anesthetic. If necessary, hair may be removed from the surgical site prior to prepping and draping the area in standard, sterile fashion.

The sequence of events performed in a typical Mohs surgical procedure is outlined below and depicted in Fig. 11.2. The actual surgical procedure used to remove a skin cancer may vary somewhat depending on the surgeon's preferences, and the tumor type and location. The tumor is usually removed and reconstructed on the same day, with suture removal 1–2 weeks thereafter (Fig. 11.3a, b, c).

The visible lesion depicted in Fig. 11.2, Step 1, may be debulked preoperatively to remove obvious tumor. Since tumors are much softer than healthy tissue and are easily scraped away, preoperative curettage may help to define tumor margins and reduce the number of stages required for tumor clearance.[20–23]

Figure 11.2, Step 2: The remaining defect is excised with a narrow margin around and under it using a scalpel to remove a saucer-shaped disk of tissue (First stage, or Layer 1). Hatch marks are made (usually at 12, 3, and 9 o'clock) to orient the specimen with respect to the tissue map. Blood vessels are cauterized and the patient receives a temporary bandage. The tissue is mapped, frozen fresh, and sectioned for microscopic examination. The Mohs surgeon examines the tissue to determine whether microscopic tumor is present at any of the surgical margins (Fig. 11.4).

Figure 11.2, Step 3: If tumor is present at any microscopic margin, the patient returns to have tissue removed only from the mapped site where tumor remains (Second stage, or Layer 2). The procedure continues in this fashion until there is no remaining tumor and the margins are clear.

Figure 11.2, Step 4: The final defect is measured and photographed and the Mohs surgeon typically reconstructs the wound on the same day. As mentioned previously, healing by second intention may

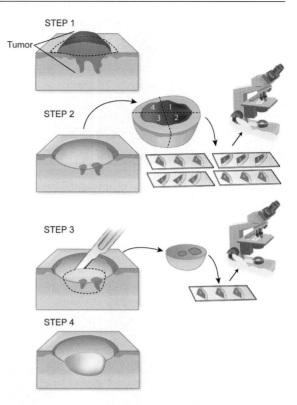

Fig. 11.2 Guide to the Mohs surgery procedure: Step (1) Preoperative lesion. The dotted line depicts the portion of the tumor that is debulked prior to surgery. Step (2) After the visible lesion has been debulked to remove obvious tumor, the remaining defect is excised with a narrow margin around and under it using a scalpel to remove a saucer-shaped disk of tissue. Step (3) The tissue is oriented, mapped, sectioned, and placed on slides for microscopic examination. Step (4) Remaining tumor is removed only from the mapped site in the second stage and placed on the slide for examination. The procedure continues in this fashion until there is no remaining tumor and margins are clear

occasionally be preferable to reconstruction. For complex tumors, subsequent management by a plastic or oculoplastic surgeon, otolaryngologist, or neurosurgeon may be required. This is generally arranged prior to the planned procedure.

Slide Preparation

Once the tissue is removed, oriented with hatch marks, and mapped, it will be processed by a histotechnician working within the surgical facility. The tissue is pressed down to flatten the skin so that the

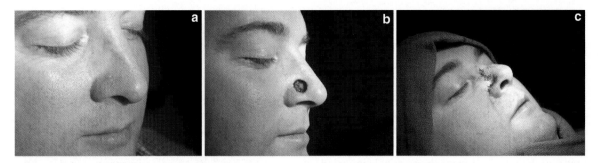

Fig. 11.3 (**a**) Basal cell carcinoma on the nasal sidewall. (**b**) Surgical defect following microscopic tumor clearance. (**c**) Same-day reconstruction with rhombic flap

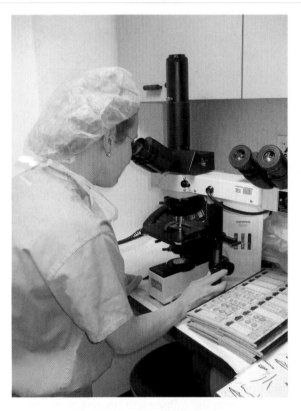

Fig. 11.4 Microscopic examination of stained frozen sections is performed by the Mohs surgeon.

entire tissue margin is leveled for even sectioning, with preservation of the epidermis around the entire periphery of the specimen. The tissue is divided and the ends of the pressed tissue specimen are dyed with colored inks to maintain orientation. These colors and the division of the specimen are also marked on the map so that orientation is coordinated between the patient (hatch marks), the specimen sections (hatch marks and colored dyes), and the written map. The tissue is embedded, frozen, sectioned, and mounted on slides (Fig. 11.5a, b), which are then stained, most commonly with hematoxylin and eosin and occasionally with toluidine blue or immunostains. The horizontal frozen sections are immediately examined under the microscope by the Mohs surgeon. It is important to mention that consistent high-quality slide preparation is essential to the success of the Mohs technique. While there may be some variability in tissue preparation or staining, if slide quality is poor, or if portions of the epidermis or deep tissue are missing, the processing must be repeated to ensure examination of 100% of the peripheral and deep tissue margins (Fig. 11.6a, b, c).

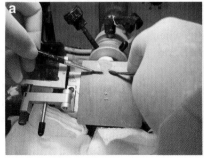
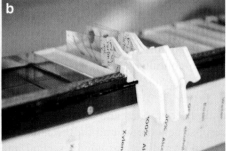

Fig. 11.5 (**a**) Frozen tissue is sectioned and placed on a slide. (**b**) These slides are then stained; in this image, an automatic stainer is being used

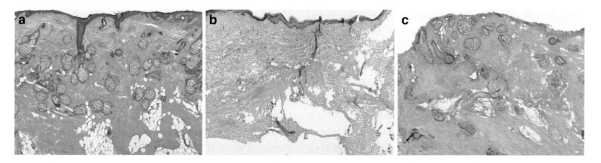

Fig. 11.6 Variations in histological slide preparation (**a**) Good quality frozen section stained with hematoxylin and eosin. (**b**) This poor quality section would be difficult to interpret. Note that it has no clear adnexal structures and fat is not visible. (**c**) Section missing epidermis

Variations on the Mohs Surgery Technique

Classical Mohs surgery is performed with a scalpel beveled at 45°—a technique that is helpful for flattening the epidermis against a glass slide, but less ideal for wound reconstruction. Once a tumor-free margin is achieved, the surgeon may de-bevel, or re-cut the defect at 90° prior to reconstruction. Conversely, there are surgeons who use a 90° angle for Mohs layers and avoid this step.

Several situations may require permanent, delayed formalin-fixed paraffin embedded sections to confirm tumor-free margins. Tumors with histology that can be difficult to interpret on frozen sections, such as sebaceous carcinoma, often necessitate permanent sections with tissue mapping. This "slow Mohs" procedure allows for confirmation of histology, while still allowing for tissue mapping and several stages with delayed repair. Another situation in which the surgeon may employ permanent sections to confirm frozen section findings is in the delineation of tumor margins in the setting of a dense inflammatory infiltrate, or in further characterizing basaloid proliferations encountered incidentally on microscopic examination.

Some have advocated the use of immunohistochemical stains to define tumor margins on frozen sections.[24] These include: anticytokeratin stains for BCC and SCC, MNF116 for BCC, and CD34 for DFSP.[25] The use of immunostains may also be used to evaluate melanoma in Mohs surgery, but use of these stains is still somewhat controversial. Studies exist regarding the use of HMB-45, MEL-5, S-100, and MART-1 for evaluation of melanoma on frozen section slides.[26–30] However, the standard surgical treatment of melanoma is wide local excision, where surgical margins are determined by the Breslow depth of the tumor.[31] The role of Mohs surgery in this setting is not yet well defined. In cases in which tumors are known to be locally aggressive or recurrent, including dermatofibrosarcoma protuberans, Merkel cell carcinoma, and melanoma, the Mohs surgeon may take an extra margin of tissue around the microscopically clear defect to be sent for permanent section processing. This "wide Mohs" variation is similar to wide local excision, with the added reassurance of 100% examination of all peripheral and deep tissue margins.

Lentigo maligna (LM) and lentigo maligna melanoma (LMM) have been managed with Mohs surgery. Owing to the difficulty in assessing melanocytic atypia on frozen sections, evaluation of melanoma specimens is typically performed using permanent histological confirmation and/or adjunctive use of immunostains. In a recent study directly comparing Mohs surgery to staged surgical excision, the Mohs-treated patients experienced higher local rates of recurrence (6/18 patients or 33%) compared to those treated by staged excision (3/41 or 7.3%),[32] although in this study immunohistochemical stains were not used. Zitelli et al. reported large prospective studies of Mohs surgery for head and neck melanoma and found recurrence rates comparable or even superior to historic recurrence rates with standard excision, particularly for in situ and thin melanomas (<0.76 mm) on the head and neck.[26,27] The technique has been described and refined to include removal of a 3-mm margin surrounding the clinically apparent tumor, which was sent for permanent examination. An additional 3-mm Mohs layer was removed for 100% margin examination in frozen sections with immunohisto-chemical staining. Although the authors used both HMB-45 and MART-1, they found that the latter stained more consistently and reliably.[27]

For the majority of Mohs surgeons, however, LM and LMM may be best managed using staged surgical excision with rush permanent specimens, or the "square" procedure described by Johnson et al. in 1997.[33] In the "square" technique, a square or rectangular outline 0.5–1.0 cm around the clinical Wood's lamp margins is marked and a 2–4-mm wide strip of tissue is excised, tagged for orientation, and sent for permanent sections. The lesion is left intact on the patient while the cutaneous strip from the margin is being assessed, leaving the patient with a smaller wound while awaiting the histological interpretation. The geometric angles of the speci-men are reported to increase accuracy of orientation for both the surgeon and the dermatopathologist. Geometric strips can be removed from any areas with positive tumor on subsequent permanent sec-tions (similar to the "slow Mohs" technique). After confirmed marginal clearance, the entire lesion can be excised and the defect repaired.

Complications and Follow-Up

Serious complications following Mohs surgery are rare and generally avoided by completing a meticu-lous preoperative evaluation as outlined previously. With any surgery there is potential for infection, hematoma/seroma formation, dehiscence, necrosis, scarring, and asymmetry. Fortunately, most Mohs surgeons do their best to perform meticulous recon-struction of their surgical defects—both on the head and neck and elsewhere—and are often able to achieve reconstruction with excellent preservation of facial symmetry and minimal scarring.

Wound infection following dermatologic surgery is low, with reported incidence rates averaging <3%.[34,35] Patients at higher risk for infection include those who are immunosuppressed, diabetic, smo-kers, or elderly. Patients undergoing long proce-dures, procedures requiring delayed repair or under significant tension, or repairs in contaminated or clean-contaminated locations (leg, groin, etc.) are also at higher risk for infection. These patients may require oral antibiotics to prevent postoperative wound infection. Some surgeons prescribe topical antibiotic ointment for wound care, although it has been shown that white petrolatum can be used with-out an increase in infection rate.[36] Complications are minimized by tailoring treatment to the individual needs of the patient, using sterile surgical technique, performing meticulous hemostasis following tumor removal, and choosing the best reconstructive option to optimize healing and minimize the potential for necrosis and scarring. Postoperative pain is typically minimal and easily managed with acetaminophen and/or other oral analgesics.

The surgical dressing generally remains in place for 24–48 h. The patient is then responsible for wound care involving twice-daily cleansing, appli-cation of ointment, and covering the wound with a nonstick dressing. Sutures are typically removed in 1–2 weeks (depending on the surgical site), although certain flaps will require subsequent pedicle division after 3 weeks, prolonging the wound-healing pro-cess. Second intention healing also requires addi-tional dedication to wound care for a longer period of time. However, most patients can resume normal activities within 2–3 weeks following surgery and may be evaluated thereafter to ensure that the wound is healing properly. Patients may return thereafter to their primary dermatologist for fol-low-up skin examinations.

Mohs Surgery Pearls

1. It is essential to pinpoint the biopsy site accu-rately before proceeding with surgery. Taking a photograph or making a diagram at the time of the initial biopsy or consultation visit may be helpful. Measuring the distance from the lesion to nearby anatomic land-marks can be useful as well. Allowing the patient to confirm the biopsy site by looking in the mirror and asking them to use a cotton-tipped applicator to point to the site at the time of surgery may be necessary if uncer-tainty remains regarding the exact location.

2. Correct orientation of the specimen with respect to the patient is critical. Making a pronounced double hatch mark at the

12 o'clock position facilitates orientation and mapping of the specimen.

3. If a biopsy slide is not available at the time of surgery, it may be helpful to take a frozen section biopsy of the tumor prior to debulking. Doing so enables the surgeon to compare suspected areas of positivity on the Mohs surgical slides with a known positive tissue sample and may provide additional important information regarding the histopathologic characteristics of the tumor.

4. Buffered lidocaine may be infiltrated nearly painlessly, but bupivacaine is extremely painful when infiltrated. If longer-acting anesthesia is required for patient comfort—as, for example, if tissue processing is expected to take several hours—be sure the patient has been completely numbed with lidocaine prior to infiltration of bupivacaine.

5. Be certain that your technician is proficient at preserving epidermis around the entire tissue specimen, that there are no holes in the center of the specimen, and that subcutaneous fat is not missing at the deepest portion of the specimen. If tissue dye is seen along the entire base of the specimen, the entire depth of the specimen has been preserved and the deep margin can be adequately visualized.

References

1. Mohs FE. Chemosurgery: a microscopically controlled method of cancer excision. *Arch Surg.* 1941;42:279–295.
2. Drake LA, Dinehart SM, Goltz RW, et al. Guidelines of care for Mohs micrographic surgery. *J Am Acad Dermatol.* 1995;33:271–278.
3. Rowe DE, Carroll RJ, Day CL. Mohs surgery is the treatment of choice for recurrent (previously treated) basal cell carcinoma. *J Dermatol Surg Oncol.* 1989;15(4):424–431.
4. Leibovitch I, Huilgol SC, Selva D, et al. Basal cell carcinoma treated with Mohs surgery in Australia II. Outcome at 5-year follow-up. *J Am Acad Dermatol.* 2005;53(3):452–457.
5. Smeets NWJ, Kuijpers DIM, Nelemans P, et al. Mohs' micrographic surgery for treatment of basal cell carcinoma of the face—results of a retrospective study and review of the literature. *Br J Dermatol.* 2004;151: 141–147.
6. Rowe DE, Carroll RJ, Day CL. Prognostic factors for local recurrence, metastasis, and survival rates in squamous cell carcinoma of the skin, ear, and lip. *J Am Acad Dermatol.* 1992;26:976–990.
7. Leibovitch I, Huilgol SC, Selva D, et al. Cutaneous squamous cell carcinoma treated with Mohs micrographic surgery in Australia I. Experience over 10 years. *J Am Acad Dermatol.* 2005;53(2):253–260.
8. Mohs FE. Chemosurgery: microscopically controlled surgery for skin cancer—past, present and future. *J Dermatol Surg Oncol.* 1978;4:41–54.
9. Mohs FE. Chemosurgery for the microscopically controlled excision of cutaneous cancer. *Head Neck Surg.* 1978;1:150–163.
10. Robins P, Dzubow LM, Rigel DS. Squamous-cell carcinoma treated by Mohs surgery: an experience with 414 cases in a period of 15 years. *J Dermatol Surg Oncol.* 1981;7:800–801.
11. Dzubow LM, Rigel DS, Robins P. Risk factors for local recurrence of primary cutaneous squamous cell carcinoma: treatment by microscopically controlled excision. *Arch Dermatol.* 1982;118:900–902.
12. Holmkvist KA, Roenigk RK. Squamous cell carcinoma of the lip treated with Mohs micrographic surgery: outcome at 5 years. *J Am Acad Dermatol.* 1998;38:960–966.
13. Mehrany K, Weenig RH, Pittelkow MR, et al. High recurrence rates of squamous cell carcinoma after Mohs surgery in patients with chronic lymphocytic leukemia. *Dermatol Surg.* 2005;31(1):38–42.
14. Kirkorian AY, Moore BL, Siskind J, et al. Perioperative management of anticoagulant therapy during cutaneous surgery: 2005 survey of Mohs surgeons. *Dermatol Surg.* 2007;33(10):1189–1197.
15. Alcalay J, Alkalay R. Controversies in perioperative management of blood thinners in dermatologic surgery: continue or discontinue? *Dermatol Surg.* 2004;30(8): 1091–1094.
16. Dixon AJ, Dixon MP, Dixon JB. Bleeding complications in skin cancer surgery are associated with warfarin but not aspirin therapy. *Br J Surg.* 2007;94:1356–1360.
17. Wilson W, Taubert KA, Gewitz M, et al. Prevention of Infective Endocarditis Guidelines From the American Heart Association. *Circulation.* 2007;116:1736–1754.
18. American Academy of Orthopaedic Surgeons Advisory Statement on Antibiotic Prophylaxis for Dental Patients with Total Joint Replacements. http://www.aaos.org/about/papers/advistmt/1027.asp. Accessed 1/21/09.
19. Wright TI, Baddour LM, Berbari EF, et al. Antibiotic prophylaxis in dermatologic surgery: Advisory statement. *J Am Acad Dermatol.* 2008;59:464–473.
20. Ratner D, Bagiella E. The efficacy of curettage in delineating margins of basal cell carcinoma before mohs micrographic surgery. *Dermatol Surg.* 2003;29(9): 899–903.
21. Lee DA, Ratner D. Economic impact of preoperative curettage before mohs micrographic surgery for basal cell carcinoma. *Dermatol Surg.* 2006;32(7):916–923.
22. Huang CC, Boyce S, Northington M, et al. Randomized, controlled surgical trial of preoperative tumor curettage of basal cell carcinoma in Mohs micrographic surgery. *J Am Acad Dermatol.* 2004;51(4):585–591.

23. Chung VQ, Bernardo L, Jiang SB. Presurgical curettage appropriately reduces the number of Mohs stages by better delineating the subclinical extensions of tumor margins. *Dermatol Surg.* 2005;31(9 Pt 1):1094–1100.

24. Jimenez FJ, Grichnik JM, Buchanan HT, et al. Immunohistochemical techniques in Mohs micrographic surgery: their potential use in the detection of neoplastic cells masked by inflammation. *J Am Acad Dermatol.* 1995;32:89–94.

25. Jimenez FJ, Grichnik JM, Buchanan MD, et al. Immunohistochemical margin control applied to Mohs micrographic surgical excision of dermatofibrosarcoma protuberans. *J Dermatol Surg Oncol.* 1994;20(10):687–689.

26. Zitelli JA, Brown C, Hanusa BH. Mohs micrographic surgery for the treatment of primary cutaneous melanoma. *J Am Acad Dermatol.* 1997;37(2 Pt 1):236–245.

27. Bricca GM, Brodland DG, Ren D, Zitelli JA. Cutaneous head and neck melanoma treated with Mohs micrographic surgery. *J Am Acad Dermatol.* 2005 Jan;52(1):92–100.

28. Hendi A, Brodland DG, Zitelli JA. Melanocytes in longstanding sun-exposed skin- quantitative analysis using the MART-1 immunostain. *Arch Dermatol.* 2006;142:871–876.

29. Zalla MJ, Lim KK, Dicaudo DJ, Gagnot MM. Mohs micrographic excision of melanoma using immunostains. *Dermatol Surg.* 2000 Aug;26(8):771–784.

30. Albertini G, Elston DM, Libow LF, et al. Mohs micrographic surgery for melanoma: a case series, a comparative study of immunostains, an informative case report, and a unique mapping technique. *Dermatol Surg.* 2002;28(8):656–665.

31. Melanoma clinical practice guidelines in oncology. *J Natl Compr Cancer Netw.* 2004;2:46–60.

32. Walling HW, Scupham RK, Bean AK, et al. Staged excision vs Mohs micrographic surgery for lentigo maligna and lentigo maligna melanoma. *J Am Acad Dermatol.* 2007 Oct;57(4):659–664.

33. Johnson TM, Headington JT, Baker SR, et al. Usefulness of the staged excision for lentigo maligna and lentigo maligna melanoma: the "square" procedure. *J Am Acad Dermatol.* 1997;37:758–764.

34. Hurst EA, Grekin RC, Yu SS, et al. Infectious complications and antibiotic use in dermatologic surgery. *Semin Cutan Med Surg.* 2007;26(1):47–53.

35. Furoryan T, Grande D. Postoperative wound infection rates in dermatologic surgery. *Dermatol Surg.* 1995;21(6):509–514.

36. Smack DP, Harrington AC, Dunn C, et al. Infection and allergy incidence in ambulatory surgery patients using white petrolatum vs bacitracin ointment: a randomized controlled trial. *JAMA.* 1996;25(12): 972–977.

Chapter 12
Cutaneous Flaps

Tatyana Humphreys

The origin of cutaneous flaps dates back to 600 BC in India when crimes such as adultery were punished by amputation of the nose. Indian physicians such as Sushruta Samita were called upon to correct the resultant deformity using cheek flap procedures.[1] Nasal reconstruction using the forehead flap evolved centuries later in India[1] and continued to be used in Europe through the fifteenth century. In the late sixteenth century, Italian surgeons such as Tagliacozzi also utilized pedicled flaps from the arm for nasal reconstruction.[1] It was not until the nineteenth century that further refinements in flap surgery occurred in England, France, and Germany. By the twentieth century, the appearance of new suture materials and local anesthesia brought further innovations in closure of skin and soft tissue defects. The development of the fresh tissue technique of Mohs micrographic surgery in the 1950s provided prompt evaluation of tissue margins following skin cancer removal and allowed for immediate wound closure using local cutaneous flaps.

The blood supply to the skin consists of two vascular networks, the deep and the superficial plexus (Fig. 12.1). The deep plexus lies at the junction of the dermis and the subcutaneous fat, while the super-

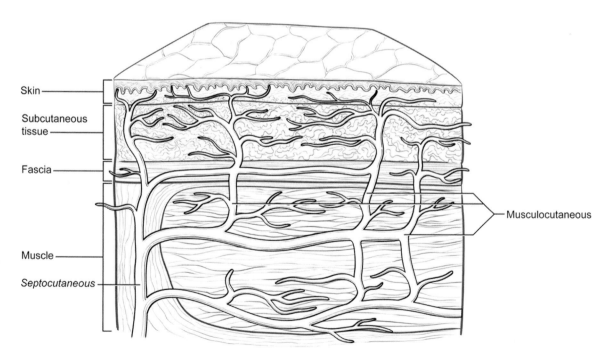

Fig. 12.1 Vascular supply of the skin (Illustration by Alice Y. Chen)

D.F. MacFarlane (ed.), *Skin Cancer Management*, DOI 10.1007/978-0-387-88495-0_12,
© Springer Science+Business Media, LLC 2010

ficial plexus is located in the superficial portion of the reticular dermis supplying the capillary loops of the dermal papillae. Subcutaneous perforating vessels emanating from the main arteries that supply the skin of the face connect with the deep vascular plexus.[2,3] Cutaneous flaps can be classified based on their vascular supply: random pattern, axial, fasciocutaneous, and musculocutaneous (Fig. 12.2).

Random pattern flaps derive their blood supply from the subdermal plexus supplied by musculocutaneous perforators. In contrast, axial flaps obtain their blood supply from a specific fasciocutaneous artery that runs beneath the longitudinal axis of the flap. Fasciocutaneous flaps are composed of skin, fat, and deep fascia, while musculocutaneous flaps include the same tissue layers with the underlying muscle.[2,3]

Classification of Skin Flaps based on Vascular Supply

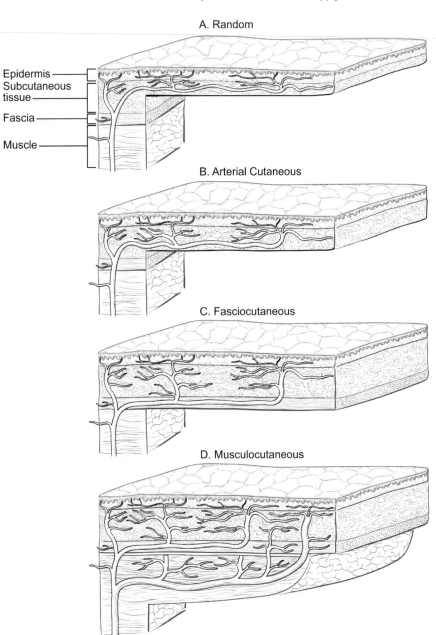

Fig. 12.2 Classification of cutaneous flaps (Illustration by Alice Y. Chen)

Random pattern and axial flaps are the most frequently employed by dermatologic surgeons. Both flap types will be discussed in this chapter with an emphasis on surgical technique and esthetic considerations. While basic flap types will be addressed, an exhaustive discussion of flap design is beyond the scope of this chapter.

Indications and Contraindications to Flap Closure

Cutaneous flaps are typically utilized to close defects when primary closure is not possible because of excess tension or distortion of free margins after adequate undermining or when secondary intention healing is likely to result in poor cosmesis or poor functional outcome. Whenever possible, primary linear or curvilinear closure should be the preferred method of closure. It is remarkable how even very large defects can be closed in this manner with adequate undermining. Whether primary closure is possible will depend on the degree of tissue laxity, which varies considerably with age and anatomic location.

> A flap should not be used because one can perform it, but because it is necessary for optimal contour and cosmesis.

Beginning surgeons are often eager to test their skills by performing a sophisticated flap, but experienced surgeons know that choosing the simplest best solution will yield the best result. A more complicated repair means greater potential for complications.

One contraindication to flap closure is failure to confirm negative tumor margins prior to closure. Immediate closure of a defect resulting from removal of skin cancer is only advised following Mohs micrographic surgery confirmation of negative margins. In situations where Mohs micrographic surgery and immediate margin confirmation is not possible, a flap closure should be delayed. Re-excision of positive margins after a flap closure is difficult at best and much more likely to result in a recurrence.

Even with confirmation of negative tumor margins, the risk of recurrence needs to be assessed routinely prior to closure. For example, one might opt for a simpler repair in the setting of a large high-risk squamous cell carcinoma with perineural invasion to allow for postoperative detection of recurrence. In some instances, skin grafts may be preferable to flaps with regard to detection of recurrent tumor because of the relative thickness of the overlying tissue.

Additional contraindications to immediate closure with a flap may include an avascular recipient bed such as exposed cartilage or bone lacking perichondrium or periosteum, respectively. In these situations, the surgeon might opt for delayed closure or use of an axial flap with its own vascular supply and less risk of ischemia.

Preoperative Considerations

Preoperative assessment and planning are essential for obtaining the best surgical results. The usual considerations in any cutaneous surgery also apply to flaps and include risk of intraoperative or postoperative bleeding, infection, and compromised wound healing. Most of these issues have been discussed in depth in preceding chapters so the emphasis here will be specific to flap-repair procedures.

Flap Design

Some general esthetic issues must be considered when designing a flap.

> The surgeon should always strive to maintain symmetry with the unaltered side since the human eye readily perceives asymmetry.

When designing a flap, the surgeon should seek to blend its borders and contours with its surroundings and recapitulate natural patterns rather than draw attention to itself.

When determining the best closure for a skin and soft tissue defect, the following algorithm can be used to guide you to the best design (Table 12.1):

1. *Identify relaxed skin tension lines and cosmetic unit boundaries.* Prior to administration of any local anesthetic, the author examines the patient in a sitting upright position to determine the location of preexisting wrinkle lines, cosmetic unit boundary lines (Fig. 12.3), and relaxed skin

Table 12.1 Considerations in flap design

Identify relaxed skin tension lines

Identify cosmetic unit boundaries

Identify reservoirs of skin laxity

Assess texture, thickness, and color of the skin surrounding the defect

Assess mobility of skin surrounding the defect and potential donor sites

tension lines (Fig. 12.4) that can serve to camouflage incision lines. *Marking of these lines with a surgical pen prior to administration of local anesthesia is highly recommended* and is performed routinely by the author.

2. *Identify reservoirs of skin laxity near the anticipated defect.* Typical reservoirs of tissue laxity are found at the glabella, melolabial crease, preauricular, and jowl regions, but the amount varies considerably with age and gender.

3. *Assess tissue mobility.* Tissue mobility varies tremendously with location of the defect and age of the patient. On the face, the greatest mobility is found on the cheek and the least on the nose and scalp. Younger skin will be tauter, less distensible, and more likely to require a flap or graft for closure of a defect than that of an older patient. Adequate undermining around the defect is important in assessing tissue mobility and determining whether a flap closure is required. *The author recommends undermining at least 1.0 cm in all directions before abandoning primary closure as an option.*

4. *Assess texture, thickness, and color of the skin around the wound.* This is especially important when considering adjacent tissue transfers to sites such as the nose where matching of the donor and recipient site is critical for optimal cosmesis. Even subtle disruption of natural patterns can draw attention to a scar.

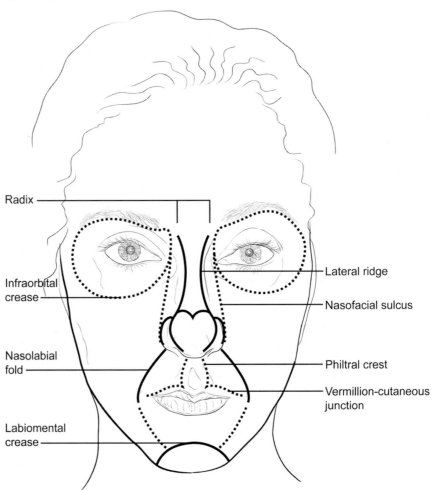

Fig. 12.3 Cosmetic unit boundaries (Illustration by Alice Y. Chen)

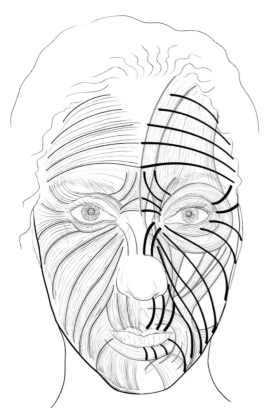

Fig. 12.4 Relaxed skin tension lines perpendicular to muscles of facial expression (Illustration by Alice Y. Chen)

5. *Assess the quality of skin at the prospective donor site.* The presence of excessive scarring or neoplasia at a potential donor site should prompt reconsideration of the flap design. The poor vascularity of scarred tissue will decrease tissue mobility and increase the risk of flap ischemia. The presence of an incipient skin cancer at the donor site of a flap can produce a recurrent skin cancer at the recipient site.

Random Pattern Flaps

Random pattern flaps can be divided into subtypes based on the principal vector of tissue movement.[3–5] Flaps can be advanced, rotated, transposed, or pedicled (Fig. 12.5 and Table 12.2). In practice, many flaps will defy precise classification since they may demonstrate several types of tissue movement. While every defect has its unique closure solutions, certain flap types work best in specific anatomic locations because of esthetic considerations and relative tissue mobility.

Advancement Flaps

Advancement flaps create tissue movement along one-directional vector, usually horizontal (Fig. 12.5). Advancement flaps can be single, double (H-plasty, A-T, O-T), or triple (Mercedes flap). While advancement flaps provide limited tissue movement relative to other types of flaps, the unidirectional movement allows incision lines to be placed easily along the boundaries of cosmetic subunits. Advancement flaps can also be used to optimize placement of incision lines resulting from the removal of redundant standing cones of tissue or "dog ears". One example is closure of a defect of the nasal sidewall (Fig. 12.6a, b). The incision line to advance the flap is placed along the alar groove. Redundant tissue must also be removed from the superior aspect of the defect to allow advancement of the flap (the so-called "Burrow's wedge") and this incision is well placed at the junction of the nasal dorsum and sidewall subunits.

The advancement flap can also be used to redirect the tension vectors from vertical to horizontal, prevent upward retraction, and facilitate alignment of free margins. The bilateral advancement flap (H-plasty type) is very useful for the realignment of the eyebrow and for placement of incision lines in prominent horizontal forehead lines (Fig. 12.7a). A Mohs defect involving the eyebrow shown in Fig. 12.7b was closed using an H-plasty in order to realign the brow (Fig. 12.7c). Another variant of the advancement flap, the O-T or A-T, also functions well for preservation of free margins (eyebrow or vermilion border) or cosmetic unit boundary lines. In Fig. 12.8a–f, a defect of the forehead is closed using an O-T advancement flap above the eyebrow. The horizontal movement of the flap prevents upward deviation of the brow.

The O-T advancement is particularly useful for closure of small- to medium-sized defects of the upper lip while preserving the position of the vermilion border as shown in Fig. 12.9a, b. The movement of an advancement flap will create small pockets of redundant tissue at the pedicle base. These can usually be eliminated extending the length of the flap and applying the "rule of halves" when suturing skin edges of unequal lengths. The horizontal line of the "T" can be extended if necessary to further distribute the dog ear along its length. The author prefers this method over excision of redundant tissue as a wedge.

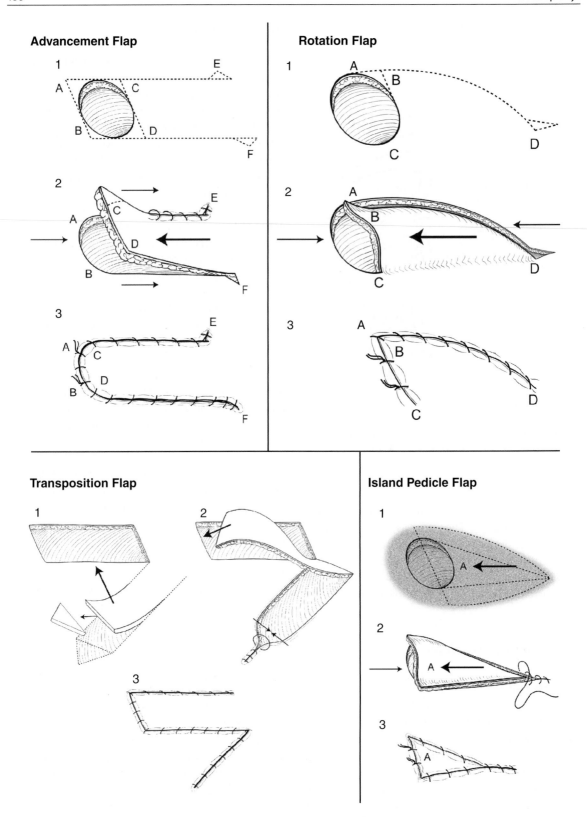

Fig. 12.5 General types of random pattern flaps. (Illustration by Alice Y. Chen)

Table 12.2 Commonly used cutaneous random pattern flaps

Advancement flap

Indications:

- To create horizontal orientation of tension vectors and avoid upward displacement of free margins (lip, eyebrow)
- To achieve favorable placement of incision lines or dog ears (forehead) for maximal camouflage

Examples:

- Forehead, eyebrow (bilateral advancement or "H-plasty")
- Medial upper lip (O-T advancement)
- Helical rim (bilateral advancement)

Rotation flap

Indications:

- Camouflage of incision lines along curvilinear RSTLs or cosmetic unit boundary lines
- Reduce risk of flap ischemia with broad-based pedicle

Examples:

- Cheek
- Chin (bilateral rotation along mental crease)
- Nasal sidewall
- Nasal ala (small defects)
- Nasal tip (bilateral rotation or Peng flap)

Transposition flap

Indications:

- Need for greater tissue movement between best donor site and defect
- Complex contour considerations
- Risk of retraction of free margin with advancement or rotation flap closure

Examples:

- Nasal ala (larger defects)—melolabial transposition
- Nasal tip/medial tip defects—bilobed flap
- Large defects of proximal helix, temple (preauricular sulcus)
- Lateral lower eyelid (upper eyelid transposition)

Island pedicle flap

Indications:

- Need for greater unidirectional tissue movement and preservation of subunit boundaries or free margins

Examples:

- Lateral upper lip- large defects (nasolabial crease and vermilion border)
- Anterior pinna (trap door island pedicle from postauricular sulcus)

Fig. 12.6 Advancement flap on nose. (**a**) Defect of nasal sidewall with outline of advancement flap along alar groove and anticipated standing cone of redundant tissue superior to the defect. (**b**) Final appearance at closure

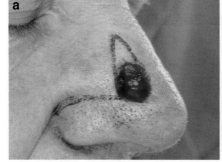
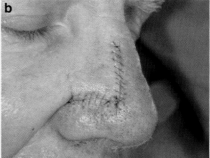

Fig. 12.7 Advancement flap (eyebrow). (**a**) "H-plasty" type double advancement flap. (**b**) Defect of eyebrow following Mohs micrographic surgery. (**c**) Advancement flap incised and closed along superior and inferior borders of eyebrow to maintain brow position

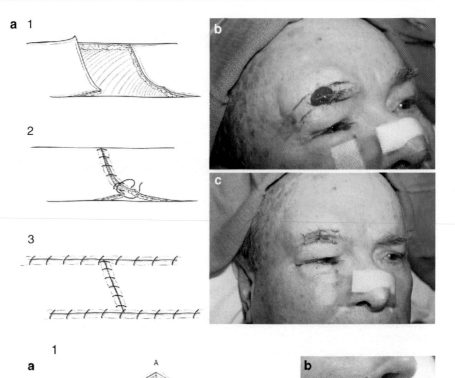

Fig. 12.8 O-T advancement flap of upper lip. (**a**) Design of "O" or "A" to "T" bilateral advancement flap. (**b**) Defect of cutaneous upper lip. Design of "O-T" advancement flap with the base placed horizontally along the vermilion border and vertically along relaxed skin tension lines of the upper lip. (**c**) After undermining both flaps, the skin edges are advanced to the midline of the defect and a subcutaneous suture placed. (**d**) A standing cone of redundant tissue (dog ear) is noted at the superior pole. (**e**) After dog ear excision. (**f**) Final appearance after placement of subcutaneous and superficial sutures

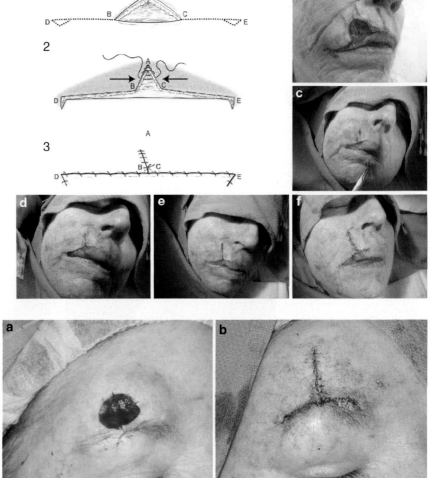

Fig. 12.9 Advancement flap (forehead). (**a**) Forehead defect above eyebrow. (**b**) O-T advancement flap over eyebrow to maintain brow position

Rotation Flaps

Rotation flaps move tissue along a defined arc of rotation (Fig. 12.5b). The curved incision line of a rotation flap is easily camouflaged within curvilinear relaxed skin tension lines in areas such as the cheek. In general, but particularly in this location, curves are much more natural and pleasing to the eye than straight or angular lines. Other advantages are a broad pedicle with ample blood supply and a relatively low risk of ischemia compared to other flap types. Because of these factors, the author utilizes rotation flaps whenever possible in locations such as the cheek and chin.

Figure 12.10a–i demonstrates the use of a rotation flap to close a Mohs defect along the orbital rim that could not be closed primarily without creating excess tension along the lower eyelid. The rotation flap redirects the tension of closure horizontally. Large defects of the zygoma or lateral cheek are very well suited to closure with a rotation flap that can be extended onto the lateral cheek and preauricular sulcus. A lentigo maligna was excised using Mohs margin control and subsequently

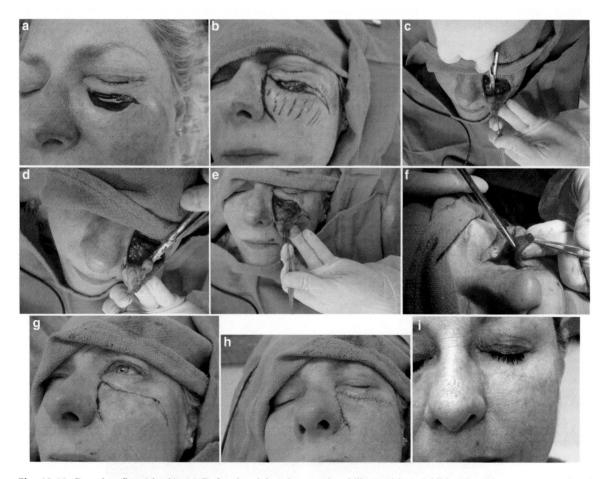

Fig. 12.10 Rotation flap (cheek). (**a**) Defect involving the upper cheek along the orbital rim. (**b**) A rotation flap is planned using the boundary line of the nasofacial sulcus as the incision line and primary arc of rotation. The anticipated position of the standing cone resulting from rotation and the suggested area of undermining are drawn. (**c**) Undermining is performed at the subcutaneous fat using iris scissors. (**d, e**) Defatting of the flap to reduce bulk along the orbital rim. (**f**) Deep subcutaneous tacking sutures are placed to create lift and stabilize position. Additional tacking sutures are placed between base of flap and recipient bed to eliminate dead space and optimize contour. After flap is anchored in place with subcutaneous sutures, redundant tissue is identified and excised. (**g**) Flap appears well positioned before placement of superficial sutures. No alteration in the position of the lower eyelid is noted. (**h**) Superficial sutures (6.0 nylon) are placed to precisely align skin edges. (**i**) Appearance at 2 months postoperatively

closed using a large rotation flap (Fig. 12.11a, b, c). The closure is well camouflaged at 4 weeks (Fig. 12.11d).

The mental crease is another curved cosmetic boundary line. Chin defects below the mental crease can be closed seamlessly using unilateral or bilateral rotation flaps as shown in Fig. 12.12a, b. Rotation flaps are not only indispensable for closing larger defects of the cheek and chin, but also very useful for smaller defects where curved subunit boundaries allow optimal camouflage of the incision. Figure 12.13a, b, c demonstrates a small alar defect that is closed with a "spiral" variant of a rotation flap[6] placed along the alar groove. Small- to medium-sized defects of the nasal sidewall may also be closed using a rotation flap along the junction of the superior nasal sidewall and dorsum.

Rotation flaps may be slightly oversized at the leading edge to compensate for the loss of height with the movement of the flap and reduce the amount of tension at the tip. This is particularly useful for cheek defects near the orbital rim. Contrary to conventional teaching, the author generally avoids the use of a superficial "positioning stitch," which places undue tension at the most vulnerable site. When executing a rotation flap, the arc must often be extended much further than initially expected to achieve the required amount of tissue movement. This can create opposing skin edges of unequal lengths, which can be blended applying the rule

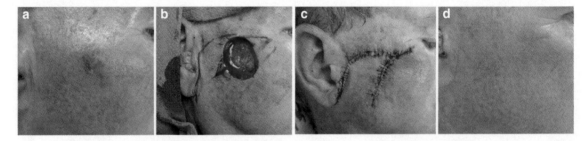

Fig. 12.11 Rotation flap lateral cheek. (**a**) Lentigo maligna lateral cheek. (**b**) Defect following Mohs micrographic surgery. (**c**) The defect is closed using rotation flap repair. The arc of rotation is placed as far laterally as possible for best camouflage. (**d**) Appearance at 4 weeks postoperatively. Note the relatively large scar is almost invisible because of the placement along relaxed skin tension lines

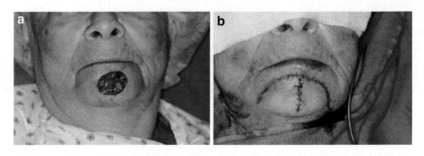

Fig. 12.12 Rotation flap, bilateral (chin). (**a**) Defect on chin below mental crease and proposed bilateral rotation flap along mental crease. (**b**) Final closure after suture placement

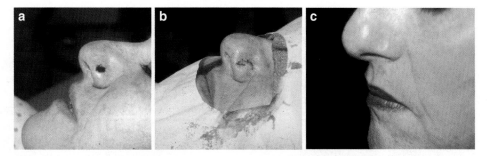

Fig. 12.13 Rotation flap, spiral (ala). (**a**) Small defect of nasal ala. (**b**) A small rotation flap is incised along the alar crease and base. Rotating the flap over itself in a spiral fashion prevents formation of a standing cone along the alar rim. (**c**) Appearance 4 weeks postoperatively. Reproduced with permission from Humphreys TR[6]

of halves with subcutaneous and superficial sutures. If the rotation pucker cannot be divided in this manner, a standing cone of tissue at the base of the flap will need to be excised.

Transposition Flaps

Transposition flaps move tissue from recipient to donor site by crossing over intervening tissue (Fig. 12.5c and Table 12.2). They enable the surgeon to utilize reservoirs of tissue laxity not directly adjacent to the defect, such as the melolabial crease for nasal defects and the preauricular sulcus for auricular defects. Since they can be easily manipulated to restore contour, the author uses transposition flaps most frequently to close defects located on sites with complex topography such as the nose and the ear. Figure 12.14a–h shows a basal cell carcinoma at the base of the helical rim. The defect after Mohs excision involves the surface of the proximal helix, scalp, and cheek. Because of the complex contour and the reservoir of laxity at the preauricular sulcus, a transposition flap was used to close the defect. Tacking sutures from the base of the flap to the base of the defect were used to recreate natural creases and areas of concavity. In the case of transposition flaps, it is usually easier to close the secondary defect first to reduce the tension when closing the primary defect.

The nasolabial or melolabial flap is a dependable flap for reconstruction of mid-alar defects. A basal cell carcinoma of the ala was excised using Mohs surgery (Fig. 12.15a). A transposition flap based on the tissue laxity of the melolabial crease was used to close the resultant defect (Fig. 12.15b–f). Tacking sutures at the alar groove are placed to preserve natural concavity and prevent tenting. Additional fat is removed at the base of the secondary defect to help recreate the natural crease. Cosmesis is excellent and the closure of the secondary defect is well camouflaged within the nasolabial crease.

The use of multi-lobed transposition flaps used in succession can increase the distance of tissue transfer. The bilobed transposition flap as described by Zitelli[7] (Fig. 12.16a) is a masterful design and usually the author's first choice for closure of medium-sized defects involving the medial ala and nasal tip (Fig. 12.16b–k). When properly designed, the contour results are outstanding and removal of any standing cone of tissue is well hidden in the alar groove.

Potential disadvantages of transposition flaps include greater likelihood of flap tip ischemia with a greater length-to-width ratio and "pincushioning" or "trapdooring" with peripheral contracture of the flap. The author generally avoids the use of angular transposition flaps such as the rhombic flap and its variants (i.e., Webster 30 degree angle, Dufourmental) because angular scars tend to stand out rather than blend on most parts of the face.

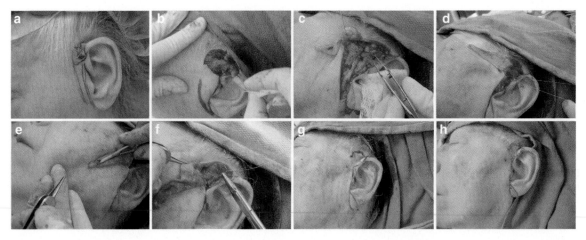

Fig. 12.14 Transposition flap repair (scalp and proximal helix). (**a**) A basal carcinoma on the proximal helix was removed using Mohs micrographic surgery. Prior to surgery, a reservoir of laxity was identified at the preauricular sulcus and relaxed skin tension lines marked. (**b**) The resulting defect involved the proximal helical rim, scalp, and lateral cheek. The proposed transposition flap was designed based on available tissue laxity and best camouflage of the incision lines. (**c**) The flap is incised at the flap borders. Using a skin hook to retract the edge of the secondary defect, undermining is performed using iris scissors in the subcutaneous plane 2–3 cm to achieve adequate mobility. (**d**) The secondary defect is closed with subcutaneous sutures so that all of the edges appear to be completely opposed. (**e**) The flap tip is selectively defatted to better approximate the thickness of the recipient sites. Note that the defect involves sites of varying skin thickness (scalp, helix). (**f**) The flap is opposed to the recipient bed using deep basting or tacking subcutaneous sutures. Basting sutures are placed in areas of natural concavity or depression or to avoid tenting of the flap at the junction of the helix to the scalp. Basting sutures should be placed parallel to the direction of blood flow to minimize vascular compromise to the flap. (**g**) Flap edges are completely opposed after placement of subcutaneous sutures. (**h**) Superficial sutures are then placed in the absence of surface tension to assure seamless closure. The result is a repair with excellent contour and virtually invisible suture lines

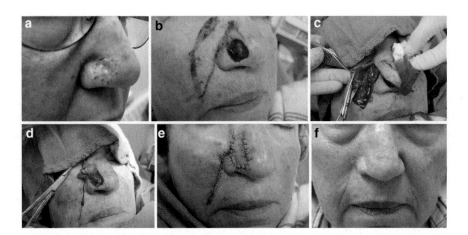

Fig. 12.15 Transposition flap (melolabial flap) closure of alar defect. (**a**) Basal cell carcinoma of the nasal ala. (**b**) Defect of the mid-nasal ala following Mohs micrographic surgery. The outline of the proposed melolabial flap and Burrows triangle (redundant tissue) above defect are drawn. (**c**) Flap borders are incised as drawn and Burrows triangle excised and discarded. The flap tip is defatted to approximate the thickness of the defect. (**d**) The secondary defect is closed first to minimize tension on the flap and allow for more precise placement. Defatting along the newly created nasolabial crease prior to approximation helps maintain normal contour and symmetry. Subcutaneous tacking sutures are placed to recreate the alar groove. Additional tacking sutures placed to oppose underside of flap to recipient bed. (**e**) Appearance after placement of superficial sutures. (**f**) Appearance 4 weeks postoperatively

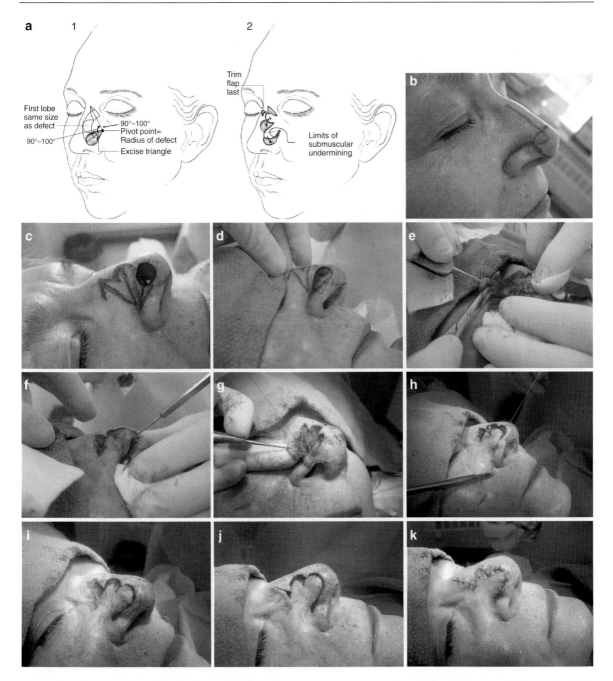

Fig. 12.16 Transposition flap, bilobed type (medial ala/nasal tip defect). (**a**) Design of a bilobed flap repair. The pivot point of the flap is identified by approximating the Burrows triangle along the alar groove. A *line* is drawn from the tip of the standing cone to bisect the defect. A *second line* is drawn from the pivot point at a 90° angle or slightly less for optimal placement. A *third line* is drawn at approximately 45° between line one and two. The two lobes of the flap are then placed centered on lines two and three. The first lobe adjacent to the defect is the size of the defect while the second lobe may be undersized and triangulated. (**b**) Basal cell carcinoma of the nasal tip with preoperative markings of the cosmetic unit boundaries of the nose. (**c**) Defect involving the nasal tip and medial ala. Design of bilobed flap is marked with surgical marker. (**d**) Removal of dog ear at alar groove is performed first to allow movement of the flap. (**e**) The flap is incised and the distal portion defatted using Westcott scissors. (**f**) The mobility of flap is assessed with skin hook. Additional undermining can be performed toward nasal facial sulcus as needed. (**g**) Deep tacking sutures from underside of flap to nasofacial sulcus and nasal sidewall are placed to increase opposition and prevent tenting. (**h**) Closure of secondary defect along alar crease. (**i**) Undermining at periphery of defect. (**j**) Appearance after placement of subcutaneous sutures (5.0 monocryl). (**k**) Final closure after superficial sutures (6.0 Ethilon)

Island Pedicle Flap

The island pedicle flap is completely incised along its periphery and derives its blood supply via the attached subcutaneous tissue (Fig. 12.5d and Table 12.2). Because the skin edges are detached from the recipient site, they may provide greater mobility in certain anatomic locations than flaps with cutaneous pedicles. Island pedicle flaps can be advanced or transposed, tubed, or tunneled. When used to advance tissue along one-directional vector they can achieve increased movement while preserving cosmetic subunit boundaries and position of free margins such as the upper lip.

In Fig. 12.17a, a basal cell carcinoma of the upper cutaneous lip was excised using Mohs micrographic surgery, creating a defect of the cutaneous lip and alar base. Because of the laxity and prominent melolabial crease, the defect was closed using an island pedicle flap from this region (Fig. 12.17b–d). The pedicle should be released from the surrounding subcutaneous tissue enough to allow movement but not so much as to compromise the vascular supply of the underlying pedicle.

Upper lip defects that are too large to be closed using a single or double advancement flap without compromising the contour of the philtral columns can often be closed using an island pedicle flap whose borders lie along the vermilion and nasolabial crease. A large Mohs defect on the upper lip is shown in Fig. 12.18a. It is closed easily using an island pedicle flap (Fig. 12.18b, c), which preserves the position of the vermilion border.

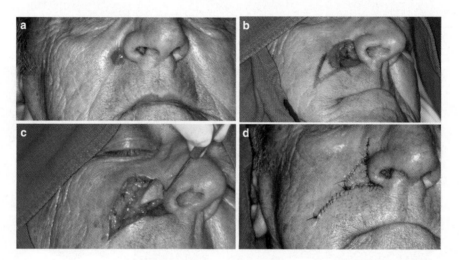

Fig. 12.17 Island pedicle flap repair (alar/cheek defect) (**a**) BCC at alar base and cheek. (**b**) Defect of the alar base and cutaneous upper lip with Island pedicle flap drawn along the melolabial crease. (**c**) The flap is incised along its entire periphery though the subcutaneous fat and the pedicle is released from the surrounding subcutaneous tissue using iris or Metzenbaum scissors. The pedicle is narrowed at the advancing and trailing edges. Mobility is assessed using a skin hook and additional releasing cuts made in the subcutaneous tissue as needed to permit movement to the recipient site. The surgeon must take care to ensure the thickness of the pedicle is sufficient to maintain viability while minimizing tension at the leading edge. (**d**) Final appearance after deep and superficial closure

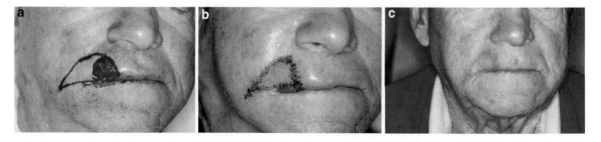

Fig. 12.18 Island pedicle flap closure (upper lip). (**a**) Defect of upper lip and outline of island pedicle flap. (**b**) Closure using an island pedicle flap. (**c**) Appearance at 1 week postoperatively. Note that the position of vermilion border is not altered

Large defects of the anterior pinna that are at risk for infection or prolonged wound healing can be closed effectively by utilizing an island pedicle flap from the posterior surface of the ear along the postauricular sulcus.[8] In this variant, the island of tissue is passed through an incision in the cartilage from the posterior to the anterior surface of the ear (Fig. 12.19a–g). This repair is best limited to defects

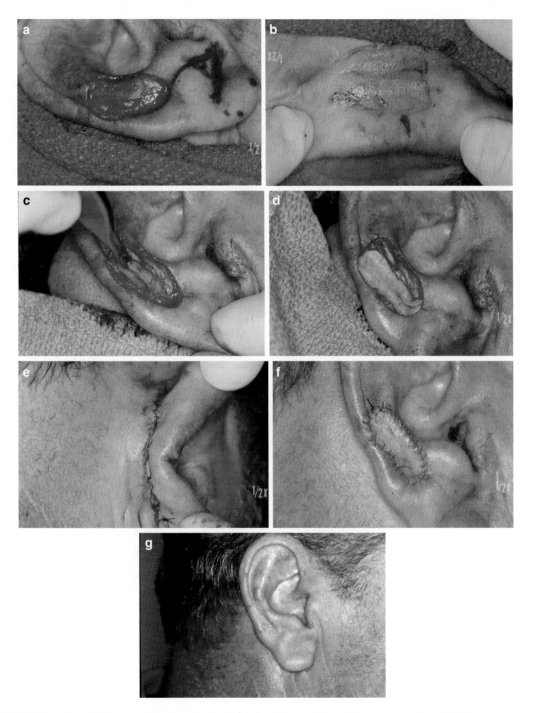

Fig. 12.19 "Trapdoor" island pedicle flap (ear). (**a**) Mohs defect of the right anterior pinna. (**b**) Flap design on the postauricular surface. (**c**) An incision is made through cartilage to allow passage of the flap. (**d**) Flap passed through incision in cartilage from posterior to anterior surface of ear. (**e**) Closure of postauricular donor site.(**f**) Closure of recipient site anteriorly. (**g**) Appearance at 12 months postoperatively. Reproduced with permission from Humphreys TR[6]

of the concha or antihelix, since pinning of the ear can occur with defects located near the helical rim.

Axial Flaps

Because axial flaps are supplied by a specific arterial branch they are less vulnerable to ischemia than random pattern flaps and can be moved a greater distance from donor to recipient site.[2] The most common axial flap used in dermatology is the paramedian forehead flap, which is typically used to reconstruct large defects of the nose, especially the nasal tip. The texture match is excellent and the cosmetic results are usually superior to that of random pattern flaps. Several factors must be considered to determine whether a forehead flap is appropriate for the individual patient. Physical or psychological inability to undergo a multi-stage procedure may preclude the use of a forehead flap. Many patients are reluctant to have a tubed pedicle in place for the 3 weeks required for revascularization, despite the usual superior long-term result compared to other closure choices. The availability of tissue on the forehead may be inadequate due to a small forehead, excessive scarring, or skin cancer present in the donor region.[9]

The forehead flap is based on the vascular path of the supratrochlear artery, which lies just medial to the eyebrow (Fig. 12.20). The paramedian design based on one supratrochlear artery has the advantages of a narrower pedicle base and a greater arc of rotation than the traditional midline forehead flap.[1,10] The path of the supratrochlear artery from the medial eyebrow onto the forehead can be confirmed by Doppler.[9] In cases where Doppler flow is undetectable or unavailable, the supratrochlear artery is located at the glabellar furrow 50% of the time.[11] The remainder of the time it lies between 1 and 6 mm lateral to the crease created by the movement of the procerus and corrugators muscles. When designing a paramedian forehead flap, the pedicle should thus include the glabellar furrow and extend 6 mm laterally toward the medial brow.[11] For optimal vascularity, the flap should extend onto the forehead directly superior to the pedicle rather than obliquely crossing over the midline.[10]

Figure 12.21a demonstrates the resultant cutaneous defect of the nasal tip following Mohs excision of a basal cell carcinoma. A forehead flap was

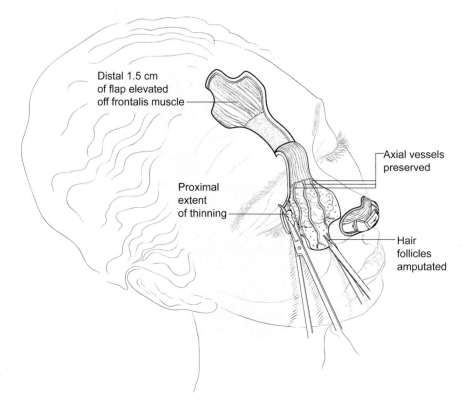

Distal 1.5 cm of flap elevated off frontalis muscle

Axial vessels preserved

Proximal extent of thinning

Hair follicles amputated

Fig. 12.20 Axial (paramedian) forehead flap design (Illustration by Alice Y. Chen)

Fig. 12.21 Paramedian forehead flap closure of nasal tip defect. (**a**) Large defect involving the entire nasal tip and proposed design of a paramedian forehead flap repair. The pedicle is designed to include the supratrochlear artery located between the glabellar furrow and the medial brow. (**b**) The flap is incised down to periosteum. After conservative thinning of the flap tip, the pedicled flap is transposed inferiorly to cover the nasal tip defect. (**c**) Flap after suturing of primary and secondary defect. (**d**) After 3 weeks, the flap is divided from its distal attachment and site of origin and inset

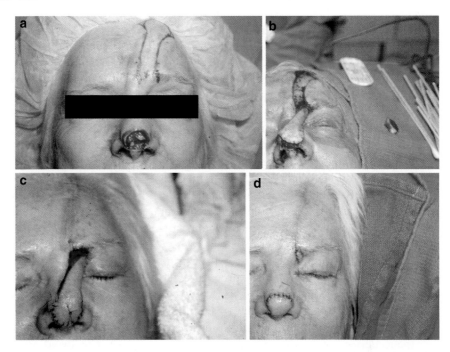

felt to be the best repair option (Fig. 12.21b, c, d). To design the flap, the distance from the pivot point at the origin of the pedicle at the medial brow to the nasal tip was measured and the flap length slightly oversized to compensate for length lost from movement from donor to recipient site. A template of the nasal tip unit can be fashioned from Telfa or aluminum foil and flattened onto the superior forehead to outline the flap. While the actual defect may not encompass an entire subunit of the nose, a superior esthetic result may be obtained by enlarging the defect and replacing the entire subunit.[1,10]

The flap is incised to the periosteum and the flap tip can be thinned for best contour. After suturing the flap in place, the muscular underside of the pedicle is lightly cauterized and wrapped in Vaseline gauze. After 3 weeks, neovascularization at the recipient site is usually sufficient to support the donor tissue.[1] The flap pedicle can then be divided and inset at its origin and insertion. Excellent cosmetic results can be achieved even with large skin and subcutaneous defects as seen in Fig. 12.22a–f. Large full thickness defects involving the cartilage or mucosa will require additional structural support and lining for best results.[1,10]

Fig. 12.22 Paramedian forehead flap closure of nasal tip defect. (**a**) Large basal cell carcinoma of nasal tip. (**b**) Mohs defect and design of a paramedian forehead flap repair. (**c**) Closure of the defect using the paramedian forehead flap. (**d**) Appearance at 3 weeks postoperatively with pedicle intact. (**e**) Closure after completion of division and inset. (**f**) Appearance 5 months postoperative

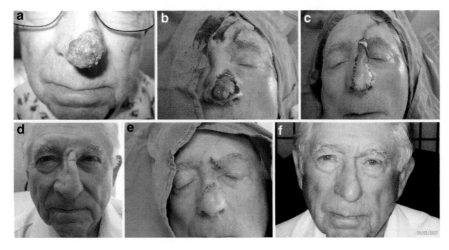

Technical Pearls for Cutaneous Flap Surgery

- Preoperative marking of cosmetic boundaries and contour lines as described earlier in the chapter is a critical step in flap planning and should be performed prior to the administration of local anesthetic, which can distort skin and soft tissue.

   This is especially important for structures with more complex topography such as the nose, ear, or lip where restoration of contour is essential to maintaining symmetry and normal appearance.
- An adequate skin prep with a broad-spectrum antiseptic is critical for flap procedures to reduce the risk of infection.

   The author does not routinely give antibiotics unless there is a specific indication (prosthetic device, immunosuppression, prolonged Mohs surgery preceding the repair). Instead she relies on chlorhexidine (4%) solution to disinfect the surgical site. Chlorhexidine offers broad bactericidal spectrum and longer duration of action than other antiseptics since it binds to the stratum corneum.[12] Contraindications to chlorhexidine are use on the eyelids and ear canal since prolonged exposure can lead to corneal and inner ear toxicity.

   The author also relies on the generous use of local anesthetic, which is advantageous for several reasons. Diffuse infiltration of the tissue with local anesthetic promotes ease of incision and less bleeding, resulting in better visibility and less tissue injury due to cautery.[13] Allowing the infused anesthetic to sit for 10–15 min prior to the flap procedure can help maximize the vasoconstrictive effect of the epinephrine.[14]

   Some undermining of a flap and the surrounding tissue is usually required to reduce tension, facilitate movement, re-drape, or redistribute tissue. Undermining should be performed prudently to minimize tissue injury and optimize flap movement.
- Inadequate undermining will result in excess tension on the flap tip and poor contour, while excessive undermining can result in reduced blood supply and increased risk of bleeding and tissue injury due to cautery.

   Generally, little additional mobility is gained and the risk of cutaneous necrosis increases by undermining more than 4.0 cm.[2,3] The ideal tissue plane for undermining will depend on the location of the flap and the underlying vascular supply. On most areas of the face, it will be in the subcutaneous fat. Submuscular undermining can sometimes be advantageous on the nose to increase the blood supply to the flap. Undermining in the subgaleal level of the scalp minimizes bleeding since it is a relatively avascular plane that separates easily.
- Good flap design and gentle tissue handling are the best insurance against disaster.

   Tissue handling should always be gentle and the amount of manipulation should be minimized to avoid crush injury, especially at the flap tip, which is the most vulnerable portion. Skin hooks are very useful for manipulating tissue with minimal trauma but can be hazardous to the inexperienced user. Tissue forceps must be used for guiding not for grabbing to prevent inadvertent crush injury.

   The amount of cautery used should be minimized to reduce the risk of thermal injury and loss of perfusion.
- Cautery should be used only sparingly to focal areas of bleeding at the wound depth and not to the skin edge, since bleeding usually resolves with suturing and overly aggressive cauterization can result in ischemia and tissue necrosis.

   Radiofrequency electrosurgical units are especially effective for precise coagulation with minimal surrounding thermal injury.
- It is critical for both flap survival and optimal cosmesis to minimize excess tension on the flap edges and especially the tip, which is the most vulnerable portion.

   To achieve fine minimally perceptible scars, any tension present at the wound edges should be borne by the subcutaneous and not the superficial sutures. Superficial sutures should be secure but not tight, which can result in "cutting in" with flap edema, which in turn can lead to infection or wound-edge necrosis.

In addition to meticulous suturing technique, the use of a carefully applied pressure dressing for 24–48 h postoperatively can greatly reduce swelling and fluid collection below the flap that can put the flap at risk.

Defatting of the flap tip, especially in the case of transposition flaps, can improve contour, prevent trapdooring, and reduce the need for secondary revision. Recent literature also suggests that it can increase flap survival[15] by diverting blood flow cutaneously to the distal flap tip.

- The use of tacking sutures to oppose the undersurface of the flap to the defect is critical for optimal contouring, and it also reduces the amount of dead space and risk of hematoma.

Deep "basting" or "tacking" sutures from the underside of the flap to the wound base should be placed parallel to direction of blood flow from the flap pedicle and never perpendicular so as not to compromise perfusion. The author often relies on the use of subsurface tacking sutures rather than horizontal subcutaneous sutures at the opposing wound edges for optimal closure.

Any type of tissue movement or transfer will create standing cones of redundant tissue (Burrow's wedge). Advancement and rotation flaps will create pockets of redundant tissue away from the defect site, while transposition flaps will require removal of additional tissue adjacent to the defect for placement. Skin edges of unequal length should be divided over the length of the incision using the rule of halves whenever possible. If a rotation or advancement pucker is still present then a standing cone of tissue can be removed.

- With a few notable exceptions (such as the bilobed flap), excision of redundant tissue is best performed toward the end of the procedure after tissue redistribution has been completed.

Frequently, standing cones of tissue are smaller than anticipated after undermining and applying the rule of halves. Alternatively, tissue mobility and flap movement may be less than anticipated and discarding tissue prematurely may cause unnecessary difficulty in closing the wound. As a rule, never discard tissue until you are sure that you do not need it.

Postoperative Dressings and Wound Care

After completion of the procedure, the area is cleaned with sterile saline. Because of the increasing incidence of sensitization and risk of contact dermatitis, as well as lack of demonstrated efficacy in preventing infection, the author prefers to apply plain white petrolatum ointment to the surgical site and cover it with Xeroform™ gauze. On top of that, gauze and dental rolls are placed to apply gentle pressure.

> A well-designed pressure dressing can reduce postoperative swelling and oozing, which both contribute to flap failure.

The pressure dressing can be secured with Hypafix™ tape (Smith & Nephew, London, UK), which is secure yet flexible enough to conform to curved surfaces. Patients are instructed to leave the pressure dressing in place for 24–48 h depending on the extent of the flap. Ice or cold packs can also be applied for 10 min every 2 h for the first day to help reduce swelling.

After the pressure dressing is removed, the patient is instructed to clean the area twice daily with hydrogen peroxide-soaked cotton-tipped applicators and reapply the petrolatum. Additional cleanings can be done to avoid the accumulation of crust and scab.

> The importance of meticulous wound care is stressed since poor wound care and the accumulation of debris can lead to skin breakdown and subsequent infection.

If a flap is particularly large or not easily dressed by the patient, we will ask them to return in 24–48 h to have the dressings removed and the area cleaned in the office. Visiting nurse care can also help ensure adequate wound care for patients unable to perform it well by themselves.

Complications in Cutaneous Flap Reconstruction

Adverse sequelae such as infection, bleeding, and hematoma are risks of any cutaneous flap repair. Flap complications can be categorized as acute or delayed (Table 12.3). The ability to identify patients or repairs that are at greater risk for complications is critical to managing them effectively with early intervention. The author's surgical patients are routinely contacted by the office 24 h postoperatively and inquiries made regarding pain, bleeding, and understanding of wound care instructions. Patient complaints should carry a low threshold for re-evaluation in the office since problems such as seroma, hematoma, or ischemia can be minimized by early intervention and supportive care. Patients with flap repairs at locations at risk for delayed complications should be seen at 4–6 weeks postoperatively for evaluation and early intervention.

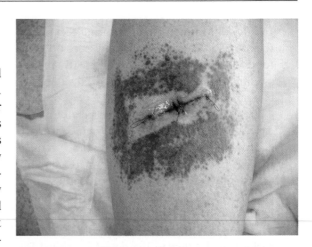

Fig. 12.23 Contact dermatitis secondary to adhesive used for postoperative dressing. – need to crop tighter right side

of contact dermatitis to topical antibiotics, the author instructs patients to apply white petrolatum to the wound after cleaning. Triamcinolone ointment applied to the wound site can hasten resolution.

Table 12.3 Causes of flap ischemia

Cause	Prevention
Excess tension at flap tip or edges	Optimize flap design, use tension bearing sutures subcutaneous tissue not surface
Tissue trauma	Gentle handling of tissue, minimize cautery
	Use of correct suturing technique
Nicotine–induced vasoconstriction	Smoking cessation 2–4 weeks preoperatively
Avascular wound bed	Delayed closure

Acute Complications

Contact Dermatitis

Contact dermatitis can occur postoperatively from a variety of topical antibiotics including neomycin, bacitracin, and Polysporin.[16] It may also occur secondary to adhesive used to secure the postoperative dressing (Fig. 12.23). Contact dermatitis is not only distressing to the patient but can lead to more serious complications because of secondary edema and superinfection. Because of the increasing incidence

Infection

Wound infection is a risk of any cutaneous surgical procedure. The infection rate with Mohs micrographic surgery is remarkably low (0.7%)[17] but increased with flap reconstruction (2.4%). Prevention of infection should be the first-line approach and should include use of broad-spectrum topical antisepsis and good hand hygiene by personnel. The use of sterile versus clean non-sterile gloves does not seem to influence infection rate.[18] The author does not routinely give postoperative antibiotics, but certain clinical scenarios may be associated with an increased incidence of infection such as eroded tumors, prolonged procedures, iatrogenic immunosuppression, or endogenous immune dysregulation (chronic myelogenous leukemia, myelodysplasia, etc.).

The most frequent pathogenic organism seen with postoperative skin infection is *Staphylococcus aureus*. The incidence of methicillin-resistant staph aureus (MRSA) in hospitals and communities varies considerably by location. Figure 12.24 demonstrates a wound infection in an MRSA carrier following Mohs and a nasolabial flap repair. Facial infections need to be treated aggressively with frequent follow-up to assure resolution. Wound

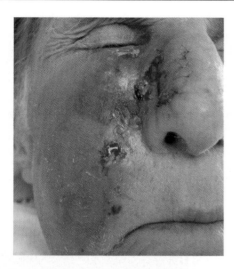

Fig. 12.24 Postoperative infection associated with chronic MRSA colonization

culture of any discharge should be taken and purulent material evacuated and drained. Culture results will dictate the choice of antibiotic. The author's first-line antibiotic is usually cephalexin for an uncomplicated wound infection. If MRSA is suspected or confirmed, then Bactrim DS or doxycycline provides better coverage. If the patient is suspected to be a chronic staph carrier then mupirocin or retapamulin ointment can also be applied to the nares and axilla twice a day for a month to eradicate reservoirs of colonization.

Bleeding Complications

Pharmacologic agents known to inhibit clotting are numerous and include both over-the-counter products (herbal supplements, tocopherol, aspirin, nonsteroidals) and prescription drugs. The most frequent prescription drugs encountered by the dermatologic surgeon include warfarin and clopidogrel. It is controversial whether the use of warfarin increases the risk of postoperative bleeding.[19–22] Since bleeding complications are uncommon, it is generally agreed that if the risk of a thromboembolic event is significant then anticoagulants should not be discontinued. This determination is best left to the discretion of the patient's primary physician. A bleeding time or international normalized ratio (INR) can be obtained to assess the risk of bleeding complications

preoperatively and is best obtained as close to the time of surgery as possible. A bleeding time greater than 8 min[23] or INR greater than 3.0[21] may warrant postponement of the procedure until levels are within therapeutic range. Excessive anticoagulation can lead to postoperative bleeding and hematoma in the perioperative period (Fig. 12.25).

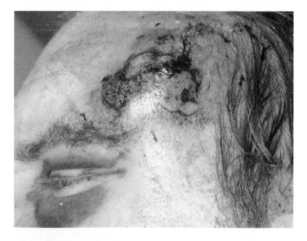

Fig. 12.25 Postoperative ecchymoses and hematoma associated with excessive anticoagulation in a patient with a prosthetic heart valve

Intraoperative bleeding that obscures visibility can be managed with generous use of local anesthetic with epinephrine. Application of epinephrine-soaked gauze can help dampen areas of diffuse bleeding as with exposed muscle. Regardless of what supplemental agents are used, meticulous hemostasis should be applied in each case and patients at risk for postoperative bleeding should be contacted or seen within 48 h postoperatively. Active bleeding should be investigated to determine the source, with take down of the flap and cauterization if necessary. Any fluid collection beneath a flap should be evacuated as early as possible to avoid vascular compromise due to increased flap tension and infection. This can be done using a syringe and 18-gauge needle acutely. Older more viscous collections will require use of a larger bore needle for evacuation.

Flap Ischemia

Flap ischemia, perhaps the most feared acute complication, is due to decreased blood flow and inadequate perfusion pressure. Tissue changes due to ischemia range from relatively minor superficial sloughing (Fig. 12.26a) to partial thickness necrosis (Fig. 12.26b, c) to full thickness eschar formation (Fig. 12.26d). Random pattern flaps are at greatest risk because they are initially dependant on blood flow from small arterioles that are more easily compromised. Flap ischemia can be caused by a variety of factors that include surgical technique and intrinsic patient factors (Table 12.4). With regard to flap design and surgical technique, random pattern flaps are typically thought to be at risk for ischemia if the ratio of the flap length to the width of the pedicle

Table 12.4 Salvage of ischemic flaps

Mild ischemia (superficial denudation/epidermal sloughing)
• Early removal of constricting sutures
• Supportive wound care until re-epithelialized
• Consider antibiotics
Severe ischemia (partial or full thickness skin necrosis)
• Gentle conservative debridement of necrotic tissue
• Antibiotics
• Supportive care with frequent follow-up

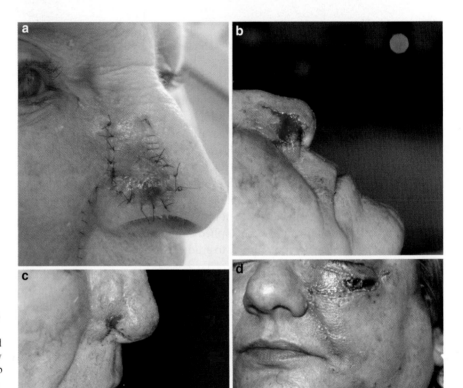

Fig. 12.26 Flap ischemia. (**a**) Mild flap ischemia with superficial epidermal sloughing at flap tip. (**b**) Tip necrosis of nasal labial transposition flap associated with smoking. (**c**) Secondary notching of alar rim. (**d**) Flap tip necrosis of transposition flap associated with diabetes and smoking

exceeds 4:1, but venous congestion may also be a cause of poor flow.[2] Excess tension at the flap tip or edges is a common cause of tissue ischemia, as is tissue injury due to rough handling or excessive cauterization.

Patient risk factors for flap ischemia include smoking and diabetes as shown in Fig. 12.26b, c, d. Smokers should be encouraged to stop or decrease their smoking for a minimum of 2–4

weeks before surgery in order to reverse the vaso-constrictive effect.[24] Another option is delaying the reconstruction for several weeks to allow the wound to granulate and reduce the risk of flap necrosis. Inadequate vascularity of the recipient bed as is seen with cartilage lacking in perichondrium or exposed bone can also lead to flap failure, which can be prevented by the development of granulation tissue at the wound bed.

Management of the Ischemic Flap

Patients with flap repairs that are deemed to be at increased risk for ischemia should be re-evaluated early (24–48 h) so that a timely intervention can be made. If evidence of ischemia is present, the cause should be identified and corrected. Any tight or constricting sutures can be removed and any fluid collection beneath the flap evacuated. In the case of mild ischemia manifested by epidermal sloughing (Fig. 12.26a), supportive care with topical antibiotics and a dressing should be used until the surface re-epithelializes. Antibiotics are indicated if secondary infection is present or likely to occur. Management of full thickness tissue necrosis as seen in Fig. 12.26b, d is more controversial. Traditional surgical teaching instructs the surgeon to avoid debridement and allow an eschar to form and separate. The author believes that conservative debridement of obviously nonviable tissue can facilitate wound healing and remove a potential reservoir of bacterial colonization. Patients can be seen at weekly intervals to facilitate wound debridement and reinforce wound care. The placement of focal guiding sutures (5.0 Prolene) can help re-oppose separated edges more quickly. Full thickness necrosis will likely result in contraction or notching, which may require later revision.

Delayed Complications

Wound contracture that alters the flap contours is the most common delayed complication. The delayed manifestations of scar contracture usually begin to appear at 4 weeks postoperatively. These include trapdooring or pincushioning, ectropion, and displacement of other free margins such as the alar rim and lips with the contractile phase of wound

healing. Pincushioning occurs most frequently with transposition or interpolated pedicle flaps (Fig. 12.27a). While scar contracture is the main cause of pincushioning, it can also be caused by the use of an excessive bulky flap that is too thick for the recipient site as in the case of the melolabial transposition flap. The risk of pincushioning can be reduced by sizing the flap appropriately to the recipient site (same size or slightly smaller), undermining the periphery of the recipient site. Nasal defects repaired with transposition flaps frequently demonstrate some degree of pincushioning. The author always instructs patients to begin gentle massage of the nasal flap 2–3 weeks postoperatively to reduce swelling and maintain tissue suppleness. Patients with nasal flap repairs also return for a postoperative check 4–6 weeks after surgery, when one would expect to first see signs of contracture and pincushioning. Mild induration or pincushioning is usually reversed with focal use of intralesional Kenalog (10 mg/ml), which can be repeated monthly as needed.

Contraction of a flap can also cause displacement of other free margins such as the alar rim, vermilion border, and eyelid margin. Tip necrosis is also a common cause of exaggerated scar contracture leading to distortion of normal contour. Optimal flap design and suturing techniques are the best prevention of margin displacement. In the case of the alar rim, adequate replacement of nasal lining in the case of full thickness defects and the use of cartilage grafts along the ala for stabilization of large repairs[1] can help reduce the risk in the case of large or full thickness defects. Failure to adequately repair lost nasal lining or provide structural support can result in unopposed wound contracture and a poor cosmetic result that requires revision (Fig. 12.27b). For repairs near free margins, the author routinely asks patients to follow up at 4 weeks postoperatively. Early contracture can be

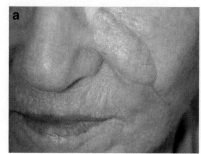 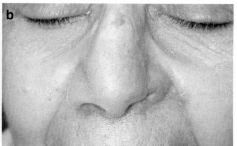

Fig. 12.27 Manifestations of wound contracture. (**a**) "Trap door" deformity of interpolated pedicle flap at 4 weeks. (**b**) Delayed retraction of nasal ala due to insufficient cartilaginous support

reversed with intralesional Kenalog given at monthly intervals, while contracture resulting from tissue ischemia or inadequate support will often require secondary revision.

The lower eyelid is a free margin often affected by scar contracture. Although excess tension on the lid margin may not be apparent at the time of the repair, subsequent maturation and contracture of the scar can produce displacement of the eyelid at around 4 weeks postoperatively, as shown in Fig. 12.28a. This is particularly true in the case of

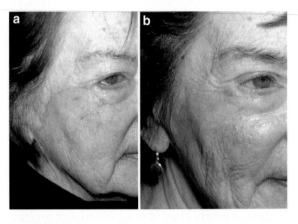

Fig. 12.28 Ectropion. (**a**) Delayed ectropion associated with large cheek rotation flap, 4 weeks postoperatively. (**b**) Correction of ectropion following a transposition flap from the upper eyelid

elderly patients whose lid laxity should be assessed preoperatively using the "snap" test. If a significant lid lag is noted, one should consider additional means of support to resist the forces of contracture such as a canthopexy, suspension, or fixation of the lateral canthus to the lateral orbital rim or adjacent soft tissue, or even cartilaginous support.[25]

When repairing defects adjacent to the orbital rim, the flap repair should always be designed to avoid and redirect downward pull on the lower lid. Anchoring sutures placed in the subcutaneous tissue are often useful to lift the flap and reduce downward tension. Tension on the subcutaneous sutures should always be directed along a horizontal rather than vertical orientation. Mild ectropion can often be ameliorated with intralesional Kenalog at the site of contraction, while those cases that fail to correct with conservative measures will require a revision procedure to restore volume and lid position, such as a transposition flap from the ipsilateral upper eyelid (Fig. 12.28b) or skin graft.

Since angiogenesis is part of the tissue reparative process, prominent telangiectasia or erythema can persist in vascular areas such as the nose or in those prone to rosacea (Fig. 12.29a). The author generally advises patients to wait 3 months for postoperative erythema to resolve spontaneously. If it fails to do

Fig. 12.29 Persistent postoperative telangiectasia. (**a**) Persistent telangiectasia at site of advancement flap along nasal sidewall (shown in Fig. 12.8) 2 months postoperatively. (**b**) Early scar contracture and telangiectasia 6 weeks following a cheek rotation flap. (**c**) Resolution of induration and erythema after intralesional Kenalog and long-pulsed dye laser therapy (two sessions 4 weeks apart)

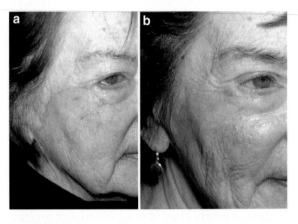
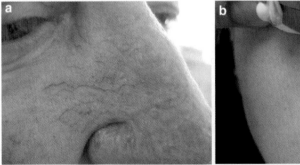
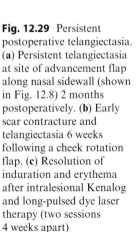
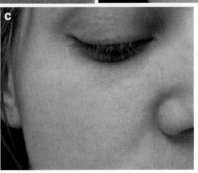

so, treatment of the surgical site with a long-pulsed dye laser at monthly intervals is usually corrective. Figure 12.29b demonstrates telangiectasia and induration around a rotation flap on the cheek at 6 weeks that resolved with ILK and long-pulsed dye laser treatment (Fig. 12.29c).

Prominent scarring or ridging is more common on sebaceous areas of the nose, especially male patients with preexisting rosacea and sebaceous hyperplasia. If meticulous suturing fails to produce a cosmetically acceptable result, resurfacing by laser or manual dermabrasion after 4–8 weeks postoperatively can greatly improve the appearance of a prominent scar.[26] For severe ridging, the author uses a 15c scalpel blade to re-contour the edges adjacent to the scar. More subtle textural problems can be addressed with manual dermabrasion, which is easily performed using a 2 mm curette or medium-grade sandpaper that has been sterilized and wrapped around a 3 cc syringe. CO_2 laser can also be used to resurface surgical scars with excellent results.

Summary

Flap repairs of cutaneous and subcutaneous defects can yield excellent results in restoring contour and appearance. Preoperative planning with regard to flap design and placement is critical to success. Meticulous surgical technique is essential for maintaining flap viability. Despite proper planning and technique, complications can occur, and surgeons performing flap repairs should be thoroughly prepared to manage them (Table 12.5).

References

1. Burget G, Menick F. *Aesthetic Reconstruction of the Nose*. St Louis, Missouri: Mosby-Yearbook; 1994.
2. Gaboriau H, Murakami C. Skin anatomy and flap physiology. *Otolaryngol Clin North Am.* 2001;34(3): 555–569.
3. Baker S. *Local Flaps in Facial Reconstruction*. Philadelphia, Pennsylvania: Mosby-Elsevier; 2007.
4. Salasche S, Bernstein G, Senkarik M. *Surgical Anatomy of the Skin*. Norwalk, Connecticut: Appleton and Lange; 1998.
5. Tromovitch T, Stegman S, Glogau R. *Flaps and Grafts in Dermatologic Surgery*. Chicago, IL: Yearbook Medical; 1989.
6. Humphreys TR. Use of the "spiral" flap for closure of small defects of the nasal ala. *Dermatol Surg.* 1997;27(4):409–410.
7. Zitelli JA. The bilobed flap for nasal reconstruction. *Arch Dermatol.* 1989;125(7):957–959.
8. Humphreys TR, Goldberg L, Wiemer DR. The postauricular (trap door) island pedicle flap revisited. *Dermatol Surg.* 1996;22:148–150.
9. Brodland D. Paramedian forehead flap reconstruction for nasal defects. *Dermatol Surg.* 2005;31:1046–1052.
10. Menick F. Aesthetic refinements in the use of the forehead for nasal reconstruction: the paramedian forehead flap. *Clin Plast Surg.* 1990;17(4):607–622.
11. Vural E, Batay F, Key I. Glabellar frown lines as a reliable landmark for the supratrochlear artery. *Otolaryngol Head Neck Surg.* 2000;123:543–546.
12. Kaiser A, Kernoodle D, Burg N, et al. Influence of preoperative showers on staphylococcal skin colonization: a comparative trial of antiseptic skin cleansers. *Ann Thorac Surg.* 1998;45:35.
13. Behroozan D, Goldberg LH. Dermal tumescent anesthesia in cutaneous surgery. *J Am Acad Dermatol.* 2005;53:828–830.
14. Grekin RC, Auletta MJ. Local anesthesia in dermatologic surgery. *J Am Acad Dermatol.* 1988;19:599–614.
15. Chetboun A, Masquelet AC. Experimental animal model proving the benefit of primary defatting of full thickness random pattern skin flaps by suppressing "perfusion steal". *Plast Reconstr Surg.* 2007;20(6):1496–1502.
16. Gehrig K, Warshaw E. Allergic contact dermatitis to topical antibiotics: epidemiology, responsible allergens, and management. *J Am Acad Dermatol.* 2008;58:1–21.
17. Maragh S, Brown M. Prospective evaluation of surgical site infection rate among patients with Mohs

Table 12.5 Surgical pearls for successful flap closure

Choose simplest closure design to minimize complications
Make contour the primary consideration in flap design
Use broad-spectrum, long-acting antiseptic skin prep (CHG)
Generous use of local anesthetic to maximize hemostasis
Handle tissue gently
Cauterize sparingly
Selectively defat flaps to restore contour and increase vascularity
Meticulous suturing technique with use of deep tacking and basting sutures
Apply secure pressure dressing for 24–48 h
Postoperative phone call within first 24 h
Thorough patient education about wound care and potential complications

micrographic surgery without the use of prophylactic antibiotics. *J Am Acad Dermatol.* 2008;59:275–278.

18. Rhinehart BM, Murphy ME, Farley MF, et al. Sterile versus non-sterile gloves during Mohs micrographic surgery: infection rate is not affected. *Dermatol Surg.* 2006; 32(2):170–176.

19. Billingsley E, Maloney M. Intraoperative bleeding problems in patients taking warfarin, aspirin, and non-steroidal anti-inflammatory agents: a prospective study. *Dermatol Surg.* 1997;23(5):381–383.

20. Dixon AJ, Dixon MP, Dixon JB. Bleeding complications in skin cancer surgery are associated with warfarin but not aspirin therapy. *Br J Surg.* 2007;94(11): 1356–1360.

21. Blasdale C, Lawrence C. Perioperative international normalized ratio level is a poor predictor of postoperative bleeding complications in dermatologic surgery patients taking warfarin. *Br J Dermatol.* 2008;158: 522–526.

22. Ah-Weng A, Natarjan S, Velangi S, et al. Preoperative monitoring of warfarin in cutaneous surgery. *Br J Dermatol.* 2003;149:386–389.

23. Alcalay J. Cutaneous surgery in patients receiving warfarin therapy. *Dermatol Surg.* 2001;27(8):756–758.

24. Chan LK, Withey S, Butler P. Smoking and wound healing problems in reduction mammoplasty. *Ann Plast Surg.* 2006;56(2):111–115.

25. Hashikawa K, Tahara S, Nakahara M, et al. Total lower lid support with auricular cartilage graft. *Plast Reconstr Surg.* 2005;115(3):880–884.

26. Lawrence N, Mandy S, Yarborough J, Alt T. History of Dermabrasion. *Dermatol Surg.* 2000;26(2):95–101.

Chapter 13
Techniques in Skin Grafting

Deborah F. MacFarlane

Free skin grafting, defined as the severing of a piece of skin from its local blood supply and transfer to another location, is thought to have originated in India approximately 2,500 years ago. However, it was not until the nineteenth century that the first accounts appeared in Western literature.[1]

The goal of this chapter will be to provide the practitioner with an understanding of the physiological processes involved in skin grafting, be it with full thickness, split thickness, free cartilage, or composite grafts. This knowledge coupled with attention to meticulous hemostasis, careful tissue matching, and postoperative management is essential to achieving an excellent outcome.

General Principles

Graft survival is dependent upon the establishment of a blood supply from the recipient site and occurs over a series of stages. It is essential that this process is appreciated if graft survival is to be achieved.

During imbibition (from Latin *bibere* "to drink"), which occurs during the first 24–48 h, the graft absorbs transudate from the recipient bed and becomes edematous.[2] The graft is initially held in place by fibrin, which is eventually replaced by granulation tissue. Over the next 48–72 h, inosculation occurs with the development of vascular anastomoses between the recipient bed and donor site.[3] By 4–7 days, capillaries have grown from the recipient bed to the graft in the process of neovascularization and full circulation has been restored to the graft.[4] Restoration of lymphatic circulation also occurs within this period. Two to four weeks following grafting, reinnervation occurs, and full sensation may take several months or even years to return to normal.[5]

Full-Thickness Skin Grafts

Composed of epidermis and the entire dermis, including adnexal structures such as hair follicles and sweat glands, full-thickness skin grafts (FTSGs) are especially useful for the repair of defects of the nasal tip, dorsum, ala, lateral nasal sidewall, lower eyelid, and ear.[6] When close attention is paid to skin color, texture, and thickness, FTSGs can provide an excellent cosmetic result (Fig. 13.1a, b).

Wound contraction is minimal with FTSGs and dermal adnexal structures are left intact. Recipient sites must be able to provide a rich vascular supply for capillary ingrowth as well as fibroblasts for graft adherence. In general, avascular structures such as exposed bone, cartilage, tendon, and nerve, which have had their periosteum, perichondrium, peritenon, or perineurium removed, are unable to support FTSGs.[7]

Technique

Preoperative Planning

A thorough preoperative history should be taken to identify medications and dietary supplements that

D.F. MacFarlane (ed.), *Skin Cancer Management*, DOI 10.1007/978-0-387-88495-0_13,
© Springer Science+Business Media, LLC 2010

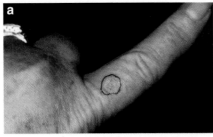
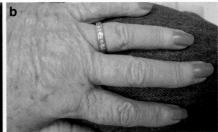

Fig. 13.1 (**a**) Squamous cell carcinoma on the base of the left index finger prior to Mohs surgery. (**b**) Appearance of FTSG 1 month postoperatively. Note careful matching of color and texture between donor skin (upper inner arm) and recipient site provides a cosmetically very acceptable result. Figures reproduced with permission from MacFarlane, D.F.[17]

may increase the risk of bleeding. It cannot be stressed enough how vital hemostasis is to graft success, and any medication or supplement that is not essential should be stopped at least 1 week prior to surgery.[8,9] Since a three-fold risk of graft necrosis has been observed in patients smoking more than one packet of cigarettes daily compared with nonsmokers or those smoking less than a packet daily,[10] all smokers should be encouraged to cease or decrease cigarette smoking markedly several days prior to surgery and to continue this for at least the first postoperative week. Patients should similarly be advised that they will need to curtail physical exercise; this is especially important when dealing with FTSGs on the lower extremities of elderly patients. One may consider hospitalization in such circumstances (Fig. 13.2a, b, c).

Donor Site Considerations

In order to maximize esthetic outcome, like skin is always best repaired with like skin.

> Time should be spent matching donor skin with that of the recipient site, taking into consideration not just color, but also texture, thickness, extent of photodamage, and degree and direction of hair growth, (Fig. 13.3a, b) if appropriate.

Skin grafts taken from excess upper eyelid skin can be used to repair lower eyelid defects. However, grafts of this especially thin skin should be oversized by at least 100% to prevent contraction and possible ectropion.[11] The preauricular region is a good source of a thicker skin with a degree of sun exposure that can be used to repair nasal defects, and the donor site heals nicely (Fig. 13.4a, b).[12]

Skin taken from the nasolabial fold may also be used to close small nasal tip defects and may often supply a degree of sebaceous quality. The donor site heals imperceptibly and the author recommends this over preauricular skin, which is less sebaceous,

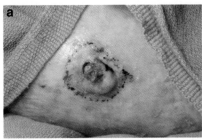
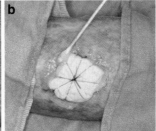
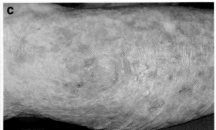

Fig. 13.2 (**a**) A large squamous cell carcinoma on the leg of a 93-year-old albino African-American woman prior to Mohs surgery. (**b**) A bolster is placed over the FTSG and the patient is hospitalized for 1 week of bed rest. The daily application of antibiotic ointment to the wound periphery, commencing on postoperative day 2, is demonstrated. (**c**) Appearance of the FTSG 89 weeks later. Note the patient's varices. Figures reproduced with permission from MacFarlane, D.F.[17]

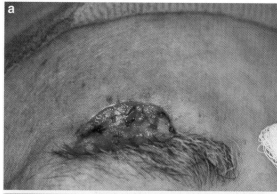

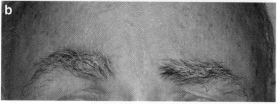

Fig. 13.3 (**a**) A large defect involving the superior aspect of the eyebrow is apparent following three stages of Mohs surgery for a recurrent SCC. (**b**) Appearance of the brow 2 months after complex linear repair and Burow's graft from the supero-medial brow and placement of the FTSG so that the eyebrow hairs are carefully aligned with adjacent hairs

may often have fine hairs, and may not provide as close a color match (Fig. 13.5a, b, c, d).

Conchal bowl grafts provide another option where a sebaceous texture is needed, as with the nasal tip on some patients;[13] however, it may take weeks for the donor site to granulate in and patients should be aware of this.

A graft taken from skin adjacent to the surgical defect, known as a Burow's graft, often provides an ideal match with respect to both color and texture.[14] As there are several reports of skin cancers being accidentally transferred in donor skin, a careful examination should be made of prospective donor skin to exclude malignancies (Fig. 13.6).[15]

Often a better color match is provided by using skin with a certain degree of photodamage. Clavicular skin, for instance, may be used for larger defects requiring FTSGs of sun-damaged skin; however, these grafts need to be carefully placed to avoid an unattractive scar.[16] Similarly, skin can also be harvested from the forearms or wrists to repair defects on the fingers or hands (Fig. 13.7a, b).

Skin may be harvested from the abdomen; however, the color and texture match may be less desirable and, for the author, this is the place of last resort. Care should be taken to place the excision in an area free from trauma due to clothing.

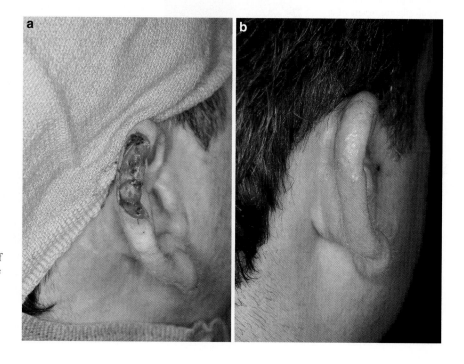

Fig. 13.4 (**a**) Defect following two stages of Mohs surgery to remove a BCC on the ear of a young male. Note some notching of the auricular cartilage where the BCC was adherent. (**b**) Appearance of the ear 2 months following surgery. There is a small crust at the preauricular donor site

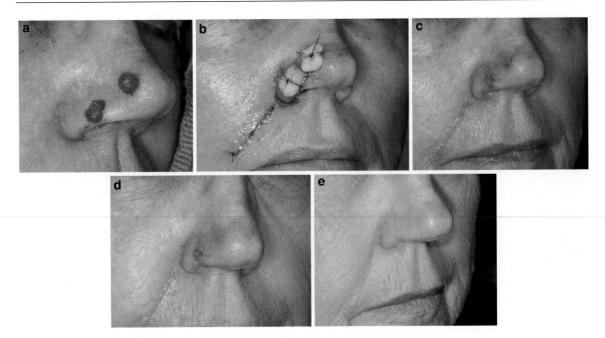

Fig. 13.5 (**a**) Defects on the nasal wall following Mohs surgery for 2 basal cell cancers. (**b**) FTSGs are taken from the right nasolabial fold. (**c**) Appearance at suture removal 7 days later. The crust is left undisturbed and the area redressed for another week. (**d**) Appearance at 2 weeks—the FTSG is left open. (**e**) Appearance 5 months following surgery

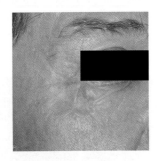

Fig. 13.6 SCC in situ has occurred within this FTSG taken from the patient's right upper eyelid after occuloplastic repair of a Mohs defect beneath the patient's eye 18 months prior. Reproduced with permission from MacFarlane, D.F.[17]

Procedure

There are many techniques used in the construction of full-thickness skin grafts. What follows is the author's personal technique.

Hemostasis of the recipient site is essential for graft survival and electrocautery must be precise and meticulous. Once the wound is dry and the recipient site chosen, a template can be manufactured from any sterile and flexible material. The author uses Telfa, which is placed on the recipient site and firmly pressed

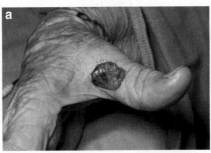
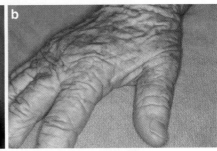

Fig. 13.7 (**a**) Wound defect following Mohs surgery for a squamous cell cancer. Note that donor site (inner wrist) has been selected for color match. (**b**) FSTG appearance 2 months later

into the contours of the bed. Any blood present is absorbed onto the Telfa, forming an outline that is then cut out. The author does not personally cut FTSGs larger than the defect, except in the ocular area as described previously. Next the template is outlined on the donor site prior to local anesthesia. The FTSG is then excised down to superficial fat, placed in a sterile saline-filled container, and the donor site is repaired. The FTSG is next defatted until the dermal surface is white and shiny. This is facilitated by placing the FTSG on a piece of gauze, dermal side up, and trimming with sharp scissors (Fig. 13.8d).

The author has observed that overly thinned FTSGs will later result in an unattractive hypopigmented appearance.

Immobilization

It is essential that FTSGs be kept in direct contact with the recipient bed if the previously described physiological processes are to occur successfully.

> "Support ties," placed at regular intervals around the perimeter of the FTSG, may be anchored to the drapes with sterile Steri-Strips, which serve to stop them from becoming tangled[17] (Fig. 13.8e, f).

Next a running suture is placed around the perimeter of the FTSG. Basting sutures are not used as

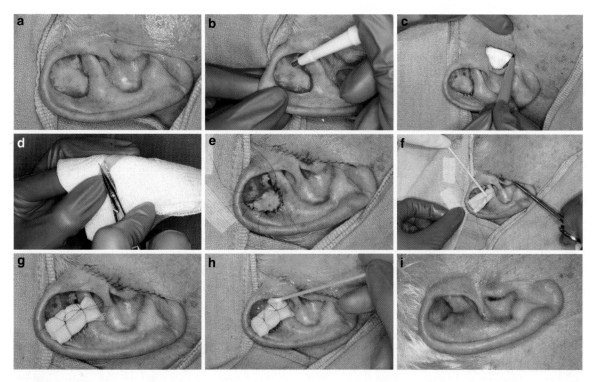

Fig. 13.8 (a) Defect following four stages of Mohs surgery for a BCC, which necessitated removal of perichondrium in the superior aspect of the defect. (b) A 2-mm punch is used to punch through the denuded cartilage to facilitate ingrowth of granulation tissue from the posterior aspect of the ear. (c) A Telfa template of the defect is outlined on the preauricular area, which has been chosen as a suitable color and texture match. (d) Gradle scissors are used to defat the graft. (e) A running 6-0 Ethilon suture has been placed around the periphery of the defatted FTSG. Long ties are placed at symmetric points on the FTSG and anchored to the drapes with Steri-Strips. (f) A Xeroform bolster is tied in place. (g) The finished bolster. (h) Antibiotic ointment is applied to the exposed cartilage and around the perimeter of the bolster. This is then covered with a protective dressing (Telfa, gauze, and Hypafix), which is left untouched for 48 h. Thereafter antibiotic ointment is applied daily and the wound dressed similarly following suture removal 7 days after surgery. (i) Appearance of the FTSG 4 weeks later—the superior aspect of the defect has granulated in fully and blends imperceptibly with the FTSG. The shape and appearance of the ear is fully restored. Figures reproduced with permission from MacFarlane, D.F.[17]

they are felt to contribute toward a "pincushion" effect. A bolster is manufactured from Xeroform and tied securely over the FTSG using the support ties, which are released sequentially from beneath the Steri-Strips (Fig. 13.8 f, g). A thick layer of antibiotic ointment is placed around the perimeter of the bolster (Fig. 13.8 h) and the entire area is covered with Telfa and Hypafix.

Post-Operative Care

The patient is instructed to change the dressing after 2 days and to apply the antibiotic ointment to the perimeter of the bolster, replace the dressing, and to continue this process thereafter until suture removal. Using this technique, bolster and suture removal are both extremely easy. It is important to caution patients that following suture removal a graft is still delicate and that trauma such as a hot shower on the area should be avoided for an additional 1–2 weeks. For this reason the author instructs patients to continue to keep the grafted area covered with antibiotic ointment, Xeroform, and an occlusive dressing for a further week.

Special Situations

Be aware that skin grafts less than 1 cm in diameter can survive due to vascular re-anastomoses, which form solely from the edges of the wound.[18] However, other solutions are needed for larger grafts. When an immediate FTSG is needed to cover bare cartilage, fenestrating the cartilage and lifting a hinge flap have been found to increase graft survival.[19]

> The author often uses a 2-mm skin punch to punch out the cartilage (Fig. 13.8b), allowing the ingrowth of granulation tissue, and then waits 2–3 weeks until sufficient granulation has occurred (Fig. 13.8i).

It is advisable to position these punches so that the support function of the auricular cartilage is not compromised, and it is essential that the patient keep the area moist with an ointment like mupirocin (less chance of contact dermatitis) and covered with a layer of Xeroform and an occlusive dressing, which is changed daily. Nonsteroidal anti-inflammatories are useful to relieve pain due to the chondritis, which often occurs following manipulation of auricular cartilage. Other authors have documented the benefits of delaying FTSGs.[20,21] The author has not uncommonly performed auricular FTSGs 2–3 weeks following surgery when sufficient granulation has occurred.

Complications

Partial or complete graft failure may be due to excessive electrocautery of the recipient bed, hematoma, infection, and disruption of graft-bed contact. Attention to hemostasis, careful bolster design, and stressing the importance of avoiding strenuous activities should help reduce the risk of such failure (Fig. 13.9a, b, c).

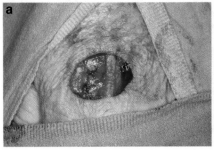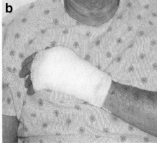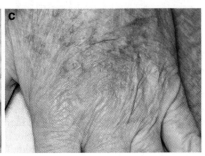

Fig. 13.9 (**a**) Defect appearance following Mohs surgical removal of a large SCC on the dorsum of the hand of a farmer. (**b**) Avoidance of strenuous activities was emphasized. (**c**) FTSG appearance 3 months following surgery

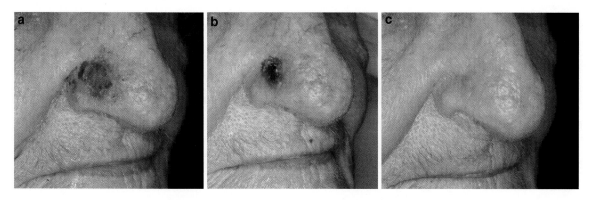

Fig. 13.10 (**a**) Appearance of FTSG on a patient's nasal ala at 1 week. The patient is reassured, and told that the area will dry out and become darker in color. (**b**) Appearance 1 week later. (**c**) Appearance 6 weeks following surgery

Another complication is necrosis; this is usually superficial and not full-thickness.

> If graft necrosis occurs, it is important not to debride the region of necrosis. Instead, advise patients that the graft is acting as a dressing, that new skin is growing underneath, and that it is important that they refrain from manipulating the area and should just let it dry out and lift off (Fig. 13.10a, b, c).

Debridement of the necrotic area will only interfere with this process. Graft elevation can be treated with intralesional corticosteroids after several months have elapsed. Duoderm or Curad scar therapy strips may be applied nightly by patients to help smooth out any contour irregularities.

Split-Thickness Skin Grafts

Split-thickness skin grafts (STSGs) consist of the epidermis and a portion of the dermis. Dependent upon the amount of dermis included in the graft, they vary from 0.25 to 0.75 mm in thickness and are categorized as thin (0.0125–0.275 mm), medium (0.275–0.4 mm), or thick (0.40–0.75 mm).

Equipment

A variety of methods and instruments are available to harvest STSGs. The simplest STSG is the pinch graft, which may be 1 cm or less in size, harvested using forceps and a scalpel blade or small scissors, and is especially useful for nonhealing leg ulcers. The Weck blade has a guard that helps the harvesting of a uniformly thick piece of skin, but requires some experience.

Powered dermatomes are used to harvest larger more uniform pieces of skin. The Davol Simon dermatome is battery operated and cuts 3-cm wide grafts at 0.015 in.[22] Larger dermatomes include the Brown and Padget dermatomes and the Zimmer dermatome. The latter is less operator-dependent, consistently harvesting grafts of predefined width and thickness (Fig. 13.11a).[23]

Technique

Following donor site selection, the area should be shaved of hair and anesthetized. Local infiltration with 1% lidocaine with epinephrine or tumescent anesthesia with 0.1% lidocaine with epinephrine (1:1,000,000) may be used. The donor site is next cleansed with an antiseptic such as povidone iodine or chlorhexidine gluconate, which should then be removed with saline, and the skin dried and draped. Typically, the skin is then coated with a thin layer of mineral oil to facilitate movement of the dermatome. The skin is pulled tightly ahead of the path of the dermatome by an assistant using dry gauze pads or special wooden paddles (tongue blades) to provide traction on the slippery skin surface.

Following harvesting, the STSG is transferred to sterile saline-soaked gauze. As the graft is so thin it is

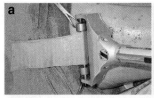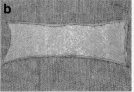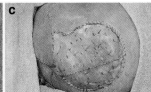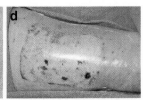

Fig. 13.11 Harvesting of an STSG using the Zimmer dermatome. (**a**) As the Zimmer dermatome glides over the donor skin of the anterior thigh, the graft emerges.[23] (**b**) Note how the edges of the STSG curl inward toward the dermal side of the graft and that the latter has a shiny appearance. (**c**) The graft is attached to the recipient bed. Note the fenestrations that allow for the drainage of any blood and serum. (**d**) An Opsite dressing is placed over the wound. Figures reproduced with permission from MacFarlane, D.F.[17]

easy to confuse the dermal and epidermal sides; the epidermal side of the graft has a duller appearance, the dermal side has a shinier appearance, and the edges of the STSG tend to curve inward toward the dermal side when the skin is lying downward (Fig. 13.11b). In order to increase the surface area of the STSG, it may be placed through a mechanical mesher.

Thorough hemostasis is essential and recipient beds should be freshened up by scoring with a scalpel. Bare cartilage can be fenestrated with a 2-mm punch as previously described, and bone lacking periosteum may be burred away to expose the blood vessels of cancellous bone.

Split-thickness skin grafts should next be attached securely to the recipient bed. The perimeter is typically secured with sutures or staples while basting sutures are placed centrally. Any overlapping skin will desiccate and drop off, so careful trimming of the STSG edges to fit the recipient bed is unnecessary. The graft can be fenestrated in several places to allow for the drainage of any blood and serum (Fig. 13.11c).

Dressing

Once secured, the graft is then dressed with a non-adhesive dressing such as N-Terface and covered by a pressure dressing or bolster. Suture and staple removal can be performed 7–10 days later.

Donor Site Care

The donor site heals by granulation and usually causes more postoperative pain than the grafted area. Once the skin around the donor site is dried,

an adhesive such as Mastisol is applied around the wound and allowed to dry; an Opsite dressing is placed over the wound (Fig. 13.11d), secured around the perimeter with paper tape, followed by a gauze dressing and Ace wrap. In the first 24 h postoperatively it is common for a large amount of serosanguinous material to accumulate beneath this dressing. This fluid can be aspirated and a new Opsite applied. Donor sites typically take 7–21 days to re-epithelialize and the dressing should remain in place for this period. Other donor site dressings include Xeroform gauze, which was one of the earliest dressings, Adaptec gauze (Johnson and Johnson, New Brunswick, NJ), Jelonet (Smith & Nephew, Montreal, Quebec, Canada), Reston (3 M Health Care, St. Paul, MN), Kaltostat (ConvaTec, Princeton, NJ), Allevyn polymer foam (Smith & Nephew, Largo, FL), and honey.[24]

Benefits of Opsite include decreased donor site pain and improved visualization of the donor site. In addition, the wound is kept moist and healing facilitated.

Postoperative Complications

Early complications, as with FTSGs, include infection, hematoma or seroma formation, and graft movement. Any infection should be cultured and treated with antibiotics. Color mismatch between the STSGs and surrounding skin is common, and STSGs and donor sites often become hypo- and hyperpigmented. Patients should be advised that this commonly occurs and that they should avoid exposure of the graft and donor site to the sun and apply broad-spectrum sunblock to both areas. Dryness of the STSG can be treated with emollients.

The very thinness of STSGs often contributes to a greater tendency to contract and a less cosmetically acceptable outcome. STSG contraction is unpredictable and they should therefore be used with caution near the eyes, oral commissure, and nasal alae. Hypertrophic scarring of the graft and donor site may be treated with intralesional steroids. The donor site often requires postoperative care to granulate and may be painful.

Vacuum-Assisted Closure (VAC)

Subatmospheric pressure dressings, commercially available as the vacuum-assisted device (VAC), have been shown to accelerate wound healing[25–28] (Fig. 13.12a). This has been especially effective in the management of skin grafts on the lower extremities. Consider VAC for the patient with poor distal circulation. The application of a negative pressure to the wound bed through a foam dressing increases dermal perfusion, promotes granulation, removes excess exudate and peri-wound edema, and reduces bacterial count. The ideal pressure setting is negative 125 mmHg on continuous or intermittent pressure. Fluid is connected in a canister and the dressing only needs to be changed every 2 days. Portable VACs are available for ambulant patients. VAC is contraindicated in malignant wounds, untreated osteomyelitis, exposed arteries or veins, or large amounts of necrosis. VAC has significantly increased skin graft take when used as a bolster over the freshly grafted wound (Fig. 13.12b).

Free Cartilage Grafts

The free cartilage graft is a portion of cartilage covered by its perichondrium and typically used for the reconstruction of cosmetic free margins such as the alar rim or lower eyelid.[29] The ear is most commonly used for free cartilage grafts in dermasurgery, and the concha and antihelix are common donor sites. The author's preferred donor site is the posterior conchal bowl, which is easily accessed without distortion of the auricular shape and the donor site scar is easily hidden.

Technique

The donor site is incised; the skin overlying the cartilage is undermined to expose the perichondrial surface of the conchal bowl (Fig. 13.13a); the desired length of cartilage, slightly oversized, is incised as a 2–3-mm wide strip, which is dissected from the anterior skin and placed in sterile saline (Fig. 13.13b); and the donor site is then sutured.

To secure the graft, the soft tissue of the recipient bed is undermined medially and laterally and the graft inserted into the pockets so that it fits snugly (Fig. 13.13c). In addition, the graft may be secured with an absorbable 5-0 suture. Once the graft has been stabilized, a nasolabial flap or FTSG is then placed (Fig. 13.13d).

Dressing

A pressure dressing over the conchal bowl will help minimize the chance of hematoma. The external

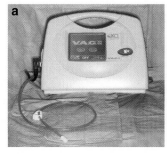
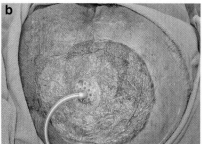

Fig. 13.12 (**a**) A wound VAC. (**b**) a VAC is used as a bolster and will stay in place for a week. Figures reproduced with permission from MacFarlane, D.F.[17]

Fig. 13.13 (a) The postauricular cartilage is exposed. Note the Hypafix tape that is used to hold the ear forward while the graft is obtained. (b) A 2–3 mm wide and slightly oversized strip of cartilage is harvested. (c) The graft is secured in place. Note an FTSG is harvested from the right nasolabial fold. (d) Appearance of the nose 6 months later

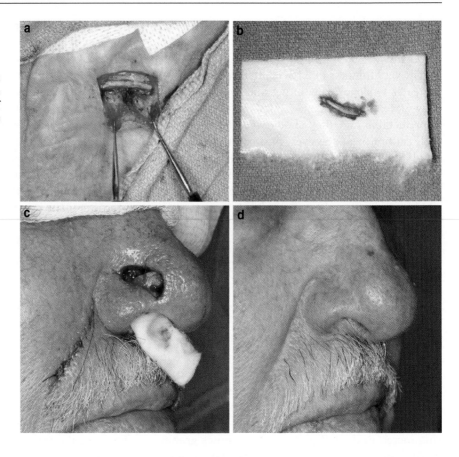

suture line is dressed with antibiotic ointment and covered with an occlusive, nonadherent dressing.

Complications

Donor site complications can include: sterile chondritis, infection, and distortion. Sterile chondritis can be treated with nonsteroidal anti-inflammatory medication. If infection is suspected, broad-spectrum antibiotics (quinolones are commonly used) should be started after cultures have been taken. Complications of free cartilage grafting include infection; hematoma; and graft displacement, distortion, and extrusion.[30]

Composite Grafts

Composite grafts contain tissue from two or more germ layers. In dermatologic surgery they generally consist of skin and cartilage, which are used in the reconstruction of full-thickness defects of the alar rim in addition to nasal tip defects with cartilage loss.[31,32] They may also comprise skin and fat, or skin and perichondrium.[33,34] Composite grafts used to repair full-thickness defects are dependent upon revascularization solely from the wound edges. It is important, therefore, that no portion of such grafts should be more than 1 cm from the vascular source and these grafts are therefore limited in size to 1–2 cm in diameter.[35]

Following graft placement the tissue undergoes a series of changes in appearance. Initially it is white in color, then after about 6 h it becomes pink as graft vessels anastomose with those of the recipient site. Between 12 and 24 h, the tissue becomes blue due to venous congestion and by 3–7 days it becomes pink again, indicating that the graft has survived.[35] Donor sites include the crus, triangular fossa, scapha, conchal cavum, and cymba of the ear, and are usually allowed to heal by secondary intention. Reconstruction of full-thickness nasal defects can be challenging. Due mainly to the presence of cartilage, the auricular chondrocutaneous graft provides structural support and has only a slight tendency to contract.

Technique

The donor and recipient sites should be anesthetized then prepped with chlorhexidine solution. Any granulation tissue should be removed from the recipient site and the edges freshened if the wound has had time to partially heal. A template is then made of the recipient site and placed onto the donor site; the graft is next harvested and placed in sterile saline. The chondrocutaneous graft may be sized to simply fill the defect or especially designed with cartilaginous wings to provide additional stability. If a winged or tongue-in-groove technique is used, then the traced graft is lengthened by several millimeters at each end and the graft including this extra tissue is excised. Once the graft is harvested, the skin is removed from each strut exposing the cartilage. Pockets are made in the alar defect and the graft is then positioned so that the cartilage wings interlock with the recipient bed. The mucosal surface is sutured first with a 6-0 absorbable suture. The skin is closed with 6-0 nonabsorbable sutures, which may be removed in 1 week's time.

Dressing

The author recommends securing the graft with intranasal packing, which can be manufactured from a Xeroform-covered dental roll.

The external suture line is dressed with antibiotic ointment and covered with an occlusive, nonstick dressing.

Donor Sites

Defects of the helical crus may be repaired in linear fashion or with rotation or transposition flaps if necessary. Defects of the helical rim may be excised in wedge fashion and grafts taken from the scapha,

triangular fossa, conchal bowl, or cymba granulate well.

Postoperative Care

Antibiotics are prescribed preoperatively and for a few days following surgery. Ice packs should be applied to the surgical site for the first 3 days. Patients should be advised as to the delicate nature of these grafts and to avoid strenuous activity. They should also be aware that these grafts have a higher rate of failure than other grafts and that multiple revisions are common. Dermabrasion or laser resurfacing may be used at 6 weeks to 6 months to improve the color and/or texture match between the graft and adjacent skin.

Complications

Composite grafts are more prone to necrosis than other graft types.[36] Disadvantages include a higher risk of failure, size limitations, and limited donor sites.

Summary

A thorough knowledge of the various techniques used in skin grafting is essential for successful soft tissue reconstruction. Careful attention to detail and planning should ensure an excellent outcome.

References

1. Hauben DJ, Baruchin A, Mahler D. On the history of the free skin graft. *Ann Plast Surg*. 1982;9:242–246.
2. Converse JM, Uhlschmid GK, Ballantyne DL Jr. 'Plasmatic circulation' on skin grafts: the phase of serum imbibition. *Plast Reconstr Surg*. 1969;43:495–499.
3. Clemmesen T, Ronhovde DA. Restoration of the blood supply to human skin autografts. *Scand J Plast Reconstr Surg*. 1960;2:44–46.
4. Smahel J. The healing of skin grafts. *Clin Plast Surg*. 1977;4:409–424.
5. Fitzgerald MJ, Martin F, Paletta FX. Innervation of skin grafts. *Surg Gynecol Obstet*. 1967;124:808–812.

6. Ratner D. Skin grafting: from here to there. *Dermatol Clin.* 1998;16:75–90.

7. Petruzelli GJ, Johnson JT. Skin grafts. *Otolaryngol Clin North Am.* 1994;27:25–37.

8. Chang LK, Whitaker DC. The impact of herbal medicines on dermatologic surgery. *Dermatol Surg.* 2001;27:759–763.

9. Collins SC, Dufresne RG. Dietary supplements in the setting of Mohs surgery. *Dermatol Surg.* 2002;6:447–452.

10. Goldminz D, Bennett RG. Cigarette smoking and flap and full-thickness graft necrosis. *Arch Dermatol.* 1991;127:1012–1015.

11. Tromovitch TA, Stegman SJ, Glogau RG. *Flaps and grafts in dermatologic surgery.* Vol 49–54. Chicago: Yearbook Medical; 1989:65–67.

12. Field LM. The preauricular site for donor grafts of skin: advantages, disadvantages, and caveats. *J Dermatol Surg Oncol.* 1980;6:40–44.

13. Rohrer TE, Dzubow LM. Conchal bowl grafting in nasal tip reconstruction: clinical and histologic evaluation. *J Am Acad Dermatol.* 1995;33:476–481.

14. Zitelli JA. Burrow's grafts. *J Am Acad Dermatol.* 1987;17:271–279.

15. Karri V, Dheansa B, Moss T. Basal cell carcinoma arising in a split skin graft. *Br J Plast Surg.* 2005;58:276–277.

16. Matheson BK, Mellette JR. Surgical pearls: clavicular grafts are "superior" to supraclavicular grafts. *J Am Acad Dermatol.* 1997;37:991–993.

17. MacFarlane DF. Current techniques in skin grafting. *Adv Dermatol.* 2006;22:125–138.

18. Gingrass P, Grabb WC, Gingrass RP. Skin graft survival on avascular defects. *Plast Reconstr Surg.* 1975;55:65–70.

19. Fader DJ, Wang TS, Johnson TM. Nasal reconstruction utilizing a muscle hinge flap with overlying Full-thickness skin graft. *J Am Acad Dermatol.* 2000;43:837–840.

20. Ceilley RI, Bumsted RM, Panje WR. Delayed skin grafting. *J Dermatol Surg Oncol.* 1983;9:288–293.

21. Thibault MJ, Bennett RG. Success of delayed full-thickness skin grafts after Mohs micrographic surgery. *J Am Acad Dermatol.* 1995;32:1004.

22. Wheeland RG. Skin grafts. In: Roenigk RK, Roegnigk HH, ed. *Dermatologic Surgery: Principles and Practice.* New York: Marcel Decker; 1996:879–896.

23. Sams HH, McDonald MA, Stasko T. Useful adjuncts to harvest split-thickness skin grafts. *Dermatol Surg.* 2004;30(12 Part 2):1591–1592.

24. Misirlioglu A, Eroglu S, Karacaoglan N, et al. Use of honey as an adjunct in the healing of split-thickness skin graft donor site. *Dermatol Surg.* 2003;29:168–172.

25. Argenta LC, Morykwas MJ. Vacuum-assisted closure: a new method for wound control and treatment: clinical experience. *Ann Plast Surg.* 1998;45:332–334.

26. Blackburn JH, Boemi L, Hall WW, et al. Negative-pressure dressings as a bolster for skin grafts. *Ann Plast Surg.* 1998;40:453–457.

27. Scherer L, Shiver S, Chang M, et al. The vacuum assisted closure device: a method of securing skin grafts and improving graft survival. *Arch Surg.* 2002;137:903–904.

28. Venturi ML, Attinger EA, Mesbahi AN, et al. Mechanisms and clinical applications of the vacuum-assisted closure (VAC) device. *Am J Clin Dermatol.* 2005;6:185–194.

29. Byrd D, Otley C, Nguyen T. Alar batten cartilage grafting in nasal reconstruction: functional and cosmetic results. *J Am Acad Dermatol.* 2000;43:833–836.

30. Otley C, Sherris D. Spectrum of cartilage grafting in cutaneous reconstructive surgery. *J Am Acad Dermatol.* 1998;39:982–992.

31. Field LM. Nasal alar rim reconstruction using the crus of the helix, with several alternatives for donor site closure. *J Dermatol Surg Oncol.* 1986;12:253–258.

32. Ratner D, Katz A, Grande DJ. An interlocking auricular composite graft. *Dermatol Surg.* 1995;21:789–792.

33. Love CW, Collison DW, Carithers JS, et al. Perichondrial cutaneous grafts for reconstruction of skin cancer excision defects. *Dermatol Surg.* 1995;21:219–222.

34. Symonds FC, Crikelair GF. Auricular composite grafts in nasal reconstruction; a report of 36 cases. *Plast Reconstr Surg.* 1966;37:433–437.

35. Ruch MK. Utilization of composite free grafts. *J Int Coll Surg.* 1958;30:274–275.

36. McLaughlin C. Composite grafts and their blood supply. *Br J Plast Surg.* 1954;7:274–278.

Chapter 14
Nail Surgery and Malignant Tumors of the Nail Unit

Deborah F. MacFarlane and Richard K. Scher

Since as many as 10% of patients seek dermatologic care for a nail disorder,[1] it is important that dermatologists be comfortable with performing nail surgery. Unfortunately, the diagnosis and treatment of nail tumors may be delayed due to a fear of causing a permanent nail dystrophy from biopsy. It is the intent of this chapter to outline the steps to an approach to nail surgery so that the clinician is able to expose subungual conditions for anatomic delineation, biopsy, or excision with as painless a technique as possible and an acceptable cosmetic outcome. This chapter will conclude with an overview of malignant tumors of the nail unit.

Anatomy

A thorough understanding of nail anatomy is crucial for successful nail surgery and will help to reduce any apprehension the clinician may have in operating on the nail unit. The components of the nail unit include the matrix, proximal and lateral folds, plate, bed, hyponychium, and four grooves—proximal, distal, and two lateral.

The most important structure in the nail unit is the nail matrix, which is found beneath the cuticle and produces the nail plate. The lunula is the distal matrix visible from the nail surface. The proximal portion of the matrix produces the upper portion of the nail plate, while the distal portion of the matrix (lunula) produces the underside of the nail plate. Therefore a distal matrix biopsy is less likely to cause onychodystrophy than a proximal one.[2]

Extreme care must be exercised when performing surgery near the proximal nail matrix. A defect will produce a deformed nail plate surface postoperatively; the split nail is an example of such a defect. The proximal nail fold is a modified extension of the finger that forms a fold over the matrix. It is continuous with the lateral nail fold that forms the side borders of the nail plate. The nail plate extends about 5 mm proximal to the cuticle where it fits into the proximal nail groove, the roof of which is the undersurface of the proximal nail fold; the floor is the matrix. The nail plate fits laterally into the lateral nail grooves formed by the junction of the lateral nail folds to the nail bed. The nail bed begins at the distal portion of the lunula (matrix) and extends distally to terminate at the hyponychium. There is no subcutaneous tissue in the nail unit, and when one is cutting through this structure the underlying periosteum of the distal phalanx may be exposed. The distance from the nail plate surface to the periosteum is only several millimeters (Fig. 14.1). The tendon of extensor digitorum communis crosses the distal interphalangeal joint (DIPJ) to insert onto the proximal dorsal portion of the terminal phalanx at a point approximately 12 mm proximal to the cuticle; incisions should be planned to avoid this area[3]. The blood and nerve supply of the nail unit run approximately the same course. It is important to remember this circulatory and neural pattern when anesthetizing and operating on the nail unit (Table 14.1).

> Vascular supply runs laterally in the finger; therefore, compress any bleeding vessels by applying lateral pressure to the finger and elevating it.

D.F. MacFarlane (ed.), *Skin Cancer Management*, DOI 10.1007/978-0-387-88495-0_14,
© Springer Science+Business Media, LLC 2010

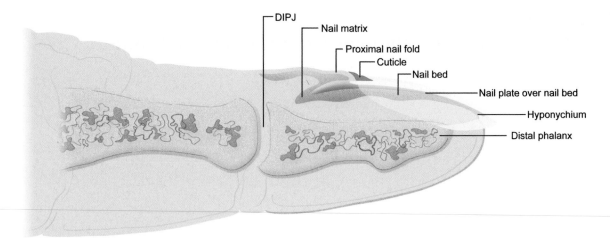

Fig. 14.1 Anatomy of the nail unit

Table 14.1 Anatomic danger areas

Matrix: beneath cuticle, damage to proximal part may cause permanent nail dystrophy
Underlying periosteum: only several millimeters beneath nail plate
Vascular and nerve supply: run laterally
Extensor Digitorum Communis tendon: inserts on proximal part of terminal phalanx, approximately 12 mm proximal to cuticle

Table 14.2 Preoperative considerations prior to nail surgery

Details of illness causing nail dysfunction
Medical history: Peripheral vascular disease, diabetes, connective tissue disease, Raynaud's, arthritis, bleeding diatheses
Previous surgical procedures
Prosthetic joints or heart valves
Drug history: Check for allergies. Monoamine oxidase inhibitors (MAOIs), B-blockers, phenothiazines may affect anesthesia. Aspirin or anticoagulants may prolong bleeding. Systemic or topical steroids may delay healing. Check for use of herbal medicine/vitamins
Anti-tetanus immunization status

Preoperative Considerations

Prior to the surgical procedure, a careful medical history and physical examination will reduce complication risks (Table 14.2). If possible, nail surgery should be avoided in those who have peripheral vascular disease, diabetes mellitus, or connective tissue disorders that compromise circulation. This includes Raynaud's phenomenon, particularly when surgery on the toenails is considered. Details of previous surgical procedures, underlying illness, current medications, and allergies should be elicited. Anesthesia may be affected by monoamine oxidase inhibitors, beta-blockers, or phenothiazines. Anticoagulants, including aspirin, may prolong bleeding. Systemic or topical steroids may delay healing. Anti-tetanus immunization status should be ascertained. The risks, benefits, and alternatives to surgery should be discussed in detail with the patient and consent obtained. Preoperative X-rays should be obtained when the condition is suspected to involve the bony phalanx.[4]

If there is evidence of active infection, elective procedures should be deferred until these are treated with antibiotics and soaks for 2 or more weeks. Nail surgery should be performed only under aseptic conditions. The surgical site should be thoroughly scrubbed with an antiseptic surgical cleanser. Many nail surgeons prefer to administer systemic antimicrobial agents prior to surgery.

Instruments

Several instruments are essential for performing nail surgery (Fig. 14.2). A Freer septum elevator or a dental spatula is useful in separating the nail plate

Fig. 14.2 From *left* to *right*:
dual action nail nipper,
English nail splitter, elevator

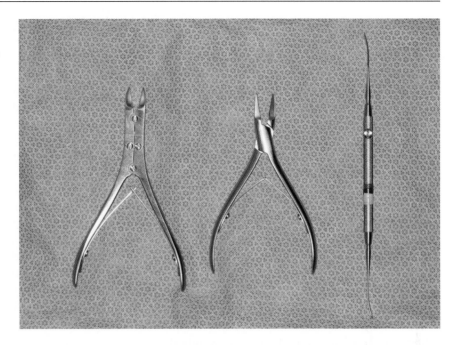

from the nail bed and the proximal nail folds. The
nail splitter is designed for partial longitudinal nail
avulsion, with its smooth lower blade for the nail
bed and a sharp upper blade for cutting through the
nail plate. The nail nipper allows close and accurate
nail cutting in an atraumatic manner. This instrument has a flexible neck that conforms to the
patient's nail and allows simple procedures to be
done painlessly without anesthesia. The ordinary
nail clipper should only be used for routine nail
trimming as it is rigid and requires the patient's
nail to conform to the instrument, often producing
pain.

A nail-pulling forceps is practical for gripping
the plate prior to avulsion once it has been separated from its attachments. A variety of rake retrac-
tors are used to retract the proximal nail fold when
one is performing matrix surgery.

Tourniquet

A Penrose drain secured with a hemostat at the
finger base will provide a safe tourniquet for the
critical 15 min that most operations take. Alternatively, a strip of rubber cut from a glove may be
used.

Radiographs

Preoperative radiographs are suggested when the
condition may possibly involve the bony structure
of the phalanx.

Anesthesia

Provision of adequate anesthesia is *vital* for successful nail surgery. Sedation is usually unnecessary. To
avoid a vasovagal response, patients should be in a
reclining position. The limb should be cleansed well
and a sterile field obtained.

A buffered solution of 1 or 2% lidocaine hydrochloride is most commonly used as a local anesthetic. Mepivacaine hydrochloride, 1 or 2%, has
also been used as an anesthetic. It may be used in
patients sensitive to lidocaine and has the added
advantage of longer action and better hemostasis.

> Bupivacaine can be added at the end of the proce-
> dure if significant postoperative pain is expected.

If a cryogen spray such as 50% ethyl chloride/
50%   dichlorotetrafluoroethane   (Fluro-Ethyl,
Gebauer Company, Cleveland, OH), ethyl chloride,

or fluoroethyl is sprayed for 1–2 s prior to needle insertion, the pain is diminished.

Traditionally, anesthesia of the nail unit has been achieved by the use of a distal or proximal digital nerve block or a combination of both. The authors more commonly use the distal wing block for most surgeries.

> Use distal wing block anesthesia when possible; it is instantaneous and aids hemostasis.

Distal Wing Block

Technique

A 30-gauge needle is used to inject at the junction of the proximal and lateral nail fold (Fig. 14.3a).

Slow infusion will help minimize pain. The injection proceeds distally and inferiorly to include the lateral digital nerve and its branches. The injection then goes across the proximal nail fold to block the transverse nerve branch at this site and then to the other side of the digit. Place each subsequent injection into a previously anesthetized site. Finally, after anesthesia is complete, additional anesthetic may be injected into the tip of the digit, particularly for procedures on the distal portion of the nail unit (Fig. 14.3b).

A sufficient quantity of anesthetic may cause moderate blanching, which aids in hemostasis. Typically between 1.5 and 3 cc of anesthesia are needed.

In the traditional digital block, anesthesia is infused into the lateral digit at the base of the finger and approximately 1 cc of anesthetic is injected into each side of the digit. With either technique the surgeon should wait for approximately 10 min for complete anesthesia. If the patient has a history of peripheral vascular disease, is elderly, or has diabetes mellitus, vasospasm due to excess anesthetic must be avoided. To ensure painless nail surgery, wait 5–10 min before performing the procedure. While anesthesia is performed under clean conditions—the skin prepped with alcohol and clean gloves used—all nail surgery including punch biopsies should be performed under sterile conditions.

Nail Avulsion

Nail avulsion may be necessary to expose the nail bed and matrix in order to perform a matrix biopsy or to excise nail unit tumors. Nail avulsion may be partial or total. The nail plate is attached to the digit at two locations: the nail bed and the proximal nail fold.

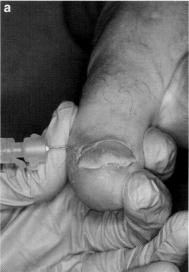 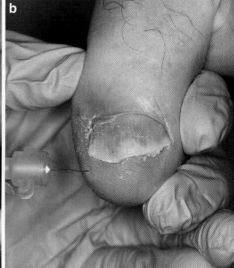

Fig. 14.3 (**a**) Local anesthetic infiltration is commenced at the junction of the proximal and lateral nail fold and then continued across the finger just below the proximal nail fold. (**b**) Additional anesthetic is injected into the digit tip

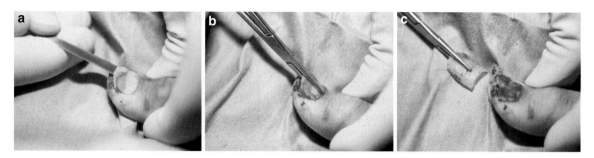

Fig. 14.4 (**a**) Nail elevator is pushed proximally to separate nail plate from nail bed. (**b**) Hemostat is used to grasp nail. (**c**) Nail plate is completely avulsed

Technique

Insert the nail elevator beneath the free edge of the nail and push it proximally (Fig. 14.4a). Resistance will be felt until the matrix is reached; do not push the elevator into the proximal nail grove as this will result in injury. Grasp the nail plate with a hemostat and remove the nail with a circular motion (Fig. 14.4b, c).

Bleeding is minimal and the patient has little discomfort once the anesthetic has worn off.

Repeated avulsion may cause a thickening of the nail plate.

Punch Biopsy of the Nail Bed

Punch biopsy of the nail bed is the most commonly performed procedure on the nail unit. A nail bed biopsy may be performed with or without avulsion of the nail bed. Sometimes partial nail avulsion is sufficient to expose the area.

Technique

To avoid nail avulsion, make a sharp 3-mm punch through the nail plate until the periosteum is met (Fig. 14.5).

It is useful to soak the nail in warm water for 10 min prior to this form of biopsy in order to soften it. Use iris or gradle scissors to recover the specimen.

Forceps are best not used as they can crush the specimen. In the two-punch technique, use a larger punch through the nail plate and a smaller punch through the nail bed. There is generally little

bleeding as the anesthetic bolus tends to compress the arteries in the operative field. A small, temporary focus of onycholysis occasionally may result.

To provide better visualization or to perform a larger nail bed biopsy, the nail may be avulsed. It is useful to score the area to be biopsied first with the punch. Once the exact location has been confirmed, the punch is placed back onto the scored area and twisted until periosteum is hit.

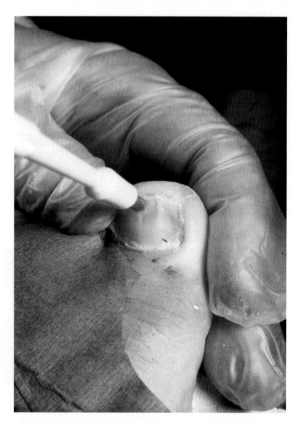

Fig. 14.5 Punch biopsy through nail plate. Photograph courtesy of Richard K. Scher, M.D.

For larger lesions, an elliptical excision can be used. Orient the ellipse longitudinally, no greater than 3-mm wide, and take care to avoid the matrix. After the specimen is removed, 35% aluminum chloride in 50% isopropyl alcohol or oxidized cellulose is applied to the site for hemostasis. Monsel's solution may cause a tattoo effect that can affect pathologic interpretation. Suturing is not necessary since the biopsy site granulates quickly without nail distortion.

Nail Matrix Biopsy

Indications for nail matrix biopsy include longitudinal hyperpigmented streaks in the nail plate, full-length nail plate deformities, and matrix tumors. Nail matrix biopsies are most commonly performed for longitudinal melanonychia, and the various techniques and their indications will be presented. Be aware that permanent nail dystrophy is much less likely to occur with 3-mm punch biopsies of the distal matrix. The proximal matrix is more susceptible to scarring and the development of a split nail even with a 3-mm punch.

Punch Biopsy of the Nail Matrix

Indications

Pigmented bands less than 3-mm wide originating in the distal matrix.

Technique

Perform anesthesia as previously described. If a Hutchinson's sign is present, a shave biopsy of the sliver of pigmented tissue can be performed.

> Always reflect the proximal nail fold for nail matrix biopsies for melanonychia.

In this technique, an elevator is first used to loosen the attachment of the proximal nail fold to the underlying nail plate (Fig. 14.6b). The proximal nail fold is then reflected to expose the matrix (Fig. 14.6c).

The site of origin of the pigmented band is identified in the matrix. In order to position the biopsy

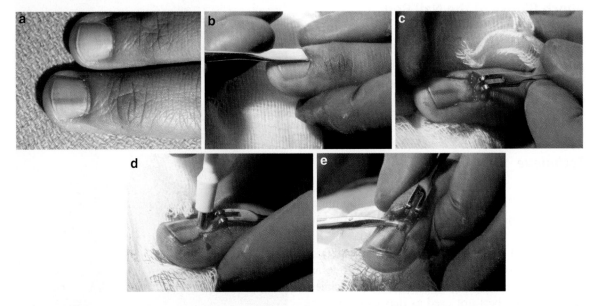

Fig. 14.6 (a) Longitudinal melanonychia striatum in the nail plate of the middle finger. (b) An elevator is used to loosen the attachment of the proximal nail fold to the underlying nail plate. (c) The proximal nail fold is reflected to expose the matrix. (d) A 3-mm punch is used to biopsy through the nail plate and through the matrix down to the underlying periosteum. (e) The biopsied nail matrix is then sent to pathology. Photographs courtesy of Richard K. Scher, M.D.

accurately, mark the proximal nail fold in line with the lesion. A 3-mm punch is used to score the overlying nail plate and then carried through matrix down to bone (Fig. 14.6d).

The specimen is then obtained as previously. Examine the punch to make sure that the nail plate is not still in it, and send to pathology as it may contain melanocytic pigmentation, blood, or even fungi.[5] The proximal nail fold may be repaired with sutures.

Lateral Longitudinal Excision

Indication

For laterally located longitudinal melanonychia (LM).

Technique

The digit is soaked in antiseptic solution to soften the nail plate. A #15 scalpel blade is inserted half way between the cuticle and the distal interphalangeal crease, 1–2-mm medial to the pigmented band, and an incision is performed through the skin and soft tissue down to bone extending through the nail plate distally to the hyponychium and then 3–4 mm distally onto the tip of the digit. The blade is then inserted in the starting point and moved laterally around the matrix horn into the nail sulcus, curving medially at the hyponychium to meet the end of the first incision. The specimen is thus an ellipse with narrow margins taken around the pigmented band and the laterally located matrix horn included. The lateral matrix pocket can be debrided with a curette to remove any residual matrix fragments, which could cause postoperative spicules, cysts, or pain.

Repair

The lateral nail wall may be repaired with 4-0 nylon and a half-buried horizontal mattress suture can be placed from the lateral nail fold through the nail plate to help stabilize the tissue. A request for longitudinal sectioning should be specified on the pathology slip.

Complications

Debridement of the lateral matrix pocket does increase the possibility of periostitis and postoperative pain.[6,7]

Shave Biopsy of the Nail Matrix (Tangential Matrix Excision)

This technique was originally described by Baran and Haneke in 2001.[5]

Indications

LM originating in the proximal matrix; LM greater than 3-mm wide in the mid-nail plate.

Shave biopsy may not provide accurate Breslow depth for invasive melanoma.

Contraindications

Those situations where clinical suspicion is high for invasive melanoma.

Technique

Reflect the nail fold to visualize the matrix. Use a nail splitter to cut the nail transversally at the level of the lunula border. Reflect the proximal part of the plate and reflect to one side like a hinge. Identify the origin of the pigmented band and score with 1–2-mm margins using a #15 blade; then turn the blade horizontally so that it is parallel to the matrix surface to shave the scored specimen. Place the specimen upside down on some wet filter paper and transfer to the formalin jar.

Some advocate longitudinal trimming of the lateral plate by 2–3 mm to avoid postoperative edema.[8]

Lay the reflected plate back over the matrix and repair with a mattress suture. Suture the proximal nail fold. Sutures may be removed at 7–10 days.

En Bloc Nail Unit Biopsy

This is a biopsy of the entire nail unit and involves removal of a tissue wedge that includes the nail fold, matrix, bed, and hyponychium. This may be used to diagnose and treat neoplastic processes.

Technique

Obtain anesthesia as previously described. Using a #15 scalpel, make two parallel incisions no more than 3 mm apart from the proximal nail fold to the finger tip. To prevent marked scarring, the blade is gently slid over the bony phalanx and the specimen dissected out with a pair of iris scissors. Sutures are unnecessary and may distort the normal nail shape. Alternatively, the nail can be avulsed, the specimen excised, then the edges undermined; and the proximal nail fold, matrix, and hyponychium repaired with fine sutures.

Dressings

To obtain hemostasis: gelatin sponges or collagen matrix sponges are useful. For minor surgical procedures: cleanse with dilute hydrogen peroxide, and apply an antibiotic ointment and a simple adhesive dressing, which is changed daily. For more extensive procedures: cleanse with dilute hydrogen peroxide or chlorhexidine solution. Dress with antibiotic ointment. Vaseline gauze is especially useful in more extensive nail surgery because it keeps the wound moist and can be easily removed. This can be covered with a layer of Telfa, and this in turn can be secured by the longitudinal placement of surgical tape (Table 14.3).

> The finger should never be wrapped circumferentially, as this may produce vasoconstriction, edema, and vascular compromise.

Table 14.3 Dressings

Cleanse area with dilute hydrogen peroxide of chlorhexidine
Apply antibiotic ointment
Cover with Vaseline gauze and then layer of Telfa secured with paper tape
Outer dressing may include surgical tape placed in longitudinal fashion
Surgitube may be used to make a protective, bulky dressing
Sling, Reese, or Zimmer boot immobilize and protect

Several layers of Surgitube dressing may then be applied and secured. Bulky dressings will absorb external trauma and reduce excessive movement. Where appropriate, use of a sling or orthopedic boot may provide additional protection and immobilization. The patient should be instructed to keep the arm elevated as much as possible and to avoid using this hand. If unusual pain, edema, throbbing, or bluish discoloration is noted, the dressing should be removed at once and the surgeon contacted immediately.

Complications

Complications are uncommon in nail surgery. These may include hematoma, infection, and nail deformity. Postoperative infection in the distal phalanx may cause superficial infection, acute purulent tenosynovitis, osteomyelitis, and septic arthritis. When infection occurs, culture the organism and treat with appropriate antibiotics and soaks. Most complications of nail surgery may be avoided by paying careful attention to sterile technique and gently handling the tissue, in particular the germinal matrix.

Malignant Tumors of the Nail Unit

The clinical appearance of the nail unit may be similar for injury, infection, benign, and malignant neoplasms. A brief overview of malignant tumors of the nail will follow. Please note that discussion of treatment will refer to surgical options. Some nail tumors including verrucae may be amenable to topical and intralesional treatment. For further discussion of these modalities see Chapters 2 and 5.

Verrucae

Although it is rare that a verruca may transform into a squamous cell cancer, the clinical appearance may be similar for the two. Various case reports exist of SCC either treated as verrucae or left untreated for long periods of time.[9,10]

Any lesion on the nail unit that does not respond appropriately to treatment, is long-standing, or has an unusual presentation should be biopsied.

Bowen's Disease

Bowen's disease, or squamous cell carcinoma in situ, is an uncommon condition and usually seen on the thumb, index, and middle fingers of men older than 60 years. It can occur in both a periungual and ungual location and primarily affects nail folds with potential extension into the rest of the nail unit. Primary involvement of the nail bed is rare.[11] Bowen's disease of the nail is human papillomavirus (HPV)-associated in 60% of cases[12] and exposure to radiation, chemicals, and arsenic ingestion have also been implicated.[13] Patients with epidermodysplasia verruciformis and dyskeratosis congenita are at increased risk.[12] This is a low-grade malignancy with moderate potential for recurrence and low potential for metastasis.

Treatment

Mohs surgery has been reported to have a recurrence rate of 33%; therefore some authors suggest an additional surgical margin.[12] Photodynamic therapy (PDT) has been successfully used.[14,15]

Follow-up to check for recurrence is essential and one should examine all 20 digits and perform a lymph node exam. The anogenital area should also be examined and female patients should be monitored for cervical cancer.[16]

Squamous Cell Cancer

Squamous cell cancer is the most common malignant tumor of the nail unit.[17] It occurs most commonly in men after the fifth decade on the thumb and index finger and, rarely, on the toes[18] (Fig. 14.7). SCC may arise in any part of the nail unit however. As this entity is often slow growing with subtle clinical findings, it can therefore be misdiagnosed as onychomycosis, onycholysis, verruca, nail deformity, subungual exostosis, chronic osteomyelitis, paronychia, or onychogryphosis.[19–21] Unresponsiveness to treatment, bleeding, and ulceration should raise suspicion.[22] Metastasis is rare. Risk factors are similar to those for Bowen's disease. Subungual SCC may involve the bone in 18–60% of patients[23] and it is important to obtain an X-ray prior to surgery.

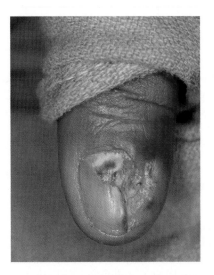

Fig. 14.7 A 45-year-old Hispanic male presented with a 2-year history of a lesion on the left thumbnail, which had been treated with over-the-counter antifungal creams. Biopsy confirmed SCC and the patient underwent Mohs surgery

Fig. 14.8 (a) A 47-year-old female with a 1-year history of a suspected wart on the right ring finger. Biopsy confirmed SCC and Mohs surgery was performed. (b) Appearance 6 months following surgery

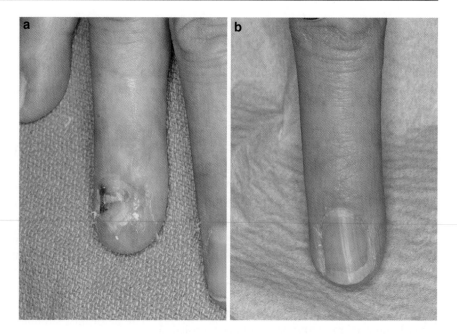

Treatment

The treatment of choice is Mohs surgery with cure rates of 92–96%[24] (Fig. 14.8a, b).

Amputation at the interphalangeal joint proximal to bone invasion is recommended for SCC with bony involvement.[25] Long-term follow-up is important as late metastasis has been reported.[18]

> Obtain an X-ray prior to surgery on SCC involving the nail unit.

Due to the common histology between a keratoacanthoma and a well-differentiated SCC, both authors feel that a subungual keratoacanthoma should be treated surgically.

Verrucous Carcinoma

This rare subtype of SCC may mimic a verruca clinically and histologically. Involvement of the nail unit is extremely rare.[26] This may transform to high-grade SCC following radiation, and may cause local destruction and can potentially metastasize.[27] Osseous involvement has been observed in 10% of cases.[28]

Treatment

Mohs surgery is recommended if there is no osseous involvement.[18] Amputation or disarticulation has been the most commonly used forms of treatment.[26]

Basal Cell Carcinoma

Basal cell carcinoma (BCC) of the nail unit is rare and has a wide variety of presentations—infectious, inflammatory, and neoplastic.[29]

Treatment

There have been no reports of metastases and Mohs surgery is recommended for treatment.[29]

Metastatic Tumors

Subungual tumors are most often due to an extension from a bony metastasis.[30] Primary tumors of the lung account for the majority of subungual metastases (41%), followed by tumors of the genitourinary system (17%) and breast (9%).[30] These typically cause pain due to their rapid growth. An X-ray will often show radiologic changes.

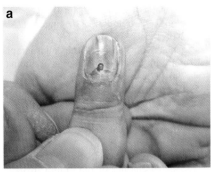
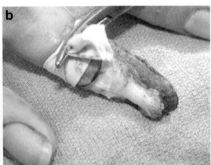

Fig. 14.9 (**a**)Appearance of the nail in an Asian female who presented with a biopsy-proven melanoma in situ. Given the clinical appearance, which was suspicious for invasive melanoma, the case was referred to melanoma surgery. (**b**) Following intraoperative lymphatic mapping and sentinel lymph biopsies (negative), an initial 5-mm margin was taken and sent for rapid pathologic interpretation, which confirmed an acral lentiginous melanoma 0.85-mm Breslow depth. A complex 1-cm wide excision was performed and this photo was taken prior to amputation of the distal phalanx. The finger tip was later repaired

Treatment

These lesions have a very poor prognosis, and treatment includes systemic therapy or radiation.[30]

Melanoma

Melanomas are more commonly seen in non-Caucasians in their 5th–7th decades, and occur most commonly on the thumb and great toenail where they usually presents as longitudinal melanonychia.[31] Hutchinson's sign, where the pigment extends onto the cuticle and proximal nail fold, may be present. This sign is certainly not diagnostic and in one series of melanoma in situ, Hutchinson's sign was observed in only four of seven patients.[32] Melanoma may account for as much as 25% of the cutaneous melanomas seen in non-Caucasians[31] and only 2–3% of cutaneous melanomas seen in Caucasians.[33] Up to a third of nail unit melanomas are amelanotic.[31]

The presence of a pigmented streak greater than 3-mm wide with color variation and proximal widening in any patient warrants a diagnostic nail biopsy including the nail matrix.[34]

Treatment

The treatment of melanoma in situ is surgery, and Mohs surgery is able to provide margin control without amputation.[32,35,36]

Invasive melanoma requires surgery and often distal amputation (Fig. 14.9a, b). The use of sentinel lymph node biopsy for nail unit melanomas is based on the same criteria for melanomas elsewhere in the body. Advanced disease is treated with chemotherapy or immunotherapy.[37]

Summary

For a variety of reasons discussed, the diagnosis of malignancy in the nail may be difficult and/or delayed. Practitioners, however, should have a very low threshold for performing biopsies on those tumors that have failed to respond to treatment or where malignancy is suspected.

References

1. Scher RK. The nail. In: Roenigk RK, Roenigk HH, eds. *Dermatologic Surgery Principles and Practice*. 2nd ed. New York, NY: Marcel Dekker Inc; 1996:389–400.
2. Krull EA. Longitudinal melanonychia. In: Krull EA, Zook EG, Baran R, et al., eds. *Nail Surgery: A Text and Atlas*. Philadelphia: Lippincott Williams & Wilkins; 2001:239–274.
3. MacFarlane DF, Scher RK. Nail Surgery. In: Ratz JL, ed. *Textbook of Dermatologic Surgery*. Philadelphia: Lippincott-Raven Publishers; 1998:621–629.
4. MacFarlane DF, Scher RK. Nail Surgery. In: Nouri K, ed. *Techniques in Dermatologic Surgery*. St. Louis Mosby Elsevier Ltd 2003, 195–201.

5. Haneke E, Baran R. Longitudinal melanonychia. *Dermatol Surg.* 2001 June;27(6):580–584.

6. Moossavi M, Scher RK. Complications of nail surgery: a review of the literature. *Dermatol Surg.* 2001;27:225–228.

7. De Berker DA, Baran R. Acquired malalignment: a complication of lateral longitudinal nail biopsy. *Australas J Dermatol.* 2001;42:142–144.

8. Jellinek N. Nail matrix biopsy of longitudinal melanonychia: diagnostic algorithm including the matrix shave biopsy. *J Am Acad Dermatol.* May 2007;56:803–810.

9. Robinette JW, Day F 3rd, Hahn P Jr. Subungual squamous cell carcinoma mistaken for a verruca. *J Am Podiatr Med Assoc.* 1999;89:435–437.

10. Fleckman P, Bernstein G, Barker E. Squamous cell carcinoma of the nail bed treated as chronic paronychia and wart for fourteen years. *Cutis.* 1985;36:189–191.

11. Mirza B, Muir JB. Bowen's disease of the nail bed. *Australas J Dermatol.* 2004;45:232–233.

12. Sau P, McMarlin SL, Sperling LC, et al. Bowen's disease of the nail bed and periungual area. A clinicopathologic analysis of seven cases. *Arch Dermatol.* 1994;130:204–209.

13. Ongenae K, Van De Kerckhove M, Naeyaert JM. Bowen's disease of the nail. *Dermatology.* 2002;204:348–350.

14. Usmani N, Stables GI, Telfer NR, et al. Subungual Bowen's disease treated by topical aminolevulinic acid-photodynamic therapy. *J Am Acad Dermatol.* 2005;53: S273–S276.

15. Tan B, Sinclair R, Foley P. Photodynamic therapy for subungual Bowen's disease. *Australas J Dermatol.* 2004; 45(3):172–174.

16. Kaiser JF, Proctor-Shipman L. Squamous cell carcinoma in situ (Bowen's disease) mimicking subungual verruca vulgaris. *J Fam Pract.* 1994;39:384–387.

17. Kovich OI, Scher RK. Tumors of the nail unit. In: Nouri K, ed. *Skin Cancer.* New York, NY: McGraw Hill Medical; 2008:264–276.

18. Virgili A, Rosaria Zampino M, Bacilieri S, et al. Squamous cell carcinoma of the nail bed: a rare disease or only misdiagnosed? *Acta Derm Venereol.* 2001;81: 306–307.

19. Dominguez-Cherit J, Garcia C, Vega-Mernije ME, et al. Pseudofibro-keratoma: an unusual presentation of subungual squamous cell carcinoma in a young girl. *Dermatol Surg.* 2003;29:788–789.

20. Obiamiwe PE, Gaze NR. Subungual squamous cell carcinoma. *Br J Plast Surg.* 2001;54:631–632.

21. Figus A, Kanitkar S, Elliot D. Squamous cell carcinoma of the lateral nail fold. *J Hand Surg.* 2006;31B:216–220.

22. Yip KM, Lam SL, Shee BW, et al. Subungual squamous cell carcinoma: report of two cases. *J Formos Med Assoc.* 2000;99:646–649.

23. Bui-Mansfield LT, Pulcini JP, Rose S. Subungual squamous cell carcinoma of the finger. *AJR Am J Roentgenol.* 2005;185:174–175.

24. Zaiac MN, Weiss E. Mohs micrographic surgery of the nail unit and squamous cell carcinoma. *Dermatol Surg.* 2001;27:246–251.

25. Peterson SR, Layton EG, Joseph AK. Squamous cell carcinoma of the nail unit with evidence of bony involvement: a multidisciplinary approach to resection and reconstruction. *Dermatol Surg.* 2004;30: 218–221.

26. Sheen MC, Sheen YS, Sheu HM, et al. Subungual verrucous carcinoma of the thumb treated by intra-arterial infusion with methotrexate. *Dermatol Surg.* 2005;31; 787–789.

27. Dobson CM, Azurdia RM, King CM. Squamous cell carcinoma arising in a psoriatic nail bed: a case report with discussion of diagnostic difficulties and therapeutic options. *Br J Dermatol.* 2003;148:1077–1078.

28. Tosti A, Morelli R, Fanti PA, Morselli PG. Carcinoma cuniculatum of the nail apparatus: report of three cases. *Dermatology.* 1993;186:217–221.

29. Martinelli PT, Cohen PR, Schulze KE, et al. Periungual basal cell carcinoma: case report and literature review. *Dermatol Surg.* 2006;32:320–323.

30. Cohen PR. Metastatic tumors to the nail unit: subungual metastases. *Dermatol Surg.* 2001;27:280–293.

31. Thai KE, Young R, Sincalir RD. Nail apparatus melanoma. *Australas J Dermatol.* 2001;42(2):71–81.

32. High WA, Quirey RA, Guillen DR, et al. Presentation, histopathologic findings and clinical outcomes in 7 cases of melanoma in situ of the nail unit. *Arch Dermatol.* 2004;140:1102–1106.

33. de Georgi V, Sante M, Carelli G, et al. Subungual melanoma: an insidious erythematous nodule on the nail bed. *Arch Dermatol.* 2005;141:398–399.

34. Levit EK, Kagen MH, Scher RK et al. The ABC rule for detection of subungual melanoma. *J Am Acad Dermatol.* 2000;42:269–274.

35. Brodland DG. The treatment of nail apparatus melanoma with Mohs micrographic surgery. *Dermatol Surg.* 2001;27:269–273.

36. Banfield CC, Dawber RP, Walker NP, et al. Mohs micrographic surgery for the treatment of in situ nail apparatus melanoma: a case report. *J Am Acad Dermatol.* 1999;40:98–99.

37. O'Leary JA, Berend KR, Johnson JL, et al. Subungual melanoma: a review of 93 cases with identification of prognostic variables. *Clin Orthop Relat Res.* 2000;378: 206–212.

Chapter 15
Practical Management of Melanoma

Mark F. Naylor

Melanoma incidence continues to rise at an alarming rate. More than 62,000 new cases and over 8,000 deaths were predicted for 2008 in the United States.[1] Today, approximately one out of every six cancer survivors is a melanoma survivor.[1] This chapter presents a broad and practical approach to the subject of treating a patient with suspected or proven melanoma.

Medical History

A thorough history should be taken from the patient with a suspected melanoma. This should focus upon established risk factors for the development of melanoma including a personal or family history of melanoma, skin type I or II, a childhood history of sunburns, the presence of large numbers of melanocytic nevi, atypical nevi, the presence of congenital nevi, extensive use of sun beds, extensive history of sunburns or sun exposure, or genetic syndromes associated with a melanoma predisposition.

A detailed history of the lesion should be obtained. How long has the lesion been present? Was the lesion present at birth? Did the lesion arise in a preexisting mole? Was there a change in shape, size, or color? Did the lesion ulcerate or bleed? Has the lesion enlarged in the last 6 months? A systems review also should be performed checking for the presence of night sweats, fatigue, weight loss, change in bowel habit, cough, shortness of breath, headache, unusual pain, or any recent symptom, particularly if it is persistent or worsening.

Physical Examination

A complete physical examination should be performed, including a skin examination of the whole body with examination of the mucous membranes and scalp. The "ABCD" mnemonic has been found to increase sensitivity when performed by individuals who have been trained in the technique, with "E" for "evolving" (enlargement) being added more recently.[2,3] Those lesions that are suspicious but do not meet the clinical criteria for melanoma may be biopsied, photographed or diagramed, and followed up. If the lesion is at all morphologically suspicious, biopsy is usually the wiser course. A lymph node exam should be routinely performed.

Imaging and Laboratory Tests

In Vivo Imaging

In vivo imaging in the clinic can be useful in the diagnosis of melanoma. Traditional oil/glass or polarized light dermoscopy are particularly cost-effective aids in deciding whether or not to perform an excisional biopsy. One or more dermoscopic features suggestive of melanoma would influence the decision toward biopsy.[4]

Radiologic Imaging

Imaging has limited value in the initial workup of patients with primary cutaneous melanomas with a

D.F. MacFarlane (ed.), *Skin Cancer Management*, DOI 10.1007/978-0-387-88495-0_15,
© Springer Science+Business Media, LLC 2010

thickness of 4 mm or less.[5] In a study of 876 patients who were asymptomatic and with localized melanomas who underwent chest radiography, an unsuspected metastasis was found in only one patient.[6] More recent studies support the idea that chest X-rays are not a useful screening tool.[7] However, some physicians will obtain a baseline chest X-ray for later comparison if one has not been done in the last 3 years, since chest X-rays are a relatively cheap and safe way to follow the progress of known pulmonary involvement.

The work up of patients with suspected stage III/IV melanoma may include magnetic resonance imaging (MRI) of the brain with contrast and extracranial imaging with positron-emission tomography/computed tomography (PET/CT) or CT with contrast.[7,8] Please see Chapter 18 for a discussion of the strengths and limitations of these modalities. Fine needle aspiration (FNA) is used in the cytological diagnosis of melanoma metastases and may be used in combination with ultrasound, CT, or PET/CT (see Chapter 18).

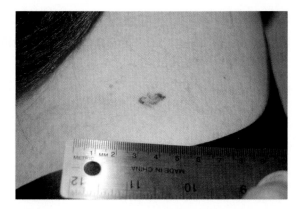

Fig. 15.1 Stage 0. The macular character and variations in color are apparent in this melanoma in situ on a patient's neck

Laboratory Investigations

Similarly, bloodwork is of limited value in the initial workup of asymptomatic patients with primary melanomas 4 mm or less in thickness.[5] However, some physicians will obtain baseline general laboratory tests against which changes can be measured in the future. In patients with melanomas larger than 4 mm, general blood chemistries, including lactate dehydrogenase (LDH) are routinely ordered. LDH is usually elevated when a significant mass of metastatic melanoma is present, and is now included as a prognostic parameter in stage IV melanoma patients.[8]

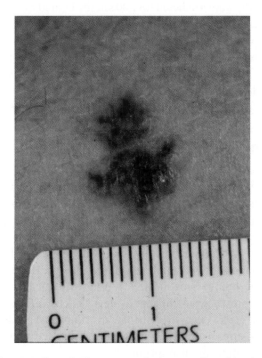

Fig. 15.2 Stage I. The asymmetric shape, scalloped borders, and variety of colors typical of a superficial spreading melanoma are seen on this patient's shoulder

Staging of Melanoma

Management of melanoma is dependent on staging. Stage 0 lesions are in situ (pre-invasive) (Fig. 15.1); stage I lesions are low risk,[a] thin primaries (Fig. 15.2);

stage II lesions are higher risk, thicker primaries (Fig. 15.3); stage III refers to regionally metastatic melanoma, and stage IV refers to spread of melanoma beyond the regional lymph nodes (Fig. 15.4). For details of staging melanoma, refer to Balch et al.[8]

---

[a] Referring to risk of progression or recurrence.

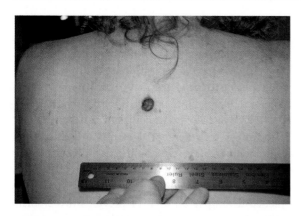

Fig. 15.3 Stage II. A nodular melanoma is apparent on the back of this middle-aged male

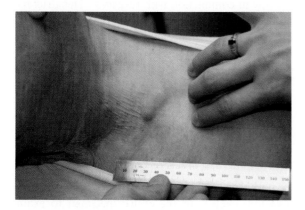

Fig. 15.4 Stage IV. This 72-year-old male had an occular primary, hepatic, and dermal metastases

Management of Melanoma In Situ (Stage 0)

In situ melanoma (MIS), also known as lentigo maligna, Hutchinson's melanotic freckle, or simply Hutchinson's freckle, is a locally aggressive tumor with a much better prognosis than invasive melanoma. Fatalities do not normally occur unless it transforms into an invasive melanoma. Although growth of MIS is usually slow, it can spread laterally at an impressive rate, as much a 1.0 mm per month or more.[b] Most cases will produce a measurable increase in diameter in a 6-month period.[2] MIS always has the potential to become invasive, particularly if left untreated for

[b] Personal observation.

many years, and perhaps more so if there is significant ongoing sun exposure to induce a transforming genetic event. The lateral spread of these lesions can be quite extensive, and lesions can be many centimeters in extent. This makes it technically and esthetically difficult to obtain and examine the entire primary tumor pathologically. An important guiding principal when dealing with suspected stage 0 lesions is to try and exclude invasive melanoma. For this reason it is best to obtain the entire lesion as an excisional biopsy with at least 1–2-mm margins of clinically normal skin for pathological evaluation, or with very large lesions, to biopsy several areas within the lesion that are the most suspicious for invasive melanoma.

In situations where a simple excisional biopsy is technically difficult (a very large lesion extending several centimeters), or when the resulting scarring may be unacceptable to the patient and consideration is being given to non-surgical therapy with imiquimod,[9] suspected MIS can be biopsied using an incisional or punch technique (see Chapter 1). With either technique it is imperative to try and biopsy the area most clinically suspicious for invasive melanoma; usually the thickest, or for flat lesions, the darkest areas as determined visually, or by dermoscopy or confocal microscopy, if available. While there are disadvantages to these techniques, the most notable being sampling error, advantages are that a full thickness specimen is obtained, and the pathologist is directed, by virtue of the limited area of the specimen, to the location the clinician considers most clinically suspicious. If using the punch technique, it is a good idea with an extensive lesion to sample the two or three most suspicious areas within the lesion to further reduce the possibility of missing an invasive melanoma. The small defect created by a 2-mm punch makes it easier to obtain multiple samples without producing cosmetically undesirable defects.

Excision of Melanoma In Situ

The National Institutes of Health (NIH) consensus called for 5-mm margins for MIS, which generally makes it possible to excise and primarily close lesions up to 1.5–2.0 cm.[10] Because local control is an issue when treating MIS, it is important to obtain good histological evaluation of the surgical margins of the specimen. Special stains for melanoma such as HMB 45, or Mart-1 are useful to identify individual melanoma cells and thus enhance the accuracy of pathological evaluation of the margins.

If removal with a 5-mm margin is difficult, or the scarring may be unacceptable (such as on a young adult's face), a narrower margin can be accepted. In theory, as long as the margins are clear, a very narrow margin is acceptable. In practice, even a 5-mm margin may not prevent recurrence, and so additional measures may be required to achieve an acceptable recurrence rate.

Mohs Surgery and Serial Excision of Melanoma In Situ

The standard surgical treatment of melanoma is wide local excision. However, Mohs surgery has been used to treat lentigo maligna and lentigo maligna melanoma in anatomically important areas.[11–14] MIS may also be managed using staged surgical excision.[16,17]

For a more detailed discussion of the Mohs technique refer to Chapter 11.

Medical Treatment of Melanoma In Situ (Stage 0)

A recent advance for treating MIS is imiquimod, a TLR receptor agonist that can be used to stimulate immune responses against melanoma. The topical 5% cream has been used as a monotherapy for treating these lesions.[9,18–20] A clearance rate of around 90% can be achieved with use of this drug.[9] However, it is important that patients realize that this is a non-FDA approved use of the drug and that surgery, the standard of care, is still the most reliable means of therapy in the absence of evidence to the contrary. Imiquimod does, however, offer a reasonable alternative if surgery is problematic.

Imiquimod cream is applied to the area of the MIS and for 5–10 mm beyond the visible border for a period of 2–3 months. Frequency of application can be adjusted depending on the severity of the inflammatory response and the tolerance of the patient. It is generally advisable to try and achieve a visible degree of erythema in and around the tumor. Daily application may not be tolerated by some individuals as local side effects can be considerable at this frequency. Three times a week application appears to be as effective as daily, usually with better tolerance.[c] Duration of treatment of less than 6 weeks is not recommended since relapses are more likely.[d] Fewer relapses are seen with treatment for 3 months or longer. After the completion of therapy it is good practice to biopsy an area of previous involvement and look for any persistence of lesion using special stains for melanoma such as Mart-1.

Imiquimod has also been used as an adjunctive therapy in conjunction with surgery.[21] This drug has been applied preoperatively to reduce large lesions to a more surgically manageable size,[22] or to treat the primary tumor site postoperatively with the aim to reduce recurrence rates.[e]

Challenges of Melanoma In Situ Management

A pathologist may miss a small area of early invasion, even with the entire specimen to examine.[22,23] Variations in appearance in different areas of the same tumor, not infrequently combined with a disconnect between morphology and clinical behavior, lead to pathological misdiagnosis of in situ melanomas, even with the best dermatopathologists. Given the difficulty of making this diagnosis pathologically, it is good practice to follow patients considered for this diagnosis, even in the face of a negative biopsy. In situations where the pathology belies the clinical aggressiveness of the tumor, the only way to make the correct diagnosis is to observe a growth rate or other clinical behavior that is inconsistent with a benign lentigo. Patients with MIS, treated with any method should have regular follow-up to look for recurrences and/or new primary lesions.

---

[c] Personal observation.

[d] Personal observation.

[e] Personal observation.

Management of Primary Melanoma (Stages I and II)

Surgical Management: Excisional Biopsy

The first step in the management of a clinically suspected invasive melanoma is the excisional biopsy. As discussed previously, the excisional biopsy is an attempt to completely remove the entire tumor with narrow margins. This provides the pathologist with a complete specimen for adequate diagnostic evaluation. The pathologist must establish the diagnosis, the maximum thickness of the tumor, and the presence of other factors that may influence staging or clinical decision making, such as the presence of ulceration, mitotic rate, and vascular proliferation, and/or angiolymphatic invasion at the tumor base. Ulceration, which for staging purposes is determined microscopically, will usually upstage a lesion of a given thickness.[8]

Surgicial Management: Incisional Biopsy

For larger lesions, or those that will be technically or esthetically difficult to remove as a complete specimen, it is reasonable to perform a non-excisional biopsy (such as a punch or an incisional biopsy) to first establish the diagnosis. For stage I melanoma, there is evidence to indicate that as long as an incisional biopsy is done within a month or so of the definitive excisional procedure, it does not affect prognosis.[24–26] A downside to an incisional biopsy is that the pathologist is not presented with the primary tumor as a contiguous specimen, which can potentially create difficulties in establishing the diagnosis, the maximum tumor thickness, or other important histological features of prognostic significance.[24]

Definitive Excision of Primary Melanoma

The second aspect of the initial surgical treatment of suspected primary melanoma is the definitive excision. This two-stage excision approach does not adversely affect survival, and one study suggested that it actually enhances it, although this may have been due to selection bias.[27]

Concern has been expressed that a definitive excision performed prior to a sentinel node biopsy may alter the lymphatic drainage from the primary tumor site, making the information from that sentinel node biopsy less reliable.[28] The evidence suggests that a previous wide local excision (WLE) does not appear to adversely affect the ability to detect lymphatic metastases, although the utility of lymphatic mapping and sentinel lymph node biopsy (LM/SLNB) in patients who have undergone extensive reconstruction of the primary excision site is yet to be defined.[28] However, these same authors strongly recommend that, whenever possible, patients undergo concomitant WLE and LM/SLNB as this provides the patient with a single operation for the best opportunity for lymph node staging and avoids the costs and potential-associated morbidity of two surgical procedures.[28]

The NIH consensus conference of 1992 called for a 1.0-cm margin for primary melanomas less than 1.0 mm in thickness.[10] The evidence suggests that a 1.0-cm margin may also be effective for lesions up to 2 mm in thickness.[29] In general, margins between 1.0 and 2.0 cm are commonly used for lesions between 2 and 4 mm in thickness. A 2.0-cm margin may be most appropriate for melanomas 4 mm or more in thickness.[30,31] Margins greater than 2.0 cm do not appear to contribute significantly either to survival or local control.[31,32] Margins of excision are also dictated by surgically challenging anatomical areas, such as the face for instance, and it is realized that in some areas, the NIH margins are guidelines. Heroic margins of 5.0 cm or more certainly do not contribute to overall survival and should therefore be avoided unless other considerations indicate such a procedure.[33,34] Local recurrences that occur beyond 2.0 cm—so-called "satellite metastases" or "local metastases"—may actually represent in transit metastases, and are already associated with a worse prognosis at the time of surgery than true localized stage I or II melanoma.[35,36]

It has been common practice among some surgeons to excise all primary melanomas to the level of, but not including, the underlying muscle fascia. However, unlike margins, the importance of depth has not been studied in a randomized trial and excisions to the muscle fascia may not always be necessary.[37,38]

Surgical Management of Regional Melanoma (Stage III)

Some of the most important advances in the surgical management of melanoma have occurred in the areas of lymphatic mapping and sentinel lymph node biopsy. Salient points of this extensive body of work are outlined as follows.

Elective Lymph Node Dissection

Based on the premise of the orderly migration of melanoma cells to the draining lymph node, elective lymph node dissection (ELND) involves the surgical resection of regional lymph nodes in patients with intermediate and high-risk primary tumors. Although it was plausible that removal of tumor-containing lymph nodes might improve survival, randomized, prospective trials have not shown a survival benefit in patients with primary melanoma treated with ELND plus wide re-excision compared to those treated with wide re-excision alone.[39–42] Complications include hematoma, wound infections, postoperative lymphedema, nerve damage, and lymphatic fistula formation.[38,43] The sentinel node biopsy, a much less morbid procedure, which shares many of the same premises and potential benefits, has supplanted the use of the elective lymph node dissection.[5,43,44]

Sentinel Node Biopsy

The sentinel lymph node (SLN) biopsy procedure has been accepted by most melanoma surgeons as the standard method for the accurate staging of clinical stages I–II melanoma and is usually performed for primaries at least 1.0 mm in thickness, as well as patients with melanomas less than 1.0 mm that have high-risk features. Sentinel node biopsy is a less traumatic technique to identify regional metastatic disease

and is also based on the concept that in most cases melanoma will first metastasize to the regional lymph nodes. The idea is that the lymphatic fluid from the tumor drains first to a sentinel lymph node(s) in one or more adjacent lymph node basins. The technique identifies the first regional lymph node in the lymphatic drainage of the primary tumor site—the "sentinel" node. Typically, 1–4 h before surgery, patients receive an intradermal injection of 0.5–1 mCi of technetium Tc 99 m sulfur colloid. A handheld gamma counter is used intraoperatively to localize the SLN. In addition, to facilitate intraoperative identification of SLNs, 1–3 ml of isosulfan blue is also injected intradermally around the tumor or biopsy site approximately 20 min before the mapping procedure. The sentinel node is then biopsied and examined histologically (Figs. 15.5, 15.6, 15.7 and 15.8). If metastatic melanoma is present, a lymph node dissection is then performed, the so-called "completion lymphadenectomy."

The *M*ulticenter *S*elective *L*ymphadenectomy *T*rial (MSLT) has provided the best evidence on the survival benefit of sentinel node biopsy.[45] Evidence from the MSLT trial suggests that *a priori* patients undergoing sentinel node biopsy have no significant overall survival benefit, although the trend is toward slightly better survival, and the 5-year disease-free survival is significantly better. A subset of patients with lymph node metastases do survive significantly better with a completion lymphadenectomy than when lymphadenectomy is performed after a period of observation and clinical nodal relapse.[45]

Nodal recurrences detected clinically are more likely to be larger and can be more difficult to control surgically than those detected with the sentinel node procedure. Early sentinel node biopsies with completion lymphadenectomy appear to reduce the rate of nodal recurrence, thus reducing or avoiding any morbid complications arising from nodal relapses.[46,47] The early evaluation and removal of lymph node metastases is therefore frequently beneficial in terms of palliation and improved survival in patients at high risk of nodal metastases.[48,49] For a more detailed analysis of the issues raised by the MSLT-I trial results, see Ross and Gershenwald.[50]

In certain areas of the body—namely the head, neck, and chest—the lymphatic drainage can be variable, making the sentinel node biopsy more difficult and less reliable than in other areas of

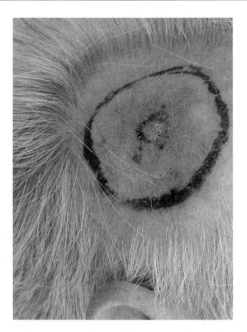

Fig. 15.5 A primary melanoma on the scalp prepped for definitive excision and sentinel lymph node biopsy. Photograph courtesy of Dr. Brad Garber

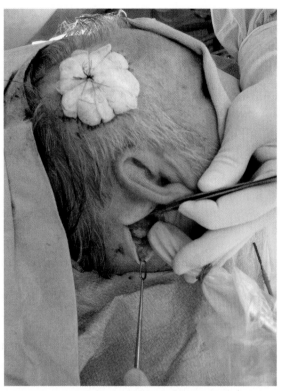

Fig. 15.7 Localized first by the Geiger counter probe, the sentinel lymph node (SLN) can be seen (*blue-yellow* nodule) in the dissection site and later confirmed by the high number of counts it emits. The primary melanoma site is seen on the scalp with a temporary packing placed after definitive excision. Photograph courtesy of Dr. Brad Garber

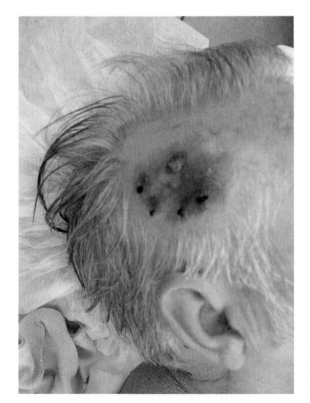

Fig. 15.6 Appearance following injection of Tc-99 and blue dye. Photograph courtesy of Dr. Brad Garber

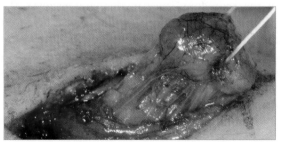

Fig. 15.8 Intraoperative identification of a sentinel lymph node (SLN). Intradermal injection of a vital blue dye around the intact melanoma or biopsy site leads to uptake of the dye by the lymphatic system and transport of the dye to the draining regional nodal basins, thereby allowing the identification of SLNs. Copyrighted photograph courtesy of Jeffrey E. Gershenwald, M.D., and the UT MD Anderson Cancer Center

better-defined drainage.[51–53] Side effects of sentinel node biopsy with completion lymphadenectomy, (beyond the immediate perioperative period) can include prolonged tenderness in the node basin area, loss of some sensation distally, and chronic lymphedema; although the lymphedema is usually less severe and less common compared to therapeutic lymph node dissections for palpable disease. Tenderness in the area of the surgery usually diminishes with time and most patients do not find that this impairs function in the affected limb.

Benefits of the sentinel node procedure in the hands of an experienced surgical team include more accurate staging and improved prognostic information together with its potential to preclude the development of regional node relapse and improved 5-year disease-free survival. These important advantages generally outweigh its potential disadvantages, especially in good surgical candidates.

Patients with primary melanomas thicker than 1.0 mm should be considered for the procedure, particularly patients with primaries between 1.2 and 3.5 mm in thickness.[45] In some situations, melanomas thinner than 1.0 mm may be considered for the procedure. These would include age between 18 and 35,[54,55] a high mitotic index in the tumor,[56,57] a microscopic designation as Clark's level III or IV,[58,59] evidence of vascular proliferation and/or angiolymphatic invasion at the base of the tumor,[60–62] and the presence of ulceration.[60,63]

The presence of a metastasis beyond the regional lymph node drainage obviates the prognostic value of the procedure, since in this circumstance, the prognosis is determined by the most advanced metastatic lesion or lesions, and not by the presence of regional disease beyond the primary. In this situation the main consideration would be the palliative value of a lymph node dissection to remove disease that may degrade quality of life.

Adjuvant Therapy for Intermediate Prognosis Melanoma (Stages IIB–III)

Patients at high risk for recurrence but without any detectable disease are in need of treatment to reduce their chance of recurrence and to enhance survival. Anti-neoplastic treatment given in this situation is termed "adjuvant therapy." Most patients with stage IIB and stage III melanoma are free of detectable disease and awaiting recurrence following surgical resection. Currently there are few good adjuvant therapy options for this situation. The large numbers of these patients emphasizes the need for more effective adjuvant treatment.

Unfortunately, cytotoxic chemotherapy, which has proven useful in other neoplastic diseases, has so far been ineffective as adjuvant therapy for melanoma.[64,65]

Radiation therapy may be useful in an adjuvant role in at least some situations. Although radiating lymph node basins after surgical clearance of stage III melanoma has not improved survival, in certain situations it may be helpful for local control in terms of enhanced relapse-free survival or beneficial palliation.[66–70] In desmoplastic melanoma, one study of postoperative adjuvant radiation has shown a benefit in relapse-free survival, although its effects on survival are still under investigation.[71]

Immunotherapy has been shown to have effects in the adjuvant setting, although no immunotherapy has yet achieved an unassailable improvement in overall survival.[72–77] The low toxicity of vaccines in particular make them ideal in the adjuvant setting, where toxicity in an otherwise healthy patient is less acceptable than when treating a symptomatic stage IV patient with a poor prognosis. The recent literature shows that some trials have come close to the goal of increased overall survival, and raise hopes that immunotherapy has a chance to succeed in the adjuvant role.

Interferon was the first, and still is the only adjuvant treatment to gain Food and Drug Administration (FDA) approval for treating melanoma in the adjuvant setting.[78,79] This was based on two key Eastern Cooperative Oncology Group (ECOG) studies that demonstrated its superiority to placebo or other regimens in terms of 5-year survival.[80] Interferon has been most widely studied in the adjuvant setting for stages II and III disease.

High-dose interferon is usually given as 12–20 million units per m^2 infused daily 5 days a week for the first month, usually given in an infusion center, and followed by thrice weekly outpatient injections of 10–12 million units per m^2.[81] This is a difficult regimen to tolerate, especially for the elderly, and it may debilitate patients to the point that they can no longer work. Influenza-like symptoms, generalized malaise, depression, and myelosuppression are among the more common side effects. More serious side effects can include suicidal ideation, seizures, psychotic reactions, stroke, thyroid disorders, hepatotoxicity, pneumonia, nephrotic syndrome, pancreatitis, renal failure, and, rarely, cardiomyopathy, myocardial infarction, life-threatening skin reactions, and autoimmune disorders.[f]

Although the high-dose interferon regimen has been associated with a slight improvement in 5-year survival, the evidence suggests that it does this primarily by delaying relapse rather than curing patients.[80] The high cost and side effects of interferon must be balanced against the modest efficacy. However, since there is no other non-experimental therapy that is effective in this role, interferon will continue to be used until more effective adjuvant treatments are available.

Melanoma Follow-Up

Follow-up is essential due to the risk of developing a second primary as well as metastasis from the original tumor. Recent studies suggest that the rate of developing a second primary melanoma is around 8% if only invasive melanoma is considered,[82] and around 12% if stage 0 (MIS) lesions are included in the calculation.[83] Second primaries tend to be thinner, earlier melanomas, and may not be as obvious to the patients as the first primary, which emphasizes the importance of skin examinations by a knowledgeable physician.[83,84]

One of the best ways to follow and manage melanoma is for physicians of various disciplines to cooperate, contributing their own skills. For example a dermatologist and an oncologist can cooperate to divide the visits with an asymptomatic patient diagnosed with stage II melanoma, each seeing the patient every 6 months, but done in phase so that the patient is seen by one or the other every 3 months. Patients can be referred for surgical, radiation therapy, or experimental therapy as needed.

[f] FDA label (package insert) for Intron-A.

Regional Recurrences

Limited regional recurrences are generally treated with surgical excision if that can be accomplished. Surgically unresectable recurrence makes this a form of advanced disease with a prognosis similar to stage IV. Such cases should probably be referred for experimental therapy.

Surgical Management of Metastatic Melanoma (Stage IV)

Evaluation of Patients with Suspected Metastatic Melanoma

Before planning therapy, it may be important to determine the metastatic burden. The periodic use of PET or PET/CT for detection of clinically occult metastases is gaining some acceptance. CT and MRI can also be used for this, and are also commonly used for evaluation of suspected or known metastases prior to surgery or radiation therapy. Bone scans may be useful if bone metastases are suspected, and in some centers, ultrasonography is used to screen lymph nodes (see Chapter 18).

Metastasectomy

Patients with stage IV melanoma have a 5-year survival between 19% for stage IV-M1a and 7% for stage IV-M1b.[8] The evidence suggests that for selected patients, complete resection of a limited number of lesions can enhance survival.[85] It is now accepted by many authorities that patients with limited numbers of surgically resectable metastases in a limited number of organs may benefit from resection.[86–90] This means that definitive surgical removal should be considered for a few (1–5) lesions that are completely resectable, especially isolated skin, lung, or brain metastases.[86] Patients with rapidly progressing disease, or with new metastases occurring weekly, will probably not benefit from this approach.

Radiation Therapy for Advanced Melanoma (Stages II–IV)

Palliative Radiotherapy

Radiation therapy may have an important role in the palliative care of symptomatic advanced melanoma patients. Painful nodules that cannot be easily removed surgically can sometimes be irradiated for pain relief. Another important role of this type of therapy is the maintenance of function. Metastases may threaten weight-bearing bones with collapse, and radiation therapy can be used to destroy such lesions and hence preserve the bone. For brain metastases larger than 1–2 cm, palliative whole brain irradiation can be tried as an alternative to surgery, although outcomes are usually less satisfactory than cases treated with focused beam radiotherapy (Gamma Knife®, CyberKnife®). Brain metastases treated with whole brain radiotherapy have a response rate of only about 15%.[91]

Curative Radiotherapy

For a limited number of small metastases to the brain, stereotactic radiosurgery techniques such as CyberKnife and Gamma Knife therapy potentially prolong and increase quality of life and occasionally can be curative if metastatic disease is limited to the brain.[92–95] This is a viable alternative to brain surgery for limited numbers of CNS metastases.

CyberKnife is more widely applicable than Gamma Knife. This newer form of stereotactic radiosurgery, in addition to treating brain metastases, can also be used to treat individual metastases located outside the central nervous system. Thus, if the clinical situation warrants it, CyberKnife can substituted for surgery for limited stage IV disease.

Chemotherapy of Advanced Melanoma (Surgically Unresectable Stages III, IV)

Dacarbazine (DTIC) is currently the only widely used chemotherapy drug that is FDA-approved for treating advanced melanoma.[96] While the initial treatment responses seen with dacarbazine were enough for approval from the FDA, it has subsequently been shown to be equivalent to supportive care in terms of survival.[96,97] Randomized trials of more toxic multidrug regimens show them to be equivalent to DTIC in terms of overall survival, meaning that they are equivalent to supportive care.[98,99] The grim reality is that there are no effective standard therapies for surgically unresectable advanced melanoma; experimental treatment is considered by many authorities the treatment of choice for this situation.[100]

Immunotherapy of Advanced Melanoma (Surgically Unresectable Stages III, IV)

Immunological therapy (immunotherapy) may increasingly be considered as an adjunctive or even as an alternative to traditional cytotoxic chemotherapy for non-resectable advanced melanoma. The combination of immunotherapy and chemotherapy, known as "biochemotherapy," has a higher response rate than chemotherapy alone, but unfortunately, this does not translate into improved survival in large studies.[101–103] Some promising, but not statistically significant reports of success in treating melanoma have come from immunological therapies, used either alone or in combination with other treatments. Some of the most common immunological treatments include vaccine strategies, cytokines, or other naturally occurring or synthetic immunostimulants. Interferon is the only treatment that is currently acknowledged to have a beneficial effect in the adjuvant setting as noted previously. IL-2, an important T-cell cytokine, is one of the few FDA-approved therapies for melanoma; the high-dose regimen has a response rate of approximately 16% and a cure rate of 6%, the highest reproducible cure rates of any currently available drug for treating stage IV.[104] Recently HSPPC-96, a heat shock protein-based vaccine, has been reported as having promising effects in early stage IV melanoma.[105]

Vaccine therapy has had some significant setbacks in the last few years. One phase III trial with Canvaxin and BCG was stopped prematurely due to reduced survival in each of the vaccine-treated groups.[106] A recent Eastern Cooperative Oncology Group GMK vaccine study was stopped early due to inferior survival in the vaccine group.[64] In spite of these reversals, dendritic cell vaccines, genetically engineered vaccines, and vaccines given together with immunostimulants such as interferon, interleukin-2, imiquimod, anti-CTLA4, and other agents may offer hope for the future.

Anti-CTLA4 is a relatively new immunological tool that may help to manipulate immune responses to benefit melanoma victims, although it has yet to be approved for use by the FDA. This drug is thought to interfere with the function of regulatory T cells (T-regs) through interaction with their CTLA4 surface receptors, although the precise mechanism of action is still disputed.[107]

Regulatory T cells are upregulated after immune stimulation by an antigen, and represent a natural suppressive regulatory mechanism that puts the brakes on the immune response at some point after it has been turned on.[108] This helps to prevent the immune system from overshooting and limits self-destructive effects, including autoimmune phenomenon.[109] Regulatory T cells are known to be involved in the suppression of the immune response against tumors.[110] Anti-CTLA4 antibodies appear to have the effect of "taking the brakes off" tumor-directed effector T cells that have been suppressed by the action of regulatory T cells.[111]

Ipilimumab is the generic drug name given by Medarex to their commercially studied anti-CTLA4 antibody. This drug produced a response rate of 13% when it was given to 56 HLA-A*0201 positive melanoma patients with two gp-100 related proteins in a dendritic cell vaccination protocol.[112] Tremelimumab, the generic drug name given by Pfizer to their commercially studied anti-CTLA4 antibody, has been reported to have beneficial effects in two phase I studies.[113,114] It is possible that anti-CTLA antibodies may have a role in treating melanoma in the future, most likely in combination with other immunotherapy strategies and with other types of anti-tumor agents. Immunotherapy is a promising area that may yet contribute significantly to our ability to treat advanced melanoma.[111] However, a better understanding of the host immune response is necessary if we are to make even greater progress in treating melanoma.

References

1. SEER Cancer Statistics Review, 1975–2005. In, Vol. 2008: National Cancer Institute 2007.
2. Abbasi NR, Shaw HM, Rigel DS, et al. Early diagnosis of cutaneous melanoma: revisiting the ABCD criteria. *JAMA*. 2004;92:2771–2776.
3. Rigel DS, Friedman RJ, Kopf AW, et al. ABCDE—an evolving concept in the early detection of melanoma. *Arch Dermatol*. 2005;141:1032–1034.
4. Braun RP, Rabinovitz HS, Oliviero M, et al. Dermoscopy of pigmented skin lesions. *J Am Acad Dermatol*. 2005;52:109–121.
5. Sober AJ, Chuang TY, Duvic M, et al. Guidelines of care for primary cutaneous melanoma. *J Am Acad Dermatol*. 2001;45:579–586.
6. Terhune MH, Swanson N, Johnson TM. Use of chest radiography in the initial evaluation of patients with localized melanoma. *Arch Dermatol*. 1998;134:569–572.
7. Morton RL, Craig JC, Thompson JF. The role of surveillance chest X-rays in the follow-up of high-risk melanoma patients. *Ann Surg Oncol*. 2008.
8. Balch CM, Buzaid AC, Soong SJ, et al. Final version of the American Joint Committee on Cancer staging system for cutaneous melanoma. *J Clin Oncol*. 2001;19:3635–3648.
9. Naylor MF, Crowson N, Kuwahara R, et al. Treatment of lentigo maligna with topical imiquimod. *Br J Dermatol*. 2003;149:66–69.
10. Diagnosis and treatment of early melanoma. NIH Consensus Development Conference. January 27–29, 1992. Consensus statement/NIH Consensus Development Conference 1992;10:1–25.
11. Bene NI, Healy C, Coldiron BM. Mohs Micrographic Surgery is Accurate 95.1% of the Time for Melanoma In Situ: A Prospective Study of 167 Cases. Dermatol Surg 2008.
12. Walling HW, Scupham RK, Bean AK, et al. Staged excision versus Mohs micrographic surgery for lentigo maligna and lentigo maligna melanoma. *J Am Acad Dermatol* 2007;57:659–664.
13. Cohen LM, McCall MW, Zax RH. Mohs micrographic surgery for lentigo maligna and lentigo maligna melanoma: a follow-up study. *Dermatol Surg*. 1998;24: 673–677.
14. Dawn ME, Dawn AG, Miller SJ. Mohs surgery for the treatment of melanoma in situ: a review. *Dermatol Surg*. 2007;33:395–402.
15. Bricca GM, Brodland DG, Ren D, et al. Cutaneous head and neck melanoma treated with Mohs micrographic surgery. *J Am Acad Dermatol*. 2005;52:92–100.
16. Huilgol SC, Selva D, Chen C, et al. Surgical margins for lentigo maligna and lentigo maligna melanoma: the technique of mapped serial excision. *Arch Dermatol*. 2004; 140:1087–1092.
17. Malhotra R, Chen C, Huilgol SC, et al. Mapped serial excision for periocular lentigo maligna and lentigo maligna melanoma. *Ophthalmology*. 2003;110: 2011–2018.
18. Chapman MS, Spencer SK, Brennick JB. Histologic resolution of melanoma in situ (lentigo maligna) with 5% imiquimod cream. *Arch Dermatol*. 2003;139: 943–944.

19. Fleming CJ, Bryden AM, Evans A, et al. A pilot study of treatment of lentigo maligna with 5% imiquimod cream. *Br J Dermatol.* 2004;151:485–488.

20. Powell AM, Russell-Jones R, Barlow RJ. Topical imiquimod immunotherapy in the management of lentigo maligna. *Clin Exp Dermatol.* 2004;29:15–21.

21. Cotter MA, McKenna JK, Bowen GM. Treatment of lentigo maligna with imiquimod before staged excision. *Dermatol Surg.* 2008;34:147–151.

22. Hazan C, Dusza SW, Delgado R, et al. Staged excision for lentigo maligna and lentigo maligna melanoma: a retrospective analysis of 117 cases. *J Am Acad Dermatol.* 2008;58:142–148.

23. Somach SC, Taira JW, Pitha JV, et al. Pigmented lesions in actinically damaged skin: histopathologic comparison of biopsy and excisional specimens. *Arch Dermatol.* 1996;132:1297–1302.

24. Lees VC, Briggs JC. Effect of initial biopsy procedure on prognosis in Stage 1 invasive cutaneous malignant melanoma: review of 1086 patients. *Br J Surg.* 1991;78:1108–1110.

25. Lederman JS, Sober AJ. Does biopsy type influence survival in clinical stage I cutaneous melanoma? *J Am Acad Dermatol.* 1985;13:983–987.

26. Bong JL, Herd RM, Hunter JA. Incisional biopsy and melanoma prognosis. *J Am Acad Dermatol.* 2002;46:690–694.

27. McKenna DB, Lee RJ, Prescott RJ, et al. A retrospective observational study of primary cutaneous malignant melanoma patients treated with excision only compared with excision biopsy followed by wider local excision. *Br J Dermatol.* 2004;150:523–530.

28. Gannon CJ, Rousseau DL Jr, Ross MI, et al. Accuracy of lymphatic mapping and sentinel lymph node biopsy after previous wide local excision in patients with primary melanoma. *Cancer.* 2006;107:2647–2652.

29. Veronesi U, Cascinelli N, Adamus J, et al. Thin stage I primary cutaneous malignant melanoma: comparison of excision with margins of 1 or 3 cm. *N Engl J Med.* 1988;318:1159–1162.

30. Balch CM, Urist MM, Karakousis CP, et al. Efficacy of 2-cm surgical margins for intermediate-thickness melanomas (1–4 mm): Results of a multi-institutional randomized surgical trial. *Ann Surg.* 1993;218:262–267; discussion 7–9.

31. Heaton KM, Sussman JJ, Gershenwald JE, et al. Surgical margins and prognostic factors in patients with thick (>4 mm) primary melanoma. *Ann Surg Oncol.* 1998;5:322–328.

32. McKinnon JG, Starritt EC, Scolyer RA, et al. Histopathologic excision margin affects local recurrence rate: analysis of 2681 patients with melanomas < or =2 mm thick. *Ann Surg.* 2005;241:326–333.

33. Kelly JW, Sagebiel RW, Calderon W, et al. The frequency of local recurrence and microsatellites as a guide to reexcision margins for cutaneous malignant melanoma. *Ann Surg.* 1984;200:759–763.

34. Aitken DR, Clausen K, Klein JP, et al. The extent of primary melanoma excision. A re-evaluation—how wide is wide? *Ann Surg.* 1983;198:634–641.

35. Ackerman AB, Scheiner AM. How wide and deep is wide and deep enough? A critique of surgical practice in excisions of primary cutaneous malignant melanoma. *Hum Pathol.* 1983;14:743–744.

36. Salopek TG, Slade JM, Marghoob AA, et al. Management of cutaneous malignant melanoma by dermatologists of the American Academy of Dermatology. II. Definitive surgery for malignant melanoma. *J Am Acad Dermatol.* 1995;33:451–461.

37. Kanzler MH, Mraz-Gernhard S. Primary cutaneous malignant melanoma and its precursor lesions: diagnostic and therapeutic overview. *J Am Acad Dermatol.* 2001;45:260–276.

38. Nestle FO, Kerl H. Melanoma. In: Bolognia JL, Jorizzo JL, Rapini RP, eds. *Dermatology.* Vol 2. 1st ed. New York, NY: Mosby; 2003:1789–1817.

39. Veronesi U, Adams J, Bandiera DC, et al. Delayed regional lymph node dissection in stage I malignant melanoma of the skin of the lower extremities. *Cancer.* 1982;49:2420–2430.

40. Veronesi U, Adamus J, Bandiera DC, et al. Inefficacy of immediate node dissection in stage 1 melanoma of the limbs. *N Engl J Med.* 1977;297:627–630.

41. Sim FH, Taylor WF, Pritchard DJ, et al. Lymphadenectomy in the management of stage I malignant melanoma: a prospective randomized study. *Mayo Clin Proc.* 1986;61:697–705.

42. Balch CM, Soong SJ, Bartolucci AA, et al. Efficacy of an elective regional lymph node dissection of 1–4 mm thick melanomas for patients 60 years of age and younger. *Ann Surg.* 1996;224:255–263; discussion 63–66.

43. Landry CS, McMasters KM, Scoggins CR. The evolution of the management of regional lymph nodes in melanoma. *J Surg Oncol.* 2007;96:316–321.

44. Bedrosian I, Gershenwald JE. Surgical clinical trials in melanoma. *Surg Clin North Am.* 2003;83:385–403.

45. Morton DL, Thompson JF, Cochran AJ, et al. Sentinel-node biopsy or nodal observation in melanoma. *N Engl J Med.* 2006;355:1307–1317.

46. Rex J, Paradelo C, Mangas C, et al. Single-institution experience in the management of patients with clinical stage I and II cutaneous melanoma: results of sentinel lymph node biopsy in 240 cases. *Dermatol Surg.* 2005;31:1385–1393.

47. Gutzmer R, Al Ghazal M, Geerlings H, et al. Sentinel node biopsy in melanoma delays recurrence but does not change melanoma-related survival: a retrospective analysis of 673 patients. *Br J Dermatol.* 2005;153:1137–1141.

48. Sabel MS, Griffith KA, Arora A, et al. Inguinal node dissection for melanoma in the era of sentinel lymph node biopsy. *Surgery.* 2007;141:728–735.

49. White RR, Tyler DS. Management of node-positive melanoma in the era of sentinel node biopsy. *Surg Oncol.* 2000;9:119–125.

50. Ross MI, Gershenwald JE. How should we view the results of the Multicenter Selective Lymphadenectomy Trial-1 (MSLT-1)? *Ann Surg Oncol.* 2008;15:670–673.

51. Willis AI, Ridge JA. Discordant lymphatic drainage patterns revealed by serial lymphoscintigraphy in cutaneous head and neck malignancies. *Head Neck.* 2007;29: 979–985.

52. Kilpatrick LA, Shen P, Stewart JH, et al. Use of sentinel lymph node biopsy for melanoma of the head and neck. *Am Surg.* 2007;73:754–758; discussion 8–9.

53. Morris KT, Stevens JS, Pommier RF, et al. Usefulness of preoperative lymphoscintigraphy for the identification

of sentinel lymph nodes in melanoma. *Am J Surg.* 2001;181:423–426.

54. Livestro DP, Kaine EM, Michaelson JS, et al. Melanoma in the young: differences and similarities with adult melanoma: a case-matched controlled analysis. *Cancer.* 2007;110:614–624.

55. Sondak VK, Taylor JM, Sabel MS, et al. Mitotic rate and younger age are predictors of sentinel lymph node positivity: lessons learned from the generation of a probabilistic model. *Ann Surg Oncol.* 2004;11:247–258.

56. Kesmodel SB, Karakousis GC, Botbyl JD, et al. Mitotic rate as a predictor of sentinel lymph node positivity in patients with thin melanomas. *Ann Surg Oncol.* 2005; 12:449–458.

57. Karakousis GC, Gimotty PA, Botbyl JD, et al. Predictors of regional nodal disease in patients with thin melanomas. *Ann Surg Oncol.* 2006;13:533–541.

58. Lowe JB, Hurst E, Moley JF, et al. Sentinel lymph node biopsy in patients with thin melanoma. *Arch Dermatol.* 2003;139:617–621.

59. Corsetti RL, Allen HM, Wanebo HJ. Thin < or = 1 mm level III and IV melanomas are higher risk lesions for regional failure and warrant sentinel lymph node biopsy. *Ann Surg Oncol.* 2000;7:456–460.

60. Cuellar FA, Vilalta A, Rull R, et al. Small cell melanoma and ulceration as predictors of positive sentinel lymph node in malignant melanoma patients. *Melanoma Res.* 2004;14:277–282.

61. Dadras SS, Lange-Asschenfeldt B, Velasco P, et al. Tumor lymphangiogenesis predicts melanoma metastasis to sentinel lymph nodes. *Mod Pathol.* 2005;18:1232–1242.

62. Paek SC, Griffith KA, Johnson TM, et al. The impact of factors beyond Breslow depth on predicting sentinel lymph node positivity in melanoma. *Cancer.* 2007;109:100–108.

63. Morris KT, Busam KJ, Bero S, et al. Primary cutaneous melanoma with regression does not require a lower threshold for sentinel lymph node biopsy. *Ann Surg Oncol.* 2008;15:316–322.

64. Eggermont AM, Gore M. Randomized adjuvant therapy trials in melanoma: surgical and systemic. *Semin Oncol.* 2007;34:509–515.

65. Shah GD, Chapman PB. Adjuvant therapy of melanoma. *Cancer J (Sudbury, Mass).* 2007;13:217–222.

66. Mendenhall W, Amdur R, Hinerman R, et al. Head and neck mucosal melanoma. *Am J Clin Oncol.* 2005;28:626–630.

67. Bastiaannet E, Beukema JC, Hoekstra HJ. Radiation therapy following lymph node dissection in melanoma patients: treatment, outcome and complications. *Cancer Treat Rev.* 2005;31:18–26.

68. Temam S, Mamelle G, Marandas P, et al. Postoperative radiotherapy for primary mucosal melanoma of the head and neck. *Cancer.* 2005;103:313–319.

69. Ballo MT, Zagars GK, Gershenwald JE, et al. A critical assessment of adjuvant radiotherapy for inguinal lymph node metastases from melanoma. *Ann Surg Oncol.* 2004;11:1079–1084.

70. Ballo MT, Gershenwald JE, Zagars GK, et al. Sphincter-sparing local excision and adjuvant radiation for anal-rectal melanoma. *J Clin Oncol.* 2002;20:4555–4558.

71. Foote M, Burmeister B, Burmeister E, et al. Desmoplastic melanoma: the role of radiotherapy in improving local control. *ANZ J Surg.* 2008;78:273–276.

72. Elias EG, Zapas JL, Beam SL, et al. Perioperative adjuvant biotherapy in high-risk resected cutaneous melanoma: the results of 5 years of follow-up. *Melanoma Res.* 2007;17:310–315.

73. Morton DL. Immune response to postsurgical adjuvant active immunotherapy with Canvaxin polyvalent cancer vaccine: correlations with clinical course of patients with metastatic melanoma. *Dev Biol (Basel).* 2004;116: 209–217; discussion 29–36.

74. Eilber FR, Morton DL, Holmes EC, et al. Adjuvant immunotherapy with BCG in treatment of regional-lymph-node metastases from malignant melanoma. *N Engl J Med.* 1976;294:237–240.

75. Davis-Daneshfar A, Boni R, von Wussow P, et al. Adjuvant immunotherapy in malignant melanoma: impact of antibody formation against interferon-alpha on immunoparameters in vivo. *J Immunother.* 1997;20: 208–213.

76. Ridolfi L, Ridolfi R, Riccobon A, et al. Adjuvant immunotherapy with tumor infiltrating lymphocytes and interleukin-2 in patients with resected stage III and IV melanoma. *J Immunother.* 2003;26:156–162.

77. Gardini A, Ercolani G, Riccobon A, et al. Adjuvant, adoptive immunotherapy with tumor infiltrating lymphocytes plus interleukin-2 after radical hepatic resection for colorectal liver metastases: 5-year analysis. *J Surg Oncol.* 2004;87:46–52.

78. Moschos S, Kirkwood J, Konstantinopoulos P. Present status and future prospects for adjuvant therapy of melanoma: time to build upon the foundation of high-dose interferon alfa-2b. *J Clin Oncol.* 2004;22:11–14.

79. Hancock B, Wheatley K, Harris S, et al. Adjuvant interferon in high-risk melanoma: the AIM HIGH Study—United Kingdom Coordinating Committee on Cancer Research randomized study of adjuvant low-dose extended-duration interferon Alfa-2a in high-risk resected malignant melanoma. *J Clin Oncol.* 2004;22: 53–61.

80. Kirkwood JM, Manola J, Ibrahim J, et al. A pooled analysis of eastern cooperative oncology group and intergroup trials of adjuvant high-dose interferon for melanoma. *Clin Cancer Res.* 2004;10:1670–1677.

81. Kirkwood JM. Studies of interferons in the therapy of melanoma. *Semin Oncol.* 1991;18:83–90.

82. Titus-Ernstoff L, Perry AE, Spencer SK, et al. Multiple primary melanoma: two-year results from a population-based study. *Arch Dermatol.* 2006;142:433–438.

83. Uliasz A, Lebwohl M. Patient education and regular surveillance results in earlier diagnosis of second primary melanoma. *Int J Dermatol.* 2007;46:575–577.

84. Francken AB, Shaw HM, Thompson JF. Detection of second primary cutaneous melanomas. *Eur J Surg Oncol.* 2008;34:587–592.

85. Wood TF, DiFronzo LA, Rose DM, et al. Does complete resection of melanoma metastatic to solid intra-abdominal organs improve survival? *Ann Surg Oncol.* 2001;8:658–662.

86. Essner R, Lee JH, Wanek LA, et al. Contemporary surgical treatment of advanced-stage melanoma. *Arch Surg.* 2004;139:961–966; discussion 6–7.

87. Hena MA, Emrich LJ, Nambisan RN, et al. Effect of surgical treatment on stage IV melanoma. *Am J Surg.* 1987;153:270–275.

88. Meyer T, Merkel S, Goehl J, et al. Surgical therapy for distant metastases of malignant melanoma. *Cancer.* 2000;89:1983–1991.

89. Gutman H, Hess KR, Kokotsakis JA, et al. Surgery for abdominal metastases of cutaneous melanoma. *World J Surg.* 2001;25:750–758.

90. de Wilt JH, McCarthy WH, Thompson JF. Surgical treatment of splenic metastases in patients with melanoma. *J Am Coll Surg.* 2003;197:38–43.

91. Boogerd W, De Gast G, Dalesio O. Temozolomide in advanced malignant melanoma with small brain metastases: can we withhold cranial irradiation? *Cancer.* 2007;109:306–312.

92. Kased N, Huang K, Nakamura J, et al. Gamma knife radiosurgery for brainstem metastases: the UCSF experience. *J Neurooncol.* 2008;86:195–205.

93. Majer M, Samlowski WE. Management of metastatic melanoma patients with brain metastases. *Curr Oncol Rep.* 2007;9:411–416.

94. Samlowski W, Watson G, Wang M, et al. Multimodality treatment of melanoma brain metastases incorporating stereotactic radiosurgery (SRS). *Cancer.* 2007;109:1855–1862.

95. Mathieu D, Kondziolka D, Cooper P, et al. Gamma knife radiosurgery in the management of malignant melanoma brain metastases. *Neurosurgery.* 2007;60:471–481; discussion 81–82.

96. Agarwala SS. Relevance and necessity of studies on second-line chemotherapy in melanoma. *Onkologie.* 2004;27:527–528.

97. Tarhini AA, Agarwala SS. Interleukin-2 for the treatment of melanoma. *Curr Opin Investig Drugs.* 2005;6:1234–1239.

98. Middleton MR, Lorigan P, Owen J, et al. A randomized phase III study comparing dacarbazine, BCNU, cisplatin and tamoxifen with dacarbazine and interferon in advanced melanoma. *Br J Cancer.* 2000;82:1158–1162.

99. Chapman PB, Einhorn LH, Meyers ML, et al. Phase III multicenter randomized trial of the Dartmouth regimen vs dacarbazine in patients with metastatic melanoma. *J Clin Oncol.* 1999;17:2745–2751.

100. Lawson DH. Choices in adjuvant therapy of melanoma. *Cancer Control.* 2005;12:236–241.

101. Lorigan P, Eisen T, Hauschild A. Systemic therapy for metastatic malignant melanoma–from deeply disappointing to bright future? *Experimental Dermatology.* 2008;17:383–394.

102. Keilholz U, Punt CJ, Gore M, et al. Dacarbazine, cisplatin, and interferon-alfa-2b with or without interleukin-2 in metastatic melanoma: a randomized phase III trial (18951) of the European Organisation for Research and Treatment of Cancer Melanoma Group. *J Clin Oncol.* 2005;23:6747–6755.

103. Bajetta E, Del Vecchio M, Nova P, et al. Multicenter phase III randomized trial of polychemotherapy (CVD regimen) versus the same chemotherapy (CT) plus subcutaneous interleukin-2 and interferon-alpha2b in metastatic melanoma. *Ann Oncol.* 2006;17:571–577.

104. Atkins MB, Kunkel L, Sznol M, et al. High-dose recombinant interleukin-2 therapy in patients with metastatic melanoma: long-term survival update. *Cancer J Sci Am.* 2000;6(Suppl 1):S11–S14.

105. Testori A, Richards J, Whitman E, et al. Phase III comparison of vitespen, an autologous tumor-derived heat shock protein gp96 peptide complex vaccine, with physician's choice of treatment for stage IV melanoma: the C-100-21 Study Group. *J Clin Oncol.* 2008;26:955–962.

106. Morton DL, Mozzillo N, Thompson JF, et al. An international, randomized, phase III trial of bacillus Calmette-Guerin (BCG) plus allogeneic melanoma vaccine (MCV) or placebo after complete resection of melanoma metastatic to regional or distant sites. *J Clin Oncol.* 2007;25:8505.

107. Comin-Anduix B, Lee Y, Jalil J, et al. Detailed analysis of immunologic effects of the cytotoxic T lymphocyte-associated antigen 4-blocking monoclonal antibody tremelimumab in peripheral blood of patients with melanoma. *J Transl Med.* 2008;6:22.

108. Cohn M. What roles do regulatory T cells play in the control of the adaptive immune response? *Int Immunol.* 2008;20:1107–1118.

109. Costantino CM, Baecher-Allan CM, Hafler DA. Human regulatory T cells and autoimmunity. *Eur J Immunol.* 2008;38:921–924.

110. Gallimore A, Godkin A. Regulatory T cells and tumour immunity—observations in mice and men. *Immunology.* 2008;123:157–163.

111. Kirkwood JM, Tarhini AA, Panelli MC, et al. Next generation of immunotherapy for melanoma. *J Clin Oncol.* 2008;26:3445–3455.

112. Attia P, Phan GQ, Maker AV, et al. Autoimmunity correlates with tumor regression in patients with metastatic melanoma treated with anti-cytotoxic T-lymphocyte antigen-4. *J Clin Oncol.* 2005;23:6043–6053.

113. Ribas A, Camacho LH, Lopez-Berestein G, et al. Antitumor activity in melanoma and anti-self responses in a phase I trial with the anti-cytotoxic T lymphocyte-associated antigen 4 monoclonal antibody CP-675,206. *J Clin Oncol.* 2005;23:8968–8977.

114. Bulanhagui CA, Ribas A, Pavlov D, et al. Phase I clinical trials of ticilimumab: tumor responses are sufficient but not necessary for prolonged survival. *J Clin Oncol.* 2006;24:8036.

Chapter 16
Skin Cancer in Skin of Color

Brooke A. Jackson

Skin cancer is the most common malignancy in the United States.[1] While skin cancer is less common in people with skin of color, it is more often associated with an increased incidence of morbidity and mortality as compared to white counterparts.[2,3] This imbalance has significant public health concerns. Current skin cancer campaigns focus on Caucasian patients in high-risk groups. There is a paucity of literature on skin cancer in skin of color. Most physicians do not immediately associate skin cancer with skin of color, and little is known about the sun-protective behaviors of those with skin of color. Similarly the collection of statistics for skin cancer in skin of color is challenging as non-melanoma skin cancer (NMSC) is not consistently reported to tumor registries, and many NMSCs in skin of color are reported as melanomas. According to the 2,000 census,[4] by the year 2050, 50% of the US population will be non-white. This changing demographic, combined with the disparate mortality, makes it imperative that physicians become familiar with skin cancer in skin of color so that they may better educate these patients on risk factors and early detection.

Unique Features of Skin of Color

While all skin, regardless of color, contains the same number of melanocytes, the melanosomes in darkly pigmented skin are larger and more evenly dispersed throughout the entire epidermis when compared to those in white skin, which are less active and grouped together.[5] The larger, more melanized epidermal melanocytes in dark skin absorb and scatter more ultraviolet (UV) light, resulting in twice as much UVB radiation filtration by dark skin than white skin.[6] Caucasian epidermal skin transmits 24% of UVB and 55% of UVA rays, whereas black epidermal skin transmits 7.4% of UVB and 17.5% of UVA rays.[6] The sun-protective factor of black skin has been estimated to be 13.1.[7] While these unique features of ethnic skin serve to protect it against actinic damage, and UV-induced skin cancers are overall less prevalent in skin of color, the incidence of NMSC in most ethnic groups is increasing,[8] suggesting that UV exposure may play less of a role in the development of certain skin cancers in skin of color. Known risk factors for non-melanoma skin cancer are listed in Table 16.1.[9]

Table 16.1 Known risk factors for NMSC[9]

UV exposure including UV light treatment
Fitzpatrick skin types I–III
Male gender
Radiation exposure
Genetic disorders (Xeroderma Pigmentosum, Basal Cell Nevus Syndrome)
Immunosuppression
Human papilloma virus
Chemical exposure (arsenic, coal tar products)
Chronic inflammation

Role of the Ozone Layer

The ozone layer has decreased over the past 20 years, allowing increased penetration of UV radiation to the earth's surface.[10] Increased risk of

D.F. MacFarlane (ed.), *Skin Cancer Management*, DOI 10.1007/978-0-387-88495-0_16,
© Springer Science+Business Media, LLC 2010

non-melanoma skin cancers have been associated with UV radiation, decreased skin pigmentation, and decreasing latitudes.[11] The role that UV exposure plays in the development of NMSC in skin of color may be correlated with the differences in the anatomical distribution of various tumors. In Caucasians, non-melanoma skin cancers occur most commonly in sun-exposed areas of the body.[12] UV radiation exposure is associated with an increased incidence of skin cancer in Asians.[13] Several studies have shown that UV radiation plays a significant role in the development of basal cell carcinoma (BCC) in blacks and these tumors are seen more commonly in sun-exposed areas of the body in blacks with fair skin tones.[14,15] Interestingly, the role of UV exposure in the development of squamous cell carcinoma (SCC) in blacks is not as clear. SCC, which occurs with equal frequency in Caucasians in sun-exposed and sun-protected areas, occurs 8.5 times more frequently on sun-protected areas in blacks, indicating that UV radiation plays a much less significant role in the development of SCC in blacks.[16]

Basal Cell Carcinoma

While the classic presentation of a solitary translucent papule with central ulceration may occur in skin of color, the presentation of BCC is more likely to be atypical in appearance[17] (Table 16.2) (Figs. 16.1, 16.2, 16.3 and 16.4). In darkly pigmented skin, rolled pearly borders and surrounding telangiectasia may be difficult to discern. Pigmented BCCs occur more frequently in skin of color,[18]

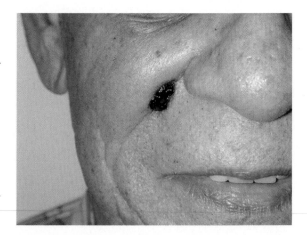

Fig. 16.1 An 80-year-old African-American man with BCC at right nasolabial fold. History of golfing

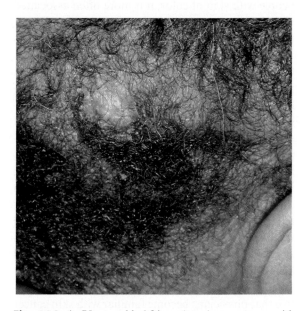

Fig. 16.2 A 75-year-old African-American woman with nodular pigmented BCC on right parietal scalp

while the morpheaform subtype is less common.[19] Many pigmented BCCs in skin of color have been diagnosed as melanoma.[20] Although the majority of BCCs in skin of color do occur in sun-exposed areas, they are seen in sun-protected areas with increasing frequency.[18]

Table 16.2 Differential diagnosis of BCC in skin of color

Seborrheic keratosis
Nevus sebaceous
Epidermal inclusion cyst
Blue nevus
Sarcoid
Melanoma
Trauma (curling iron burn)
Lupus erythematosus

Consider BCC (pigmented) in any suspicious lesion in a patient with skin of color.

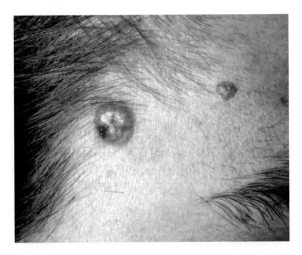

Fig. 16.3 Nodular pigmented BCC of a Hispanic female along the hairline. Photograph courtesy of June K. Robinson, MD

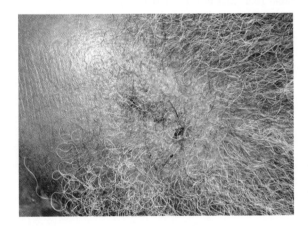

Fig. 16.4 A 70-year-old black female with multiple superficial and nodular basal cell carcinomas, each 1–2 mm in diameter in her scalp, which were initially felt to be dermatosis papula nigricans by her dermatologist

As with Caucasian patients, previous studies have documented the correlation of BCC in African-Americans to UV light exposure.[21] However, those with skin of color often have a false sense of security with regard to awareness of skin cancer risk and tend not to follow general guidelines of sun protection[22] in current skin cancer campaigns. Patients with skin of color also have a higher incidence of medical conditions such as hypertension, lupus, and diabetes, which necessitate the use of photosensitizing medications.[23] These combined factors support the need for better patient education and counseling, and perhaps a separate skin cancer campaign directed toward patients with skin of color.

Squamous Cell Carcinoma

SCC is the most common cutaneous malignancy in African-Americans[24] and the second most common cutaneous malignancy in Chinese and Japanese.[13] Of interest, actinic keratoses, the precursor lesion to SCC, tend not to occur in African-Americans,[25] but are common in Japanese[26] (Figs. 16.5, 16.6 and

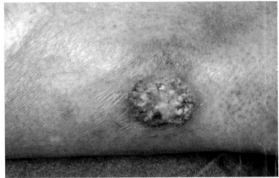

Fig. 16.5 An African-American female with SCC on her lower extremity, with a history of thermal burn to the area as a child

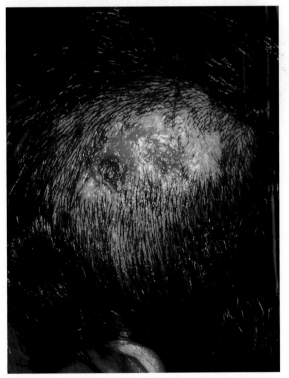

Fig. 16.6 An Indian female with SCC in nevus sebaceous of scalp. Photograph courtesy of June K. Robinson, M.D.

16.7). While most SCCs in Caucasians occur in sun-exposed areas of the head and neck, SCCs in African-Americans are found primarily in sun-protected areas,[27,28] such as the lower extremity and anogenital areas, suggesting that UV radiation plays less of a role in the development of SCCs in African-Americans. The mortality rate of African-Americans with SCC has been reported to range from 18.4 to 29%,[29,30] and is particularly high with anogenital lesions. Increased mortality may be related to both delayed diagnosis as well as the potentially more biologically aggressive nature of tumors in sun-protected areas.[30]

Bowen's disease (SCC in situ) is uncommon in African-Americans. When it does occur, it presents as a non-specific hyperkeratotic, often pigmented plaque on the lower extremity.[31,32]

Risk factors associated with the development of SCC in skin of color include chronic scarring and inflammatory processes[24] (Figs. 16.6, 16.7) as well as other disease states.

> Because of the increased mortality rate with African-Americans, surveillance of sun-protected areas with biopsy of any non-healing ulcer associated with areas of chronic inflammation or scarring is warranted.

It is also imperative that patients of color with the risk factors listed in Table 16.3 are counseled and followed up routinely for full skin examination.

Table 16.3 Risk factors for SCC in skin of color[24]

Lupus vulgaris
Scars from burn or trauma
Hidradenitis suppurativa
DLE/LE
Granuloma inguinale
Radiation sites
HPV
Immunosuppression
Albinism
Chemical exposure (tar, arsenic)
Chronic leg ulcers

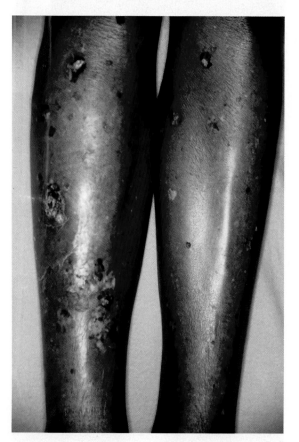

Fig. 16.7 An African-American female with SCC and arsenical keratoses on her lower extremities. History of well water ingestion. Photograph courtesy of June K. Robinson, M.D.

Malignant Melanoma

The incidence of malignant melanoma (MM) is increasing at a rate of 2.4% per year,[33] suggesting that by the year 2010, 1 in 50 Americans will be diagnosed with melanoma.

Although age-adjusted incidence rates (per 100,000) for melanoma are lower among Hispanics and blacks (4.3 and 1.0 respectively) compared to whites (20.8),[34] melanomas among darker-skinned populations are more likely to occur in sun-protected acral and mucosal areas, to metastasize, and to have poorer outcomes than among whites[35,36] (Fig. 16.8).

While family history and UV radiation exposure are risk factors for the development of malignant

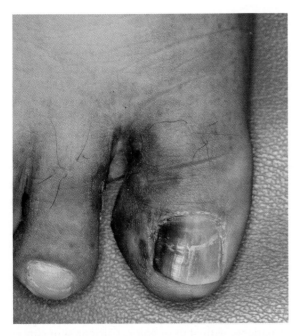

Fig. 16.8 A 43-year-old Hispanic male with a 2-year history of discoloration of right great toe and toe nail, which he treated with antifungal medication. Biopsy confirmed a melanoma

Table 16.4 Differential diagnosis for malignant melanoma in skin of color

Pigmented BCC	Tinea unguium
Seborrheic keratosis	Trauma (subungual hematoma)
Nevus	Verruca

melanoma in Caucasians, these factors do not appear to play as significant a role in the development of MM in skin of color (Table 16.4). The etiology of melanoma in non-whites, however, is still to be elucidated.

Because survival rates are directly correlated with Clark's level staging at diagnosis, early detection is critical for increased survival.

Hypopigmented Mycosis Fungoides

Mycosis Fungoides (MF), a variant of cutaneous T-cell lymphoma, classically presents as scaling plaques, nodules, tumors, or erythroderma,[37]

and occurs almost twice as often in African-Americans than in Caucasians, regardless of sex or age.[38,39] Hypopigmented MF is a variant of MF occurring almost exclusively in younger patients with skin of color (Fig. 16.9) and presents as ill-defined, hypopigmented patches.[40] Because these patients often have a history of eczema and these lesions may look similar (Table 16.5), diagnosis may be delayed from 7 months to 10 years from disease onset to histologic diagnosis.[41]

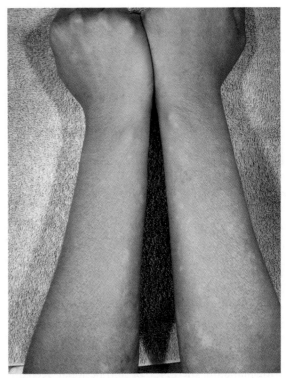

Fig. 16.9 A 37-year-old Filipino male who presented with a 2-year history of rash and was found to have hypopigmented MF. Photograph courtesy of the Section of Dermatology, Research Institute for Tropical Dermatology, Philippines, Evangeline B. Handog, M.D.

Table 16.5 Differential diagnosis for hypopigmented mycosis fungoides in skin of color

Pityriasis alba	Post-inflammatory hypopigmentation
Vitiligo	Sarcoid
Tinea versicolor	

Biopsy should be considered in those patients with skin of color whose eczema is unresponsive to standard therapies or who have an unexplained exacerbation of disease. Serial biopsies may be necessary.

Treatment Options and Operative Considerations

Treatment options for skin cancer in skin of color patients do not differ from those used in Caucasian patients and are addressed more fully in other chapters of this text.

When treating pre-cancerous lesions, this author avoids use of liquid nitrogen in skin of color in favor of imiquimod in an effort to avoid post-treatment loss of pigment.

Keloid formation can occur in any race; however, the rate in African-Americans has been reported to be from 5 to 15 times higher than that of the white population.[42] In Hawaii, keloids are found three times more commonly in the Japanese population and five times more commonly in the Chinese population than in white populations.[43] Because of this increased risk, care must be taken to minimize tension with wound closures. Patients should be counseled on the potential for hypertrophic scar and keloid formation, both of which may be treated with standard therapies of intralesional Kenalog injection and pressure. Post-operative hypertrophic scars in Caucasians and lightly complected patients of color (skin types I–IV) may be treated with the pulsed dye laser.

Several lasers may be used to improve the appearance of an erythematous scar in ethnic skin. In skin types III–IV, consider using the PDL laser with 10-mm spot, 0.5 ms, 2–3 joules, and treat every 3–4 weeks. For white or atrophic scars you may use the Affirm laser (1,440 nm, Cynosure) 10-mm spot, 2–4 joules, double pass, and treat every 2–3 weeks for a series of three to five treatments. As the Affirm laser builds collagen, the improvement may not be noticeable for 3–6 months after initiation of treatment.

Summary

Although less common than in Caucasians, skin cancer does occur in skin of color and these patients are more likely to die from their disease. This disparity is due to both delayed diagnosis and the more aggressive biologic nature of these tumors in skin of color. Pigmented BCCs are found more commonly in skin of color than in Caucasians. SCC is the most prevalent form of NMSC in skin of color. Although malignant melanoma occurs less frequently in skin of color, the aggressive acrolentiginous form accounts for poor prognosis in these patients. While sun exposure appears to play a role in the development of BCC in skin of color, there is less of a correlation with SCC and MM due to the propensity of these skin cancers to occur in sun-protected locations.

Little is known about the skin cancer awareness of patients with skin of color. Current skin cancer campaigns have focused on Caucasians in high-risk groups. Skin of color patients who do not perceive themselves as being at high risk for skin cancer development are likely to ignore early warning signs. In turn, those physicians who do not associate skin cancer with skin of color may be less likely to consider it in a differential diagnosis or to counsel patients appropriately on risk prevention, surveillance, and follow-up. A greater effort to increase public awareness must be instituted in ethnic communities. The combined efforts of physicians and an improvement in public education will result in earlier diagnosis and a better prognosis for skin of color patients with skin cancer.

References

1. US Department of Health and Human Services. Healthy People 2010. 2nd ed. Understanding and improving health and objectives for improving health. Vol 2. Washington, DC: US Government Printing Office; November 2000.
2. Gloster HM Jr, Brodland DG. The epidemiology of skin cancer. *Dermatol Surg.* 1996;22:217–226
3. Jemal A, Siegel R, Ward E, et al. Cancer Statistics, 2006. *Ca Cancer J Clin.* 2006;56:106–130.
4. US Census Bureau Population Division. Projections of the resident population by race, Hispanic origin, and nativity: middle series, 1999–2100. Washington, DC: US Census Bureau; 2000.

5. Montagna W. The architecture of black and white skin. *J Am Acad Dermatol*. 1991;24:29–37.

6. Halder RM, Bridgeman-Shah S. Skin cancer in African Americans. *Cancer*. 1995;75:667–673.

7. Halder RM, Ara CJ. Skin cancer and photoaging in ethnic skin. *Dermatol Clin*. 2003;21:725–732

8. Halder RM, Ara CJ. Skin cancer and photoaging in ethnic skin. *Dermatol Clin*. 2003;21:725–732

9. American Cancer Society, Non melanoma skin cancer detailed guide. http://documents.cancer.org/118.00. Accessed 12/19/08.

10. Naruse K, Ueda M, Nagana T, et al. Prevalence of actinic keratoses in Japan. *J Dermatol Sci*. 1997;15: 183–187.

11. Scotto J, Fears TR, Fraumeni JF. Incidence of nonmelanoma skin cancer in the United States. Washington, DC: US Government Printing Office; 1983. NIH report no. 83–2433

12. Weinstock MA. Epidemiology of melanoma. *Cancer Treat Res*. 1993;65:29–56.

13. Koh D, Wang H, Lee J, et al. Basal cell carcinoma, squamous cell carcinoma and melanoma of the skin: analysis of the Singapore Cancer Registry Data 1968–1997. *Br J Dermatol*. 2003;148:1161–1166.

14. Halder RM, Bang KM. Skin cancer in blacks in the United States. *Dermatol Clin*. 1988;6:397–405.

15. Penello GA, Devesa S, Gail M. Association of surface ultraviolet B radiation levels with melanoma and nonmelanoma skin cancer in United States blacks. *Cancer Epidemiol Biomarkers Prev*. 2000;9:291–297.

16. Sing B, Bhaya M, Shaha A, et al. Presentation, course and outcome of head and neck cancer in African Americans: a case controlled study. *Laryngoscope*. 1998;108: 1159–1163.

17. Chorun L, Norris JE, Gupta M. Basal Cell carcinoma in Blacks: a report of 15 cases. *Am Plast Surg*. 1994;33:90–95.

18. Nadiminti U, Rakkhit T, Washington C. Morpheaform basal cell carcinoma in African Americans. *Dermatol Surg*. 2004;30:1550–1552.

19. Lesher JL, d'Aubermont PC, Brown VM. Morpheaform basal cell carcinoma in a young black woman. *J Dermatol Surg Oncol*. 1988;14:200–203.

20. Cheng SY, Luk NM, Chong LY. Special features of nonmelanoma skin cancer in Hong Kong Chinese patients: 10 year retrospective study. *Hong Kong Med J*. 2001;7:22–28.

21. Matsuoka LY, Schauer PK, Sordillo PP. Basal cell carcinoma in black patients. *J Am Acad Dermatol*. 1981;4 (6):670–672.

22. Briley JJ, Chaveda K, Lynfield YL. Sunscreen use and usefulness in African Americans. *J Drugs Dermatol*. 2007;6(1):19–22.

23. Ferdinand KC, Armani AM. The management of hypertension in African Americans. *Crit Pathw Cardiol J Evid Based Med*. 2007 June;6(2):67–71.

24. Mora RG, Perniciaro C. Cancer of the skin in blacks: a review of 163 black patients with cutaneous squamous cell carcinoma. *J Am Acad Dermatol*. 1981;5:535–543.

25. Hale EK, Jorizzo JL, Nehal KS, et al. Current concepts in the management of actinic keratosis. *J Drugs Dermatol*. 2004, March–April;3(2 Suppl):S3–16.

26. Suzuki T, Ueda M, Naruse K, et al. Incidence of actinic keratosis of Japanese in Kasai City, Hyogo. *Dermatol Sci*. 1997;16:74–78.

27. Halder RM, Bang KM. Skin cancer in blacks in the United States. *Dermatol Clin*. 1988;6:397–405.

28. Mora RG, Perniciaro C, Lee B. Cancer of the skin in blacks III: a review of nineteen black patients with Bowen's disease. *J Am Acad Dermatol*. 1984;11: 557–562.

29. Mora RG. Surgical and aesthetic considerations of cancer of the skin in the black American. *Am J Dermatol Surg Oncol*. 1986;12:24–31.

30. Fleming ID, Barnawell JR, Burlison PE, et al. Skin cancer in black patients. *Cancer*. 1975;35:600–605.

31. Schamroth JM, Weiss RM, Grieve TP. Verrucous Bowen's disease in an African American patient. *S Afr Med J*. 1987;71:527–528.

32. Krishnan R, Lewis A, Orengo IG, et al. Pigmented Bowen's disease (squamous cell carcinoma in situ): a mimic of malignant melanoma. *Dermatol Surg*. 2001;27: 673–674.

33. Ries LAG, Melbert D, Krapcho M, et al. SEER Cancer statistics review, 1975–2005, Bethesda, MD: National Cancer Institute. http://seer.cancer.gov/csr/1975_2005/. Accessed 12/18/08.

34. Cress RD, Holly EA. Incidence of cutaneous melanoma among non-Hispanic whites, Hispanics, Asians and Blacks: an analysis of California Cancer Registry data, 1988–1993. *Cancer Causes Control*. 1997;8:246–252.

35. Greenlee RT, Murray T, Bolden S, et al. Cancer statistics, 2000. *CA Cancer J Clin*. 2000;50(1):7–33.

36. Washington CV, Grimes PE. Incidence and prevention of skin cancer. *Cosmetic Dermatol*. 2003;16:46–48.

37. Stone ML, Styles AR, Cockerell CJ, et al. Hypopigmented mycosis fungoides: a report of 7 cases and review of the literature. *Cutis*. 2001;67:133–138.

38. Akaraphanth R, Douglass MC, Lim HW. Hypopigmented mycosis fungoides: treatment and a 61/2 year follow up of 9 patients. *J Am Acad Dermatol*. 2000;42:33–39.

39. Wienstock MA, Horm JW. Mycosis fungoides in the United States. *JAMA*. 1988;260:42–46.

40. Stone MC, Styles AR, Cockerell CJ. Hypopigmented mycosis fungoides: a report of 7 cases and review of the literature. *Cutis*. 2001;67:133–138.

41. Whitmore SE, Simmons-O'Brien E, Rotter FS. Hypopigmented mycosis fungoides. *Arch Dermatol*. 1994; 130:476–480.

42. LeFlore IC. Misconceptions regarding elective plastic surgery in the black patient. *J Natl Med Assoc*. 1980;72: 947–948.

43. Arnold HL, Franer FH. Keloids: etiology and management by excision and intensive prophylactic radiation. *Arch Dermatol*. 1959;80:772

Chapter 17
Management of Skin Cancers in Solid Organ Transplant Recipients

John Carucci and Dariush Moussai

The number of organ transplant recipients continues to rise in the United States, with nearly 30,000 organ transplant procedures performed in 2007 and 225,000 organ transplant recipients currently living in the United States.[1] While long-term survival after organ transplantation has also increased, with the 3-year survival rate for kidney and heart transplants approaching 90%,[2] as many as 70% of organ transplant recipients will ultimately develop skin cancer.[2]

Increased longevity after transplant is attributed to optimization of immunosuppressive therapy. However, skin cancer remains a potentially devastating complication in organ transplant recipients and may account for a significant source of morbidity and mortality in these patients. Therefore, diagnosis and management of skin cancer in organ transplant recipients pose a formidable challenge.

The following chapter will discuss the epidemiology and pathogenesis of skin cancer in primarily transplant patients and then provide some practical suggestions for the management of these potentially challenging patients.

transplant recipients are nearly 100 times more likely to develop SCC than immunocompetent patients.

In a recent retrospective case-control study by Harwood et al., the histology of skin cancers in immunosuppressed organ transplant recipients was compared to immunocompetent individuals.[3] Transplant patients were younger at the time of skin cancer diagnosis, and those who were diagnosed with SCC had a worse prognosis than those diagnosed with basal cell carcinoma (BCC). Spindle cell morphology, which is mainly characterized by atypical spindle cells and can be clinically aggressive, was more common in transplant SCC cases. Histological features of human papilloma virus (HPV) infection were over-represented in transplant-related SCC as well.

Jensen et al.[4] studied 2,561 transplant recipients over a 30-year period and reported a 65-fold increase in SCC incidence. In another study by Lindelof et al.,[5] 325 patients developed SCC from a pool of 5,356 transplant recipients followed between 1970 and 1994.

Epidemiology

Squamous Cell Carcinoma Following Organ Transplantation

Squamous cell carcinoma (SCC) is the most common type of skin cancer in transplant patients and continues to be a significant cause of morbidity and mortality in these patients.[2,3] Fair-skinned

Basal Cell Carcinoma Following Organ Transplantation

Most studies show increased rates of BCC in transplant recipients, but not to the degree seen for SCC. In addition, morbidity from BCC is not necessarily greater in the transplant group. Of all BCC subtypes, superficial BCC on the trunk is over-represented in transplant recipients with an

D.F. MacFarlane (ed.), *Skin Cancer Management*, DOI 10.1007/978-0-387-88495-0_17,
© Springer Science+Business Media, LLC 2010

approximately tenfold increase.[2] A recent study suggests that increased expression of protease inhibitor TIMP1 in BCC in immunocompetent patients may limit migration through the extracellular matrix.[6]

Melanoma Following Organ Transplantation

Malignant melanoma (MM) was initially thought to be associated with greater morbidity and mortality in transplant recipients based on decreased 1-, 3-, and 5-year survival rates reported in an early study from the Penn transplant registry.[7] The average Breslow depth of MM from that study was 1.51 mm. More recent data indicates that MM is over-represented in transplant patients with a 3.5- to 8-fold increase compared with the general population.[8,9] However, the prognosis does not appear to differ significantly in this group. In a recent study of 48 consecutive MM patients from the Mayo transplant registry, there was no difference in the development of metastases or overall survival between transplant recipients with MM and otherwise prognostically matched immunocompetent patients.[10]

Skin Cancer Following Kidney Transplantation

In a prospective study (1986–2006) by Ramsay et al.,[11] the incidence of nonmelanoma skin cancer (NMSC) was approximately 8% in a cohort of 244 kidney transplant recipients. The incidence of NMSC increased with time following transplantation, with a mean incidence of 11.1% in patients 10 years postrenal transplant versus 3.3% in patients less than 5 years post-transplant. Moosa et al.[12] reviewed 542 kidney transplant patients from different ethnic groups in South Africa over a 23-year period, and found that 11 patients (5.9%) had developed skin cancer, with a mean follow-up of 6.3 years. These patients were mostly male (82%) and all were Caucasian. SCC was the most common skin cancer in this group and the majority of the lesions (84%) occurred in sun-exposed regions.

Skin Cancer Following Heart Transplantion

As with many other types of organ transplantation, SCC is also more common among heart transplant patients. Lampros et al.[13] studied 248 heart transplant patients, of which 41 (17%) developed 192 nonmelanoma skin cancers. SCCs accounted for about 90% of all the lesions and the SCC/BCC ratio was 8.6:1. In addition, skin cancer rates rise with time following heart transplantation. In a review of a cohort of 455 Australian heart transplant recipients, the reported cumulative incidence of skin cancer was 31% at 5 years and 43% at 10 years with an SCC/BCC ratio of 3:1.[14]

Other risk factors associated with skin cancer were increasing age at transplantation, Caucasian origin, HLA-DR homozygosity, and duration of follow-up.[14] Adamson et al.[15] analyzed the incidence of skin cancer in 146 heart transplant recipients in San Diego from 1985 to 1995. Aggressive skin cancer was defined as multiple recurrences with or without lymph node metastasis. In the 146 patients studied, 35 (25%) developed skin cancer and of these 16 patients had an aggressive type and 19 had a nonaggressive type of skin cancer. Of the 464 skin cancer lesions found in 35 patients, 266 were SCCs and 115 were BCCs. The reported SCC/BCC ratio was 5:1 in the aggressive group, and 3:1 in the nonaggressive group. The 7-year post-transplant survival rate was 53% versus 82% in the aggressive and nonaggressive groups respectively.

Skin Cancer Following Liver Transplantation

While SCC may be the most common skin cancer among organ transplant recipients overall, the incidence of SCC and BCC appears to be more equal for liver recipients. In a study by Perera et al.,[16] 100 liver transplant recipients were followed after transplantation for a mean period of 5.5 years. Four patients developed NMSC; among them were six BCCs and one SCC.[14] Studying malignancies following liver transplantation, Levy et al.[17] reported that the incidence of skin cancer was 1.6%. Frezza et al.[18] reviewed 1,657 liver transplant recipients and noted that 39 developed skin cancer. The SCC/BCC ratio was reported as 1:1.

Skin Cancer Following Stem Cell Transplantion

BCC may even be more prevalent than SCC among stem cell transplant recipients. Leisenring et al.[19] evaluated the incidence and risk factors of SCC and BCC in a retrospective cohort analysis of nearly 5,000 patients who had received Allogeneic Hematopoietic Stem Cell Transplants. They reported that the 20-year incidence of SCC was 3.4% while that of BCC was 6.5%. Among the 237 patients, 95 patients developed at least one cutaneous or mucosal SCC, while 158 patients had developed BCCs. Acute graft-versus-host disease (GVHD) increased the risk of SCC, while chronic GVHD increased the risk of both SCC and BCC.

Pathogenesis

Chronic sun exposure is one of the most important risk factors in developing SCC.[20] Ultraviolet radiation (UVR) in the UVB range (290–320 nm) initiates mutations in the p53 tumor suppressor gene in keratinocytes.[21] UV-mediated mutations in the p53 tumor suppressor gene prevent apoptosis of mutated cells. Uncontrolled proliferation of mutated keratinocytes drives the transition from actinic keratosis to SCC in situ and ultimately to invasive SCC. Thus, UVR acts as both a tumor initiator and promoter.[22]

HPV-driven warts are common in transplant recipients. HPV infection, particularly HPV 16, has been associated with SCC on the finger.[23] Epidermodysplasia verruciformis HPV types are prevalent in benign and malignant skin lesions in transplant recipients. It is plausible that HPV-infected transplant recipients may be at increased risk of developing actinic keratosis (AK) or SCC based on suppression of p53 mediated by HPV-derived protein E6.[24]

Ras signaling and NF-kB activation are key mediators of cell-signal transduction pathways, differentiation, and apoptosis.[25] In a study by Dajee et al., ras signal transduction pathway in association with NF-kB inhibition was sufficient to induce normal human epidermis to transform into tumor tissue, which retained cardinal features of SCC.[26]

Haider et al.[27] established a molecular fingerprint of SCC by using Microarray High Density Gene Chip Analysis. In this study, more than 12,000 genes were analyzed from surgical excisions of human SCCs. The SCC genes were compared to their adjacent site-matched, nonlesional counterparts. SCC was characterized by the upregulation of matrix metalloproteinases 1, 10, 13 (MMP1, MMP10, MMP13), cathepsin, and cystatin.

Notch-mediated signal transduction regulates cell survival, differentiation, and proliferation in development.[28] There are four different transmembrane Notch receptors, Notch1-4, which bind *Delta* and *Jagged* families of ligands. Notch1 has been described as a tumor suppressor in keratinocytes.[29] Deletion of the Notch1 gene in mice leads to extensive epidermal hyperplasia and spontaneous development of BCC. Impaired Notch signaling, created by expressing a dominant negative form of the receptor in mice, results in the spontaneous development of SCC and actinic keratosis.[30]

It is likely that catastrophic, cutaneous carcinomatosis, as observed in fair-skinned transplant recipients, represents a "perfect storm" phenomenon where long-term actinic damage provides initial hits that are compounded by HPV infection leading to extensive field disease with innumerable lesions. HPV further interferes with p53 via E6 contributing to continued proliferation of atypical cells. Transformation may be driven in part by RAS and extensive proliferation via the notch pathway. Finally, the protease expression profile suggests facilitated passage through an already weakened basement membrane. An additional, direct carcinogenic hit may be provided by the otherwise life-saving and organ-sparing immunosuppressive agents.[2] Several of these are discussed in the next section.

Immunosuppression and Skin Cancer

Immunosuppressive drug regimens are the mainstay in preventing transplant rejection. Unfortunately, however, the use of immunosuppressive regimens may play a role in the increased incidence of skin cancer in organ transplant recipients. We will briefly review the mechanism of action of some classic immunosuppressive drugs and describe their possible role in the development of skin cancer.

Azathioprine

Azathioprine is a purine analog of 6-mercaptopurine. It is metabolized in the blood to 6-mercaptopurine, which is then converted to 6-thioguanine by hypoxanthine guanosine phosphoribosyl transferase (HGPRT). Thus, azathioprine inhibits the de novo purine synthesis. Thioguanines from azathioprine metabolism are found in higher concentrations in erythrocytes of kidney transplant recipients with skin cancer.[31,32] This supports the association of higher doses of azathioprine with a higher incidence of skin cancer. In addition, azathioprine and UVA light have been shown to synergistically promote oxidative DNA damage and mutagenesis.[33] Thus, taken together these studies indicate that patients with extensive actinic damage on azathioprine may be at increased risk for skin cancer, particularly SCC.

Cyclosporine

Cyclosporine (CsA) is a macrolide isolated from the fungus *Tolypocladium inflatum*. Binding of CsA to target immunophilins inhibits calcineurin, a phosphatase enzyme critical for the production of interleukin-2 (IL-2) in T lymphocytes.[34] CsA has been shown to induce SCC-like tumor growth in severe combined immunodeficiency mice (SCID).[35,36] This is key in that it implicates direct carcinogenic effects rather than dysregulated immunity in cyclosporine-related cancers since the SCID mice have no immune systems to suppress. Hojo et al. showed that cyclosporine directly induced morphological changes in adenocarcinoma cells, which included increased cell motility and invasive growth characteristics.[35] One might postulate that cyclosporine might accelerate the development of aggressive growth characteristics in patients with extensive actinic damage prior to transplant.

Sirolimus

Sirolimus, another macrolide, was discovered from the bacterium *Streptomyces hygroscopicus* in a soil sample from Easter Island.[37] Also known as "rapamycin," it inhibits the production of IL-2 by T cells, by binding to FKBP12 or FK-binding Protein12. This complex inhibits the mammalian target of rapamycin complex 1 or mTORC1.[37] While other immunosuppressive drug regimens may promote skin cancer, rapamycin may have a protective role against skin cancer.[38] In a 5-year randomized trial by Campistol et al., the incidence of NMSC was decreased from 9.6 to 4.0% upon early withdrawal of CsA from a triple-drug regimen of CsA, sirolimus, and prednisolone, while sirolimus and prednisolone were maintained.[39]

Presentation

Primary SCC in Transplant Patients

Primary cutaneous SCC typically presents as a red scaly patch or plaque (Fig. 17.1). If isolated, it can resemble a benign inflammatory dermatosis, such as eczema or psoriasis, and the differential diagnosis may also include benign neoplasms such as irritated seborrheic keratoses or traumatized warts. Differentiation from precancerous actinic keratosis may

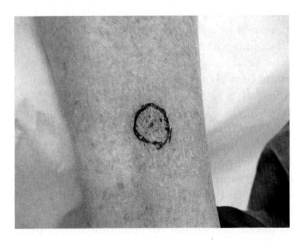

Fig. 17.1 Primary cutaneous SCC presenting as a scaly plaque

be challenging. Nodular appearing, KA-like SCC (Fig. 17.2) may resemble a subcutaneous abscess early in its course, however, a lack of fluctuance, drainage, and punctum will help to distinguish these entities. In transplant patients, SCC is more likely to be part of an overall cutaneous dysplasia (Fig. 17.3) than an isolated lesion.

> Full body exam is a must for the initial evaluation of all transplant recipients.

All SCC in transplant recipients are at high risk for local recurrence or metastasis as defined by Rowe.[40] However, risk stratification of individual SCCs becomes important when managing patients with tens to hundreds of lesions. A risk stratification algorithm was developed by the International Transplant Skin Cancer Collaborative.[41] Based on this, highest risk lesions are those that are large (>1 cm), invasive on histology, rapidly growing, located on the head and neck, poorly differentiated, perineurally invasive, and recurrent after seemingly adequate treatment. Lower-risk lesions include actinic keratoses and SCC in situ on the trunk and extremities.

Extensive Field Disease

Extensive field disease is common in transplant recipients with fair skin and chronic sun exposure. In transplant patients with extensive field disease, there may be innumerable warts, actinic keratoses, and in situ and invasive SCCs. In many cases, it is difficult to determine where one lesion ends and the adjacent one begins. This phenomenon has been described as "transplant hand."[42] The authors have observed this phenomenon on the head, neck, trunk, and extremities (Fig. 17.4). Patients with severe field disease require frequent evaluations and multimodal treatment with topical agents, destruction, shave excision, and photodynamic therapy (PDT).

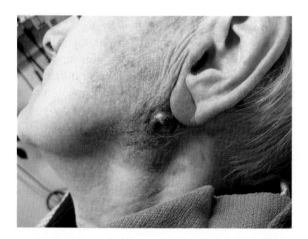

Fig. 17.2 Keratoacanthoma-like SCC presenting as a rapidly growing nodule in a transplant recipient

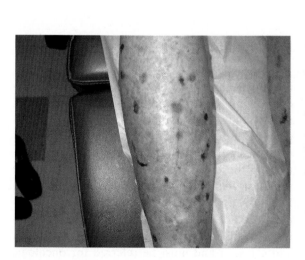

Fig. 17.3 Cutaneous dysplasia in a transplant recipient

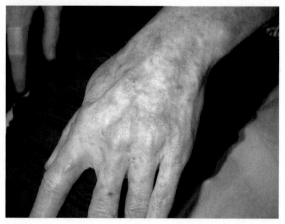

Fig. 17.4 Cutaneous dysplasia in a transplant recipient manifesting as "transplant hand"

In-Transit Metastasis

In-transit metastasis is defined as a cutaneous relapse distant to the site of the primary or recurrent tumor that occurs between the prior treatment site and the local nodal basin and that usually lacks an epidermal component.[2,43] Clinically, these present as subcutaneous or dermal papules that are not contiguous to the site of the primary or recurrent tumor and are considered satellites (Fig. 17.5). In one study, 15 organ transplant recipients with in-transit metastatic SCC were evaluated for presentation, treatment, and course. After 2 years, 5/15 were dead from the disease, 5/15 had nodal or distant organ metastases, and 5/15 showed no evidence of disease. In contrast, none of the immunocompetent patients had died of skin cancer, and 5/6 immunocompetent had no evidence of SCC. In that study development of in-transit metastasis was correlated with perineural invasiveness by SCC (Fig. 17.6).

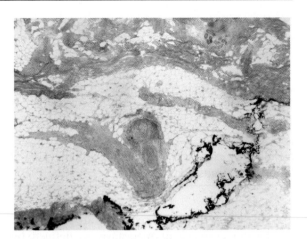

Fig. 17.6 Perineural invasion by SCC

and invasion to fat as defined by Rowe et al. in 1992.[40] Another key risk factor for metastasis of cutaneous SCC is iatrogenic immunosuppression following solid organ transplant. In-transit metastasis is associated with increased nodal metastases.[43] Thus it is essential to palpate the draining lymph nodes in any patient with a history of cutaneous SCC, particularly transplant recipients. Patients with lymphadenopathy should have magnetic resonance imaging (MRI) to evaluate the extent of involvement; a positron-emission tomography (PET) scan or PET-computed tomography (PET-CT) scan to evaluate for distant metastasis; and fine needle aspiration (FNA) for pathologic confirmation.

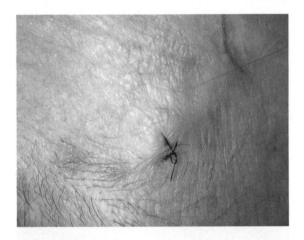

Fig. 17.5 In-transit metastatic SCC presenting as a nodule without epidermal change inferior to a previously treated site

Nodal Metastasis

Nodal metastases occur in as many as 3–5% of invasive primary cutaneous SCC and present as palpable lymph nodes. Risk factors for nodal and distant metastases include large SCC, perineural SCC, SCC on the lip or ear, poor differentiation,

Distant Metastasis

Distant metastasis of SCC is by the hematogenous route to bone, brain, lung, and the liver. In a recent study by Martinez et al. for the Transplant-Skin Collaborative, 68 organ transplant recipients with metastatic skin cancer were treated and those with distant metastasis had a poor prognosis with a 3-year survival rate of 56%. Patients with suspected distant organ involvement need to be evaluated by appropriate screening and imaging studies including PET-CT, MRI, and CT scan and must be referred for oncologic evaluation and treatment.

Basal Cell Carcinoma

BCC presents similarly in immunosuppressed and immunocompetent patients. BCC may be represented by a translucent papule (nodular BCC), pigmented papule (pigmented BCC), scar-like plaque (morpheaform BCC), or most commonly an erythematous patch on the trunk or extremities (superficial BCC) (Fig. 17.7). The incidence is increased in the fair-skinned with Fitzpatrick types I–III. The authors maintain a low threshold for biopsy for potential basal cell carcinomas in such immunosuppressed patients.

Melanoma

Melanoma presentation is similar in transplant recipients and immunocompetent patients, and may present as an irregularly pigmented macule, patch, or papule. Similarly, the appearance of pigmented lesions or change in a previously existing pigmented lesion may signal early melanoma. The authors maintain a low threshold for biopsy of new or changing pigmented lesions in transplant recipients.

Management

The management of SCC in transplant recipients should be based on risk stratification. Risk factor assessment was determined by an expert panel from the International Transplant Skin Collaborative (ITSCC), which developed clinical guidelines for the management of skin cancer in organ transplant recipients.[41] The challenge in these patients is to determine the "highest risk lesions." High-risk lesions are defined by (1) rapid growth; (2) poor differentiation; (3) invasive SCC; (4) location on scalp, lips, ears; (5) size > 1 cm; and (6) perineural invasion.

Primary Cutaneous SCC

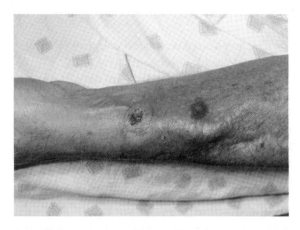

Fig. 17.7 Basal cell carcinoma over an AV fistula in the arm of a kidney transplant recipient. Photograph courtesy of Deborah F. MacFarlane, M.D.

As in the immunocompetent patient, highest risk lesions are best treated with standard excision or Mohs micrographic surgery (Fig. 17.8). Mohs

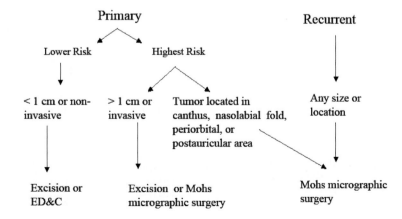

Fig. 17.8 Management of cutaneous SCC in transplant patients

surgery offers the highest cure rates with maximal tissue conservation. Moderate risk lesions, which include well-differentiated, smaller SCCs, may be treated with standard excision with postoperative margin confirmation, while lower risk AKs are treated with topical agents or destroyed by cryotherapy.

> One strategy for patients with multiple primary, lower risk SCCs is treatment by shave excision followed by electrodesiccation and curettage (ED&C). In this manner, multiple lesions can be treated in a single session under local anesthesia. Histological analysis of the tangential excision specimen will help to determine whether additional treatment is necessary.[41]

Another strategy for treating patients with multiple lesions is the so-called "megasession," where at least five larger lesions are treated by full thickness excision or Mohs surgery and repair in a single session.[44] Martinez and Otley described a series of 10 patients having an average of 8 lesions each excised in a single session. A combination of local anesthesia and sedation was used and two patients were electively hospitalized due to the extent of the surgery. Nine of ten patients in that study preferred the megasession to multiple sessions for removal of multiple lesions. In our center, we tend to limit the use of general anesthesia to cases requiring multidisciplinary management in the operating room.

Relapse

Transplant patients are predisposed to relapse via local recurrence or metastasis and frequent clinical follow-up is essential.

> Palpation of previously treated areas is crucial for evaluation for in-transit metastases from primary cutaneous SCC since these may present as subcutaneous papules with little or no epidermal change.

> Consider wide-field irradiation (3–5 cm) following removal with clear margins of in-transit metastases or deep marginal recurrences from SCC by Mohs surgery or standard excision (Fig. 17.9).

Uncomplicated peripheral marginal recurrence is best managed by Mohs surgery.

Although there is a lack of data from controlled trials, the authors tend to begin treatment 6 weeks after surgery. Treatment usually consists of 4,000–5,000 cGy delivered to a wide field (3–5 cm surrounding the site) over a 3- to 4-week period. Patients with in-transit metastases should be considered for oral retinoids and evaluated for reduction or change in their immune suppression regimen. In these cases, decreasing azathioprine or cyclosporine may be considered. In addition, changing the immunosuppression regimen to include sirolimus may be considered. Patients with nodal metastases should be evaluated

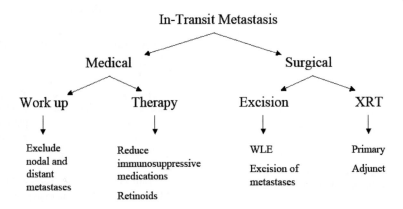

Fig. 17.9 Management of in-transit metastases from primary cutaneous SCC in transplant patients

for neck dissection followed by XRT (Fig. 17.9). Patients with distant metastases should be referred to an oncologist for evaluation for systemic chemotherapy. Platinum-based chemotherapies have been used in patients with metastatic nonmelanoma skin cancer and may be considered for transplant recipients with distant metastases from primary skin cancers. Capecitabine, a 5-fluorouracil (5-FU) pro-drug used in lung and gastrointestinal (GI) carcinomas, may be useful in this setting.[45,46]

Management of Extensive Field Disease

Extensive field disease is common in fair-skinned transplant patients with significant UV exposure histories. Initial evaluation usually may reveal several to many nodular lesions mixed in among a background of hyperkeratotic severely sun-damaged skin. One strategy includes shave excision of nodular lesions followed by ED&C with subsequent histologic evaluation as described. At this time patients are evaluated for oral retinoids.

> Hyperkeratotic, sun-damaged background skin may be treated with topical keratolytics (salicylic acid, urea) for 2–4 weeks followed by alternating 4-week courses of standard topical treatments for AKs including 5-FU, imiquimod, or diclofenac.

Standard cryotherapy may be used at follow-up visits. After 2–3 cycles of topical treatments, PDT may be considered. In cases of severe field disease unresponsive to topicals—or in cases characterized by multiple, eruptive, invasive cancers—PDT and oral retinoids and reduction or change of immune suppression may be considered. In some centers, the oral chemotherapeutic capecitabine is being evaluated for use in this context.[45,46]

The treatment modalities used in combination for extensive field disease are discussed in detail as follows.

Topical 5-Fluorouracil (5-FU)

Topical 5-FU is a competitive inhibitor of thymidylate synthase, a critical enzyme in the biosynthetic pathway of pyrimidines in DNA. Uptake of 5-FU in proliferating keratinocytes leads to termination of DNA synthesis resulting in cell death. In a study by Smith et al., five renal transplant recipients with Bowens' disease on the lower extremities were successfully treated with topical 5% 5-FU plus 5% imiquimod cream.[47] The authors of that study hypothesized that the addition of the immune response modifier imiquimod may have altered the local immune microenvironment, potentially improving the efficacy of topical 5-FU treatment.[47]

Imiquimod

Imiquimod is an immune response modifier, approved by the Food and Drug Administration (FDA) as a therapy against genital warts (condylomata acuminata), actinic keratoses, and superficial basal cell carcinomas. It binds to toll-like receptors (TLRs) TLR7, TLR8, and may enhance release of interferon-α (IFN-α).[48] In a study by Ulrich et al.,[49] the safety and efficacy of imiquimod 5% cream for the treatment of actinic keratoses in transplant recipients were evaluated. In this multicenter, randomized, placebo-controlled study, a total of 43 transplant recipients were randomized to either an imiquimod cream or placebo cream for 16 weeks. Complete clearance rate was observed in 62.1% (18/29) of the treatment group versus 0% (0/14) for vehicle alone.

Diclofenac

Diclofenac is a nonsteroidal anti-inflammatory drug (NSAID) that inhibits cycoloxygenase-2 (COX-2). In a study by Ulrich et al., six transplant recipients with numerous actinic keratoses were treated with 3% diclofenac cream, twice-daily for 16 weeks.[50] Three patients demonstrated complete clinical and histological clearance of AK lesions at the end of the 16-week treatment. Two patients demonstrated 75%

clearance reduction and one patient demonstrated 30% reduction in lesion clearance.

Photodynamic Therapy (PDT)

In PDT treatment, a photosensitizer such as 5-aminolevulinate (5-ALA) or methyl 5-aminolevulinate (MAL) is topically applied to the lesion. Subsequent activation by a red or blue light source activates the photosensitizers, which are precursors in the heme biosynthetic pathway. Production of Porphyrin IX leads to localization of this heme molecule to the plasma membrane of rapidly proliferating tumor cells and results in the production of radical oxygen species culminating in cell death (Chapter 4). In a study by Perrett al.,[51] eight organ transplant recipients with actinic keratoses were randomized to topical 5-FU or MAL PDT treatment twice daily for 3 weeks. The outcome of each treatment was evaluated at 1, 3, and 6 months. PDT was more effective than 5-FU in achieving complete resolution of lesion at all time points, with a mean lesional area reduction of 100% versus 79% in PDT and 5-FU-treated lesions respectively. In another study by Piaserico et al.,[52] PDT was successfully used to treat AKs in organ transplant recipients. The reported complete response (CR) was 71% after two treatment sessions. The response rate was higher on facial lesions (72%) versus acral lesions (40%). Pulsed dye laser (PDL, 585–600 nm) is absorbed by aminolevulinate and may provide an alternate source for treating individual lesions.

> Modified PDT consisting of Levulan application followed by local anesthesia prior to higher fluence pulse dye laser may be helpful in patients with multiple eruptive KA-like SCCs.

Oral Retinoids

Oral retinoids, such as acitretin, may decrease the incidence of primary cutaneous squamous cell carcinomas in transplant patients. Thus the authors prescribe acitretin for transplant recipients with extensive field disease.

> Consider acitretin for patients with high numbers of primary SCCs (> 10/year), extensive field disease, or metastases from primary cutaneous SCC.

A 16-year retrospective study demonstrated that low-dose acitretin significantly reduced the development of SCC in organ transplant recipients in the first 3 years of treatment.[53] Although side effects are usually limited to mucocutaneous complaints including xerosis, dry eyes and lips, and hair loss, the authors recommend discussing retinoid use with the primary transplant team prior to starting therapy. As discussed elsewhere in this text (see Chapter 21), oral retinoids including acitretin are contraindicated in pregnancy. Routine laboratory evaluation should include periodic monitoring of liver function tests and triglycerides.

Reduction of Immunosuppression

In a randomized control trial by Dantal et al.,[54] a cohort of 231 renal transplant patients were treated with two different dose regimens of cyclosporine. In the normal dose cyclosporine group, 26/115 developed NMSC, whereas in the low-dose group 17/116 developed NMSC. SCC constituted the majority of skin cancer in each group, with 15 (57%) and 8 (47%) patients in the normal and low-dose groups, respectively. Rejection episodes were more frequent in the low-dose cyclosporine group. In a study by Jensen et al.,[4] in which more than 2,500 kidney and heart transplant patients were followed for skin malignancies, patients receiving a triple-drug regimen of cyclosporine, azathioprine, and prednisolone had a higher incidence of NMSC than patients receiving a dual-drug regimen of azathioprine and prednisolone. Based on these and other studies it was thought that decreasing immunosuppression might lead to decreased incidence and severity of skin cancers.[2,54]

Otley et al.[55] reported on six solid organ transplant patients in whom immunosuppressive drug regimens had been discontinued due to graft failure. Subsequent to cessation of immunosuppressive therapy, 4/6 patients showed decreased numbers of skin cancers. The Reduction of Immunosuppression Task Force of the International Transplant Skin Cancer Collaborative recommended decreasing immune suppression in transplant recipients with severe and/or life-threatening skin cancers.[56] Reduced or decreased immunosuppression carries the risk of graft rejection; therefore, decisions regarding cessation of therapy must be made with a multidisciplinary team of transplant physicians and dermatologists.

> Discuss modification of immunosuppression with the transplant team for patients with numerous life-threatening, primary skin cancers or metastases from skin cancer.

Capecitabine

Capecitabine, a chemotherapeutic drug indicated in the systemic treatment of metastatic colon and breast cancer,[57] is a carbamate derivative of 5-FU and is converted to its active form in tumor cells. IFN-α enhances the uptake of capecitabine into tumor cells. In a report by Wollina et al.,[45] four patients with advanced SCC were treated with oral capecitabine and subcutaneous IFN-α. There was complete remission in two patients and partial response in two patients. Capecitabine has been successfully used in a small series of patients with locally aggressive cutaneous SCC.[46] Further studies are warranted to evaluate its potential safety and efficacy in the treatment of severe field disease in transplant patients. Use of capecitabine must be discussed with the primary transplant team and medical oncology team managing the patient.

Management of Basal Cell Cancer in Transplant Recipients

BCC management in transplant recipients is very similar to BCC management in the immunocompetent. Superficial lesions on the trunk may be treated by ED&C; this is especially useful in cases of multiple lesions. Mohs surgery should be considered for patients with BCC on the head and neck, recurrent BCC, or BCC with aggressive histology.

Management of Melanoma in Transplant Recipients

As with immunocompetent patients, excision with appropriate clear margins is the treatment of choice for melanoma in transplant recipients (Chapter 15). Sentinel lymph node biopsy can be considered for MM with Breslow depth > 1 mm, extension to Clarks level 4, or for lesions with indeterminate depth due to inadequate evaluation of the base. Mohs surgery or staged excision may be helpful for lentigo maligna lesions on the head and neck located on a background of extensive actinic damage (Chapter 11).

Dermatologic Follow-Up and Screening in Transplant Recipients

It has been clearly established that skin cancer is a significant cause of morbidity and mortality in organ transplant recipients. As the number of organ transplant recipients increases, screening for skin cancer remains crucial. Routine screening examination by dermatologists, along with enhanced patient education will significantly decrease morbidity and even mortality in these patients. In a report by Christenson et al. the use of an organized, established clinic model to provide ongoing educational and preventive dermatological care for transplant recipients has been advocated.[58]

In a recent study at the Mayo Clinic, 202 organ transplant patients were randomized into either a standard or an intensive educational intervention program designed to assess measurable improvement in patient knowledge and sun-protective behavior.[59] Those patients who received intensive educational training were found to be more compliant with sun-protective behavior recommendations.

High-risk patients may require long-term follow-up and treatment for their skin cancers by a multidisciplinary team that includes the dermatologist, Mohs surgeon, transplant physician, medical oncologist, and oncologic surgeon.

Summary

The increase in number of successful solid organ transplants, coupled with the ever rising incidence of skin cancer in the United States, sets the stage for a dramatic rise in skin cancer, particularly SCC, in immunosuppressed transplant patients. Based on their increased susceptibility, higher rates of morbidity, and mortality from skin cancer, we must redouble our efforts to educate these patients on photoprotection and early detection strategies. It is imperative that these patients are evaluated by dermatologists at the earliest point in their course, preferably prior to transplant surgery.

References

1. United Network for Organ Sharing (UNOS) www.Unos.org. Last accessed January 19, 2009.
2. Berg D, Otley CC. Skin cancer in organ transplant recipients: epidemiology, pathogenesis, and management. *J Am Acad Dermatol.* 2002;47(1):1–17.
3. Harwood CA, Proby CM. Human papillomaviruses and non-melanoma skin cancer. *Curr Opin Infect Dis.* 2002;15(2):101–114.
4. Jensen P, Hansen S, Moller B, et al. Skin cancer in kidney and heart transplant recipients and different long-term immunosuppressive therapy regimens. *J Am Acad Dermatol.* 1999;40(2 Pt 1):177–186.
5. Lindelof B, Sigurgeirsson B, Gabel H, Stern RS. Incidence of skin cancer in 5356 patients following organ transplantation. *Br J Dermatol.* 2000;143(3):513–519.
6. Boyd S, Tolvanen K, Virolainen S, Kuivanen T, Kyllonen L, Saarialho-Kere U. Differential expression of stromal MMP-1, MMP-9 and TIMP-1 in basal cell carcinomas of immunosuppressed patients and controls. *Virchows Arch.* 2008;452(1):83–90.
7. Penn I. Malignancies associated with renal transplantation. *Urology.* 1977;10(Suppl 1):57–63.
8. Hollenbeak CS, Todd MM, Billingsley EM, Harper G, Dyer AM, Lengerich EJ. Increased incidence of melanoma in renal transplantation recipients. *Cancer.* 2005;104(9):1962–1967.
9. Le Mire L, Hollowood K, Gray D, Bordea C, Wojnarowska F. Melanomas in renal transplant recipients. *Br J Dermatol.* 2006;154(3):472–477.
10. Dapprich DC, Weenig RH, Rohlinger AL, et al. Outcomes of melanoma in recipients of solid organ transplant. *J Am Acad Dermatol.* 2008;59(3):405–417.
11. Ramsay HM, Reece SM, Fryer AA, et al. Seven-year prospective study of nonmelanoma skin cancer incidence in U.K. renal transplant recipients. *Transplantation.* 2007;84(3):437–439.
12. Moosa MR, Gralla J. Skin cancer in renal allograft recipients—experience in different ethnic groups residing in the same geographical region. *Clin Transplant.* 2005;19(6):735–741.
13. Lampros TD, Cobanoglu A, Parker F, Ratkovec R, Norman DJ, Hershberger R. Squamous and basal cell carcinoma in heart transplant recipients. *J Heart Lung Transplant.* 1998;17(6):586–591.
14. Ong CS, Keogh AM, Kossard S, Macdonald PS, Spratt PM. Skin cancer in Australian heart transplant recipients. *J Am Acad Dermatol.* 1999;40(1):27–34.
15. Adamson R, Obispo E, Dychter S, et al. High incidence and clinical course of aggressive skin cancer in heart transplant patients: a single-center study. *Transplant Proc.* 1998;30(4):1124–1126.
16. Perera GK, Child FJ, Heaton N, O'Grady J, Higgins EM. Skin lesions in adult liver transplant recipients: a study of 100 consecutive patients. *Br J Dermatol.* 2006;154(5):868–872.
17. Levy M, Backman L, Husberg B, et al. De novo malignancy following liver transplantation: a single-center study. *Transplant Proc.* 1993;25(1 Pt 2):1397–1399.
18. Frezza EE, Fung JJ, van Thiel DH. Non-lymphoid cancer after liver transplantation. *Hepatogastroenterology.* 1997;44(16):1172–1181.
19. Leisenring W, Friedman DL, Flowers ME, et al. Nonmelanoma skin and mucosal cancers after hematopoietic cell transplantation. *J Clin Oncol.* 2006;24(7):1119–1126.
20. Goldman GD. Squamous cell cancer: a practical approach. *Semin Cutan Med Surg.* 1998;17(2):80–95.
21. Brash DE, Ziegler A, Jonason AS, et al. Sunlight and sunburn in human skin cancer: p53, apoptosis, and tumor promotion. *J Investig Dermatol Symp Proc.* 1996;1(2):136–142.
22. Leffell DJ, Brash DE. Sunlight and skin cancer. *Sci Am.* 1996;275(1):52–53, 56–59.
23. Alam M, Caldwell JB, Eliezri YD. Human papillomavirus-associated digital squamous cell carcinoma: literature review and report of 21 new cases. *J Am Acad Dermatol.* 2003;48(3):385–393.
24. Bouwes Bavinck JN, Feltkamp M, Struijk L, Schegget J. Human papillomavirus infection and skin cancer risk in organ transplant recipients. *J Investig Dermatol Symp Proc.* 2001;6(3):207–211.
25. Khavari TA, Rinn J. Ras/Erk MAPK signaling in epidermal homeostasis and neoplasia. *Cell Cycle.* 2007;6(23):2928–2931.
26. Dajee M, Lazarov M, Zhang JY, et al. NF-kappaB blockade and oncogenic Ras trigger invasive human epidermal neoplasia. *Nature.* 2003;421(6923):639–643.
27. Haider AS, Peters SB, Kaporis H, et al. Genomic analysis defines a cancer-specific gene expression signature for human squamous cell carcinoma and distinguishes malignant hyperproliferation from benign hyperplasia. *J Invest Dermatol.* 2006;126(4):869–881.
28. Lai EC. Notch signaling: control of cell communication and cell fate. *Development (Cambridge, England).* 2004;131(5):965–973.

29. Nicolas M, Wolfer A, Raj K, et al. Notch1 functions as a tumor suppressor in mouse skin. *Nat Genet*. 2003;33 (3):416–421.

30. Proweller A, Tu L, Lepore JJ, et al. Impaired notch signaling promotes de novo squamous cell carcinoma formation. *Cancer Res*. 2006;66(15):7438–7444.

31. Chan GL, Erdmann GR, Gruber SA, Matas AJ, Canafax DM. Azathioprine metabolism: pharmacokinetics of 6-mercaptopurine, 6-thiouric acid and 6-thioguanine nucleotides in renal transplant patients. *J Clin Pharmacol*. 1990;30(4):358–363.

32. Lennard L, Maddocks JL. Assay of 6-thioguanine nucleotide, a major metabolite of azathioprine, 6-mercaptopurine and 6-thioguanine, in human red blood cells. *J Pharm Pharmacol*. 1983;35(1):15–18.

33. O'Donovan P, Perrett CM, Zhang X, et al. Azathioprine and UVA light generate mutagenic oxidative DNA damage. *Science*. 2005;309(5742):1871–1874.

34. Borel JF, Di Padova F, Mason J, Quesniaux V, Ryffel B, Wenger R. Pharmacology of cyclosporine (sandimmune). I. Introduction. *Pharmacol Rev*. 1990;41(3): 239–242.

35. Hojo M, Morimoto T, Maluccio M, et al. Cyclosporine induces cancer progression by a cell-autonomous mechanism. *Nature*. 1999;397(6719):530–534.

36. Servilla KS, Burnham DK, Daynes RA. Ability of cyclosporine to promote the growth of transplanted ultraviolet radiation-induced tumors in mice. *Transplantation*. 1987;44(2):291–295.

37. Morath C, Arns W, Schwenger V, et al. Sirolimus in renal transplantation. *Nephrol Dial Transplant*. 2007;22 (Suppl 8):viii61–viii5.

38. Euvrard S, Ulrich C, Lefrancois N. Immunosuppressants and skin cancer in transplant patients: focus on rapamycin. *Dermatol Surg*. 2004;30(4 Pt 2):628–633.

39. Campistol JM, Eris J, Oberbauer R, et al. Sirolimus therapy after early cyclosporine withdrawal reduces the risk for cancer in adult renal transplantation. *J Am Soc Nephrol*. 2006;17(2):581–589.

40. Rowe DE, Carroll RJ, Day CL Jr. Prognostic factors for local recurrence, metastasis, and survival rates in squamous cell carcinoma of the skin, ear, and lip: implications for treatment modality selection. *J Am Acad Dermatol*. 1992;26(6):976–990.

41. Stasko T, Brown MD, Carucci JA, et al. Guidelines for the management of squamous cell carcinoma in organ transplant recipients. *Dermatol Surg*. 2004;30(4 Pt 2): 642–650.

42. Glover MT, Niranjan N, Kwan JT, Leigh IM. Nonmelanoma skin cancer in renal transplant recipients: the extent of the problem and a strategy for management. *Br J Plast Surg*. 1994;47(2):86–89.

43. Carucci JA, Martinez JC, Zeitouni NC, et al. In-transit metastasis from primary cutaneous squamous cell carcinoma in organ transplant recipients and nonimmunosuppressed patients: clinical characteristics, management, and outcome in a series of 21 patients. *Dermatol Surg*. 2004;30(4 Pt 2):651–655.

44. Martinez JC, Otley CC. Megasession: excision of numerous skin cancers in a single session. *Dermatol Surg*. 2005;31(7 Pt 1):757–761; discussion 61–62.

45. Wollina U, Hansel G, Koch A, Kostler E. Oral capecitabine plus subcutaneous interferon alpha in advanced squamous cell carcinoma of the skin. *J Cancer Res Clin Oncol*. 2005;131(5):300–304.

46. Petersen JE. The use of oral capecitabine chemotherapy for radioresistant and large recurrent squamous cell carcinomas of the scalp. American College of Mohs Surgery Annual Meeting 2008.

47. Smith KJ, Hamza S, Skelton H. Topical imidazoquinoline therapy of cutaneous squamous cell carcinoma polarizes lymphoid and monocyte/macrophage populations to a Th1 and M1 cytokine pattern. *Clin Exp Dermatol*. 2004;29(5):505–512.

48. Ulrich C, Busch JO, Meyer T, et al. Successful treatment of multiple actinic keratoses in organ transplant patients with topical 5% imiquimod: a report of six cases. *Br J Dermatol*. 2006;155(2):451–454.

49. Ulrich C, Bichel J, Euvrard S, et al. Topical immunomodulation under systemic immunosuppression: results of a multicentre, randomized, placebo-controlled safety and efficacy study of imiquimod 5% cream for the treatment of actinic keratoses in kidney, heart, and liver transplant patients. *Br J Dermatol*. 2007;157 (Suppl 2):25–31.

50. Ulrich C, Hackethal M, Ulrich M, et al. Treatment of multiple actinic keratoses with topical diclofenac 3% gel in organ transplant recipients: a series of six cases. *Br J Dermatol*. 2007;156(Suppl 3):40–42.

51. Perrett CM, McGregor JM, Warwick J, et al. Treatment of post-transplant premalignant skin disease: a randomized intrapatient comparative study of 5-fluorouracil cream and topical photodynamic therapy. *Br J Dermatol*. 2007;156(2):320–328.

52. Piaserico S, Belloni Fortina A, Rigotti P, et al. Topical photodynamic therapy of actinic keratosis in renal transplant recipients. *Transplant Proc*. 2007;39(6): 1847–1850.

53. Harwood CA, Leedham-Green M, Leigh IM, Proby CM. Low-dose retinoids in the prevention of cutaneous squamous cell carcinomas in organ transplant recipients: a 16-year retrospective study. *Arch Dermatol*. 2005;141 (4):456–464.

54. Dantal J, Hourmant M, Cantarovich D, et al. Effect of long-term immunosuppression in kidney-graft recipients on cancer incidence: randomised comparison of two cyclosporin regimens. *Lancet*. 1998;351(9103): 623–628.

55. Otley CC, Coldiron BM, Stasko T, Goldman GD. Decreased skin cancer after cessation of therapy with transplant-associated immunosuppressants. *Arch Dermatol*. 2001;137(4):459–463.

56. Otley CC, Maragh SL. Reduction of immunosuppression for transplant-associated skin cancer: rationale and evidence of efficacy. *Dermatol Surg*. 2005;31(2): 163–168.

57. Van Cutsem E, Van de Velde C, Roth A, et al. Expert opinion on management of gastric and gastro-oesophageal junction adenocarcinoma on behalf of the European Organisation for Research and Treatment of Cancer (EORTC)-gastrointestinal cancer group. *Eur J Cancer*. 2008;44(2):182–194.

58. Christenson LJ, Geusau A, Ferrandiz C, et al. Specialty clinics for the dermatologic care of solid-organ transplant recipients. *Dermatol Surg.* 2004;30(4 Pt 2):598–603.

59. Clowers-Webb HE, Christenson LJ, Phillips PK, et al. Educational outcomes regarding skin cancer in organ transplant recipients: randomized intervention of intensive vs standard education. *Arch Dermatol.* 2006;142(6): 712–718.

Chapter 18
Imaging of Head and Neck Skin Cancer

Komal Shah, Jane Onufer, and Deborah F. MacFarlane

It is important for clinicians to understand and to take advantage of new imaging techniques available for the management of skin cancers. There is little written in either skin cancer or radiology texts on the topic of imaging in head and neck skin cancers. This chapter is an attempt to find a common ground between the disciplines of surgery and radiology so that each may communicate more effectively with the other, thereby benefiting patient care and health-care costs.

We begin with an overview of imaging modalities such as computed tomography (CT), magnetic resonance imaging (MRI), ultrasound (US), and positron-emission tomography/CT (PET/CT) in order to clarify their specific strengths and limitations. Our next objective is to provide guidance on the indications for pre- and postoperative imaging of skin cancer and on choosing the best modality for specific clinical indications. Figures will illustrate the imaging characteristics of certain skin cancers and this will be accompanied by a review of the relevant literature. Discussion of high-resolution MRI and US imaging for diagnosis of skin cancers is beyond the scope of this chapter.

Anatomic Planes

In order to understand imaging modalities, one must first understand the anatomic planes involved. The axial plane is the plane parallel to the floor if the patient is standing up. By convention, the patient's left side is the right side of the image. If the patient

were standing in front of a window, looking out, the coronal plane could be defined as parallel to the window. Sagittal planes are parallel to the plane that would divide the body into symmetric halves, as seen in Fig. 18.1.

Imaging Techniques

Computerized Tomography

Computerized tomography (CT) is the workhorse of our imaging evaluation of skin cancers at MD Anderson Cancer Center (MDACC) because it delivers the best spatial resolution, and is also fast and relatively economical. This modality uses ionizing radiation (X-rays) to produce axial images. By convention, axial images are always shown as if the feet of the supine patient were closest to us—so the patient's left is on the right side of the image. The rotating gantry within a CT scanner houses the source of a beam of ionizing radiation, as well as multiple detectors that register the attenuation of the beam after it passes through the body. The beam is attenuated as it passes through tissue, proportional to the density of the tissue, resulting in relative values similar to that of X-ray images. For example, bone is the most attenuating (or white), water is next, then fat, and lastly air is the least attenuating (and appears black). The unit of attenuation is the Hounsfield unit (HU). Water is arbitrarily set at 0 HU; soft tissue measures 10–50 HU, and bone measures >1,000 HU. Intravenous contrast enhancement increases the X-ray

D.F. MacFarlane (ed.), *Skin Cancer Management*, DOI 10.1007/978-0-387-88495-0_18,
© Springer Science+Business Media, LLC 2010

Planes of Imaging

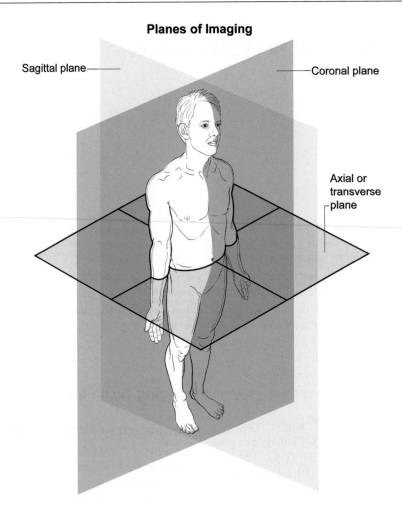

Fig. 18.1 Body planes (Illustration by Alice Y. Chen)

attenuation of blood, making vessels appear "whiter" and giving many types of pathology a characteristic enhancement pattern. For CT examinations, iodinated contrast agents are used. Unless the scan is obtained specifically to evaluate bone, administration of intravenous contrast will always provide more information than a noncontrast scan.

The first human CT scan was a brain CT performed in 1971. Each scan resulted in two contiguous slices and each scan took 4.5–20 min to acquire and 20 min to process.[1] The technical advances of helical scanning and multiple detectors have since greatly increased the rapidity of CT studies and decreased the possible slice thickness. For example, high quality CT images at 1.25-mm slice thickness, from aortic arch to the vertex, may be obtained in

30s. At this slice thickness, exquisite multi-planar reconstructions may be obtained.

Contraindications

Renal insufficiency and severe hypersensitivity are contraindications to contrast administration. Iodinated contrast can exacerbate renal insufficiency. Mild hypersensitivity reactions can be avoided by pretreatment with steroids. Consultation with the imaging facility is recommended.

During pregnancy, because of the risk of ionizing radiation to the development of the fetus, it is important to perform a thorough risk-benefit analysis when deciding whether to perform a CT study.

The same is true for children generally, especially when the orbits or thyroid gland would be included in the scan range, as these tissues are especially radiosensitive. Ultrasound or MRI would generally be a safer choice.

Strengths and Limitations

CT provides excellent spatial resolution and excellent visualization of osseous structures. For example, the question of whether a scalp mass is eroding the adjacent bone is best answered by CT. CT is also a good modality for screening lymph nodes. Because of its spatial resolution, CT is a very good tool for surgical planning. The quality of the multiplanar reconstructions obtained depends on how thin the axial slices are. The new multi-detector CT scanners easily obtain 1.25-mm images, which result in exquisite reconstructions. From a cost viewpoint, CT is considerably faster than MRI and is also much less expensive.

Artifact from metal, which is a problem with both CT and MRI, can be circumvented to some extent on CT by obtaining angled images. This is routinely done for patients with dental fillings, as seen in Fig. 18.2. CT can be less sensitive than MRI for bone metastases that are limited to the marrow, and is definitely less sensitive for perineural involvement or small brain metastases.

Magnetic Resonance Imaging

In contrast to CT, magnetic resonance imaging uses no ionizing radiation. The first requirement for MRI is a strong standing magnetic field, typically 1.0–4.0 Tesla for diagnostic medical imaging. This magnetic field aligns the spins of hydrogen protons in tissue. A radiofrequency stimulator and antenna system are used to generate a radiofrequency gradient, and superimposed radiofrequency pulses, causing a change in alignment. The prescribed set of pulses and signal acquisitions is described as a pulse sequence. The signal acquired from the realignment of the protons is processed using Fourier transformation into the MR image.

A large, and expanding, repertoire of pulse sequences allows excellent contrast resolution between different types of tissue, for example skin and subcutaneous fat, or gray matter and white matter in the brain. The pulse sequences we use most commonly for skin cancers are T1-weighted, T2-weighted, and T1-weighted with contrast and fat saturation. On T1-weighted images, materials such as fat, some blood products, some types of calcification, and the gadolinium-based contrast agents are bright. Gray matter and muscle are of intermediate signal intensity. Fluid has low signal intensity. Dense calcification, as seen in cortical bone, and blood vessels running perpendicular to the plane of the image, generate very low or no signal. On T2-weighted images, water demonstrates the

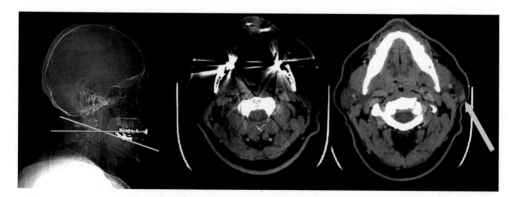

Fig. 18.2 This 70-year-old man had undergone Mohs surgery for a left preauricular squamous cell carcinoma 4 months prior to this CT. *Left*: The lateral scout image shows the planes of the axial images. *Middle*: The left parotid gland is completely obscured by streak artifact from dental fillings. *Right*: An angled image is taken, revealing a left intraparotid nodal metastasis

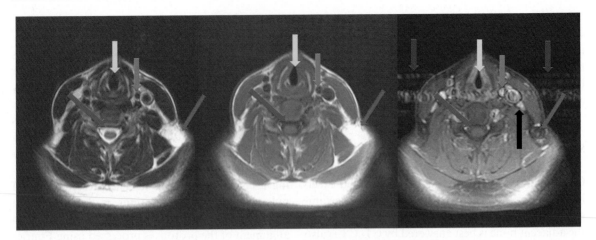

Fig. 18.3 *Left*: T2-weighted image. *Blue arrow*, CSF is bright. *Red arrow*, fat is bright. *Green arrow*, left carotid artery is black. *Yellow arrow*, air is black. *Middle*: T1-weighted image. *Blue arrow*, CSF is dark. *Red arrow*, fat is bright. *Green arrow*, left carotid artery is black. *Yellow arrow*, air is black. *Right*: T1-weighted image with gadolinium enhancement and fat saturation. CSF is dark and air is black, as on T1, middle. *Black arrow*, enhancing normal lymph node. *Red arrow*, fat is dark. *Green arrow*, left carotid artery is bright. *Purple arrows*, multiple bright linear patterns due to pulsation artifact

highest signal intensity, so cerebrospinal fluid and vitreous humor are very bright. In the case of fat suppression, a radiofrequency pulse is applied at exactly the right time to null the signal that would have been generated by fat. Fat suppression can be used with both T1 and T2 weighting. It is almost always used when gadolinium-based contrast is administered, so that enhancement can be distinguished from fat. Fat suppression is required for contrast-enhanced imaging of the orbits, as the orbital contents are surrounded by fat. See Fig. 18.3 for examples of T2-weighted; T1-weighted; and T1 gadolinium-enhanced, fat suppressed images of the neck.

Intravenous contrast administration is always preferred in cases of malignancy, as most neoplasms and nodal metastases will enhance. Most neoplasms will also demonstrate bright signal on T2-weighted images, due to their increased water content.

Contraindications

The use of Gd-based contrast agents (GBCA) is contraindicated in cases of severe renal insufficiency or acute renal failure, due to the risk of nephrogenic systemic fibrosis (NSF).[2] NSF, originally called nephrogenic fibrosing dermopathy, consists of thickening and tightening of the skin, most often the lower extremities and occasionally the trunk. Fibrosis of other organs can include the heart, lungs, bone, and skeletal muscle. As of January 2008, 215 cases had been confirmed by the International Center for Nephrogenic Fibrosing Dermopathy (NFD/NSF) Registry.[4] Guidelines vary by institution, but we withhold contrast when the estimated GFR falls to 30 or below, or if acute renal insufficiency is suspected. The FDA also recommends against using GBCA in the perioperative period of liver transplantation.[3,4] It is rare, but an estimated 3% of patients will have a hypersensitivity reaction to GBCA. In severe cases, contrast should not be administered again, but many patients with a mild reaction can be switched to a different contrast agent. Relative contraindications include pregnancy and breast feeding.

Other contraindications to MRI include the presence of ferromagnetic foreign bodies and implants, and functioning stimulators such as pacemakers and defibrillators, transcutaneous electrical nerve stimulator (TENS) devices, and cochlear implants.[5] These can be dislodged or may malfunction in the presence of the strong magnetic field. Selected patients with pacemakers and defibrillators may safely undergo MR scanning at 1.5T or lower field strength, after thorough evaluation.[6] Many aneurysm clips and stents placed within the body are nonferromagnetic and considered safe. If a patient has a history of cerebral aneurysm clipping, this potential contraindication can be addressed in advance. The MR center may request, upon the patient's medical information release, detailed information from the operative note or neurosurgeon regarding the exact type of aneurysm clip and its compatibility with a strong magnetic field. Other medical devices are only safe after a certain time period following implantation such as 6 weeks for certain types of carotid stents.

Strengths and Limitations

The major strength of MRI is the excellent tissue contrast. GBCA enhancement of the nervous system, especially cranial and peripheral nerves and brain parenchymal masses, remains far superior to iodinated contrast enhancement as seen by CT. MRI incurs none of the potential risks of ionizing radiation. MRI is much more sensitive in diagnosis of perineural involvement than is CT.[7] Although CT is better for cortical bone, MRI is better for bone metastases because they involve the marrow before they involve the cortex.

However, MRI does have diagnostic limitations and is not always superior to CT, despite the more-than-double cost. MRI is not as sensitive to subtle changes in cortical bone, which may signal involvement by, for example, a scalp tumor. Lymph nodes are difficult to evaluate by MRI, mainly because their size is quite small with respect to MRI slice thickness, and size is the main criterion by which they can be evaluated using MRI. Spatial resolution is not as good as with CT. Despite using axial T2-weighted images with fat saturation techniques through the neck, the detection of cervical adenopathy is not as good as CT or US.[8] However, at our institution, when the primary site is best evaluated by one modality, that same modality is used to screen for lymphadenopathy.

The long scan times, generally at least 45 min if contrast-enhanced sequences are performed, may result in enough patient motion to significantly degrade the images. Children may require sedation or even general anesthesia.

Ultrasound

Ultrasound (US), like MR, does not expose the patient to ionizing radiation. Frequencies higher than those we can hear are transmitted, and the time at which the reflection of the wave is received back is used to infer the location of the material that reflected the wave. The first diagnostic use of US was to distinguish solid tumors from benign cysts. This remains a primary function of ultrasound. Cysts are completely anechoic or "black" because the ultrasound waves are fully transmitted through the cyst without being reflected back to the probe. Solid tissue will reflect some or all of the waves back to the probe. As more waves are reflected, fewer waves are available to be transmitted to structures at a greater depth. Also, higher frequency waves have a decreased penetration but generate a higher resolution image. Thus, with ultrasound there is an inverse relationship between the penetration, or the depth of tissue that can be imaged, and the resolution of the images produced. Doppler ultrasound imaging is an ultrasound technique that allows characterization of vascular flow. The physical principle of Doppler shift of a waveform reflected by a moving target is used to analyze the velocity and direction of flowing blood or to detect small amounts of flowing blood.

Many tissues have a characteristic "echotexture" or pattern generated by ultrasound. For example, fat has small septations and is "echogenic" or bright. Muscle has many echogenic lines within it. Skin is typically hyperechoic. As mentioned previously, fluid-containing structures, including blood vessels, are black or anechoic. Calcified structures will also appear anechoic because all of the ultrasound waves will be reflected back to the probe. However, the edge of the calcification, where the ultrasound waves were reflected, will appear echogenic. By convention, images obtained with the probe perpendicular to the long axis of the body are labeled transverse, and those obtained with the probe parallel are labeled longitudinal. The patient's right will be on the right side of the image, as with CT.

Ultrasound is a very good choice for detection and biopsy of abnormal lymph nodes. Probably more nodal characteristics can be evaluated by ultrasound than by any other modality. A benign node typically is oval in shape, has an echogenic hilum, and demonstrates hilar blood flow, as seen in Figs. 18.4 and 18.5.

Size has traditionally been regarded as the most important nodal characteristic in CT and MRI.

Fig. 18.4 Transverse
ultrasound image of the
axilla. The *top edge* shows
the echogenic line of the
dermis. Below this is
subcutaneous fat, then the
striations of muscle. The
oval structure indicated by
the white arrow is a normal
lymph node seen in
transverse (roughly axial)
orientation. The *black arrow*
demonstrates the echogenic
hilum

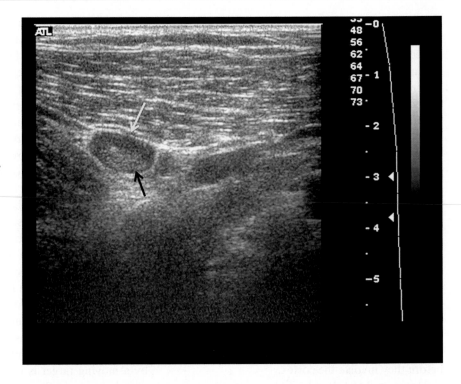

Fig. 18.5 Doppler
ultrasound imaging of a
normal cervical lymph node.
The echogenic line at the *top*
of the image represents the
dermis. The lymph node
demonstrates normal cortex
with relatively decreased
echogenicity compared to
the hilum. The *red* and *blue*
colors indicate normal blood
flow in opposite directions,
contained within the hilum

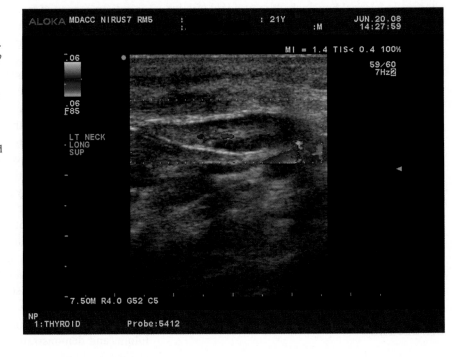

With ultrasound, measurements in three dimensions can be obtained very accurately, and an increase in node size over time is relatively straightforward to detect.

A rounded rather than oval shape, decreased echogenicity or increased "reticulated" echogenicity, the presence of necrosis, calcification, clustering, and extra-capsular spread can all be seen or assessed using grayscale ultrasound of suspicious lymph nodes (Fig. 18.6 and Fig. 18.7). Color or Power Doppler ultrasound can further contribute to the detection of suspicious lymph nodes by identifying peripheral rather than normal hilar blood flow. Diffusely increased vascularity may also be suspicious. While no single ultrasound criterion for malignancy may be specific, the combination of a rounded hypoechoic lymph node with peripheral flow outside of the hilum would be highly suspicious for a nodal metastasis.

Strengths and Limitations

An important advantage of US is that biopsy can be performed at the time of the study. Other technical advantages include mobility of the probe and machine, and the ability to scan in any plane. Patients who are unable to lie flat can be accommodated for scanning and biopsy.

As discussed above, lymph node evaluation is a strong advantage of ultrasound. While the normal neck may contain up to 300 lymph nodes, typically only 5–20 of the largest and/or most superficial nodes will be detected by ultrasound. The detection of abnormal lymph nodes is also significantly operator dependent, and requires experience and care. Ultrasound images can be difficult to use for surgical planning, unless they have been helpfully annotated. Often, an additional CT and/or intraoperative ultrasound will be useful for the surgeon.

Dressings, wounds, and sutures may interfere with the ability to place the probe and coupling gel in the appropriate area. Poor quality images may be obtained on obese patients, or if recent postoperative or postradiation changes are present.

Positron-Emission Tomography

Both positron-emission tomography (PET) and lymphoscintigraphy (discussed later) are

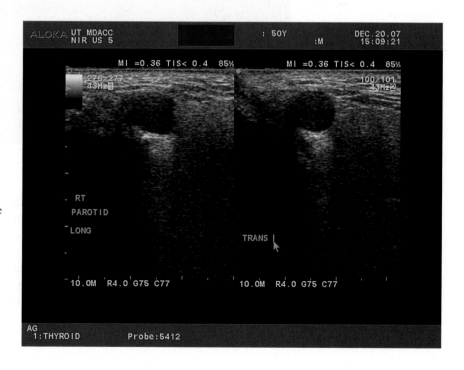

Fig. 18.6 A 50-year-old man was referred to MD Anderson Cancer Center after excision of a forehead Merkel cell carcinoma with positive deep margins. These transverse and longitudinal ultrasound images of the parotid gland were obtained as part of a staging evaluation. A 1 cm, round, hypoechoic intra-parotid lymph node is identified. Fine needle aspiration demonstrated metastatic Merkel cell carcinoma

Fig. 18.7 This 68-year-old
man with a history of chronic
lymphocytic leukemia as well
as multiple squamous cell
skin cancers, presented with
a biopsy-proven left axillary
metastasis. During
chemotherapy he developed
new right axillary
adenopathy. Prior to surgery
to excise the metastasis,
evaluation of the right
axillary node was requested.
Grayscale (*top*) and color
Doppler (*bottom*) ultrasound
images of an axillary lymph
node are shown. On
grayscale, the node is
enlarged but retains its
lobulated shape and
echogenic hilum. The cortex
demonstrates mildly
increased echogenicity with a
regular, reticular
echotexture. Color Doppler
does show increased flow,
but the flow remains
centered at the hilum. The
imaging findings suggested
leukemic involvement rather
than nodal metastasis from
the skin cancer, and this was
confirmed by biopsy

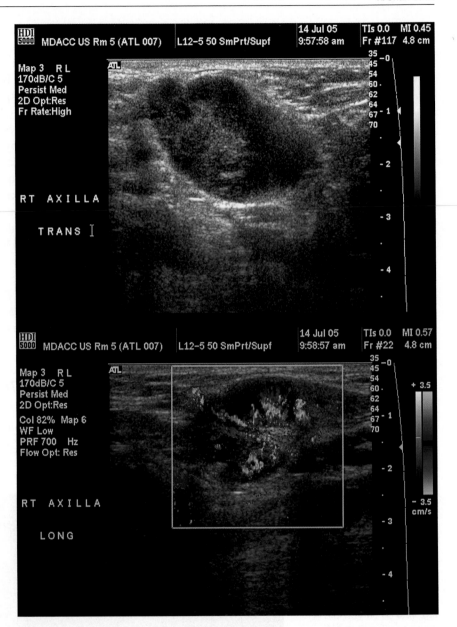

considered Nuclear Medicine procedures. The
strength of nuclear medicine is imaging structure
and function. This is achieved by attaching a radio-
nuclide, which can be imaged, to a molecule that
can participate in a targeted physiologic process.

PET images begin with the intravenous administration of 18-fluoro-deoxyglucose (18-FDG),
a molecule similar to glucose, which can be

incorporated into the same metabolic pathways
as glucose, and contains 18-Fluorine, a positron
emitter that can be imaged. Malignancies that
have a higher rate of cellular turnover will have
increased 18-FDG activity on PET scans. Modern
PET scanners are often combined with CT scanners in the same housing. This allows for the accurate fusion of CT images with PET images. In this

way, both function and structure can be imaged. The fusion of PET to CT images has greatly improved the anatomic localization of 18-FDG avid foci.[9]

The patient must fast for 4–6 h prior to an oncologic PET/CT. Plasma glucose levels are checked prior to scanning and must be within normal limits. After injection of 18-FDG, the patient must rest quietly for 1 h to allow distribution of the radiotracer. The scanning itself usually takes less than 30 min. Typically, scans are obtained from the base of the skull to the proximal thighs. For patients with, for example, melanoma of the toe, the entire lower extremity will also be scanned.

For much of this decade, PET/CT has been supplanting PET alone. With this technique, a CT scan is obtained at the same time at the PET scan, using the same equipment. Often, the CT component will be performed using a technique that results in less radiation dose but also slightly decreased spatial resolution compared to a routine CT scan, and usually will not include iodinated contrast administration. The information obtained by CT is used to process the PET information in order to display it to best advantage. This is called "attenuation correction." In addition, the CT images are fused to the PET images, allowing significantly improved localization of anatomic structures.

Benefits of PET/CT include accurate localization and staging, monitoring tumor response to therapy, and early detection of recurrence. Substantial research on PET/CT scanning in the staging of malignant melanoma and in predicting the response to treatment has found a significant benefit with the use of this modality.[10]

A disadvantage is that locoregional nodal metastases can be difficult to visualize in comparison to the highly avid uptake at a primary site. Technically, lung metastases less than 1 cm are difficult to detect due to respiratory motion. Brain metastases can be difficult to detect due to the inherent FDG avidity of gray matter.[10] Infectious and inflammatory false positives are very common; for example, acne can be mistaken for a primary skin cancer.

Lymphoscintigraphy

In this nuclear medicine study, the ability of lymph nodes to trap colloidal particles is exploited. A colloidal material, for example ultra-filtered sulfur colloid, is labeled with a radioisotope that can be imaged, such as Technetium-99m. When the 99m-Tc-sulfur colloid is injected adjacent to a primary site of tumor, the material is collected by the lymphatic system and follows the same drainage pattern as would the tumor cells. For skin cancers, the material is injected intradermally at the primary site. The 99m-Tc allows imaging of this drainage pattern, and also can be detected by gamma probe intraoperatively. Lymph nodes that are identified in this manner do not necessarily contain metastatic deposits; the imaging only serves to guide the sentinel lymph node biopsy process.

Formerly, only transmission images were obtained for lymphoscintigraphy, resulting in "2D" images without cross-sections. Today, tomographic cross-sectional images can be obtained and fused with CT images[11](Fig. 18.8). This aids in the preoperative differentiation of superficial from deeper nodes, for example, external jugular versus internal jugular nodal chains.

Strengths and Limitations

Obviously, this technique allows identification of the drainage pattern but does not indicate that the active node is actually malignant. Because head and neck drainage patterns can be variable, it offers a useful road map for the surgeon. When hybrid SPECT/CT is not available, intraoperative detection is crucial to correctly identify the sentinel nodes. Optimally, the sentinel lymph node biopsy should be performed at the time of resection of the primary site.[12]

Please see Table 18.1 for the exchange of information that may occur when speaking with your radiologist and Table 18.2 for suggested indications for imaging skin cancers.

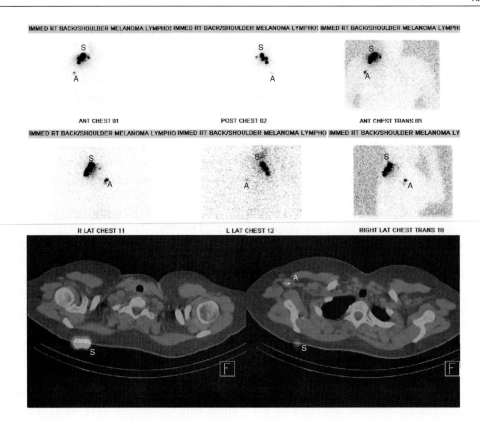

Fig. 18.8 A 36-year-old woman presented with a bleeding nodule on the right upper back. Excisional biopsy revealed a Clarks level IV melanoma, with 6.4-mm Breslow thickness. Wide local excision with sentinel lymph node biopsy was planned. Prior to surgery, lymphoscintigraphy with CT fusion was obtained. *Top row*: Anterior and posterior 2D images of the chest show a large lobulated focus of radiotracer activity at the primary site in the skin (S). Smaller adjacent foci likely represent sentinel lymph nodes. The most inferior node (A) may be an axillary or an anterior or posterior chest wall node. *Middle row*: Right and left lateral 2D images of the chest confirm that the most inferior focus of activity corresponds to a right axillary node. *Bottom*: CT images further localize the right axillary sentinel node and also confirm that all of the activity in the largest focus is in the skin rather than within nodes. At operation, the sentinel lymph nodes were negative for melanoma

Table 18.1 Speaking with your radiologist

1. What is the patient's primary malignancy and where is it located?
2. What anatomic structures would you like to include? Brain, face, neck, or sinuses?
3. What information are you interested in evaluating? Perineural spread? Skull base disease? Nodal involvement?
4. Are there any variables that may preclude certain exams? Is the patient claustrophobic? Do they have a pacemaker or other metallic foreign body?
5. Is there evidence of significant renal disease? If so, do they have a recent creatinine or calculated glomerular filtration rate (GFR)?
6. Is this a presurgical evaluation?
7. Could the radiologist correlate all the imaging modalities that have been used to assess the patient? (i.e., PET/CT/MR/US)

Table 18.2 Indications for imaging

1. Incidental perineural involvement found on biopsy
2. Clinical evidence of perineural invasion
3. Large malignancies in a nerve root distribution
4. Suspicion of bone or cartilage invasion
5. Not amenable to clinical inspection
6. Lacrimal duct involvement

Imaging Pathology

Basal Cell Carcinoma

Metastases from basal cell carcinoma (BCC) are rare, so imaging distant to the site of primary tumor is seldom necessary. Occasionally, imaging of the primary site is helpful in the assessment of nearby anatomic structures prior to surgical intervention. For example, an ulcerated basal cell cancer of the scalp may involve the skull and CT can determine whether or not cortical destruction has occurred. If perineural involvement was suspected, MRI would be the study of choice.

We have found imaging to be especially useful in cases of periorbital BCC as seen in the accompanying case illustration. Leibovitch et al. in 2005 recommended preoperative imaging for all recurrent periorbital BCC.[13] They reported 64 cases, 84% of which were recurrent and 56% of which were located at the medial canthus. Of the entire group, 21% had bony involvement seen on CT. In general, extensive orbital invasion necessitates orbital exenteration, while anterior orbital involvement alone may be treated with excision and possible radiation followed by serial MRI.

Illustrative Case 18.1

A 76-year-old man with a history of multiple basal cell carcinomas presented with a left medial canthal mass as seen in Fig. 18.9. The mass occurred 4 years following Mohs surgery at the same site, and was clinically inseparable from periosteum. The CT shown in Figs. 18.10 and 18.11 was obtained to delineate the extent of the recurrence.

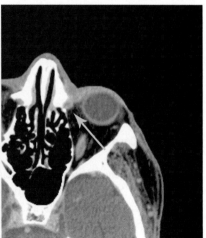

Fig. 18.9 Recurrent infiltrative basal cell carcinoma of the left medial canthus

The patient underwent resection by Mohs surgery and was referred to the oculoplastic surgery service, for further resection of the tumor. Complete resection was not possible. The patient underwent postoperative radiation treatment and continues to have imaging surveillance.

Cutaneous Squamous Cell Carcinoma

Indications for the imaging of cutaneous squamous cell (SCC) carcinoma include planning for local excision, the identification of metastatic lymph nodes, diagnosis of perineural involvement, and the early detection of recurrence. High resolution CT can provide the best spatial resolution for surgical

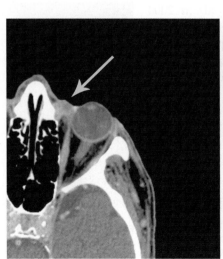

Fig. 18.10 Superior to inferior axial postcontrast images of the orbit. *Left image*: *Arrow*, left medial canthus mass, abutting the periosteum and the attachment of the medial rectus muscle on the globe. No destruction of cortical bone. *Right image*: The skin over the left side of the nose appears involved. *Arrow*, the lacrimal sac is involved

Fig. 18.11 Coronal reconstructions of the axial images seen in Fig. 18.10. Left image, *curved arrow*, normal right lacrimal sac. *Green arrows*, left lacrimal sac involved by BCC

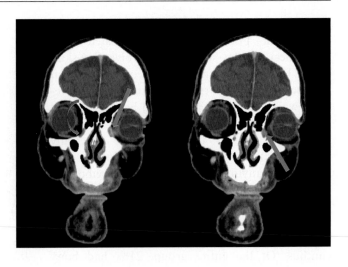

planning and for the detection of recurrence at the resection site. Nodal metastases can be seen by CT, MR, US, and PET. In a blinded, prospective study reported by Adams et al. in 1998, 60 patients underwent all four of these studies prior to neck dissection. They found 117 metastases in 1,284 lymph nodes on neck dissection.[14] PET scanning provided 90% sensitivity and 94% specificity for nodal metastases and was able to detect nodal metastases as small as 0.6 cm. However, only metastases greater than 1 cm were diagnosed as malignant by CT; in our experience, some metastatic lymph nodes smaller than 1 cm can be identified. The study found MR and CT to have similar sensitivity and specificity, ranging from 79–85%. The use of lymphoscintigraphy for sentinel lymph node localization is not currently widespread, but Wagner et al. in 2004 found a sensitivity of 89% for sentinel lymph node biopsy in a population of patients with nonmelanoma skin cancers: 17 squamous cell carcinoma, 5 Merkel cell carcinoma, and 2 adenocarcinoma.[15]

Illustrative Case 18.2

A 64-year-old man underwent excision of a left supraorbital SCC, which recurred 7 months later and was treated with a 5-week course of radiation. Seven months later, he had a second recurrence, which was treated with Mohs surgery at an outside institution. Histology demonstrated a positive margin at the supraorbital nerve. Almost a year later, he presented with headaches, blurred vision, proptosis, and paresthesias in the distribution of the ophthalmic division of the trigeminal nerve. The patient then referred himself to our institution for further management (Fig. 18.12).

The MRI shown in Fig. 18.13 was obtained to assess for perineural involvement.

Radical orbitectomy was performed. Pathology confirmed recurrent squamous cell carcinoma with perineural involvement of CN V1. The patient underwent stereotactic radiosurgery and continues to be followed with imaging.

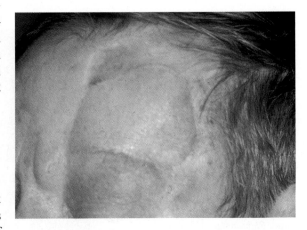

Fig. 18.12 Clinically, no tumor was apparent at the surgical site. Photograph courtesy of Charles Butler, M.D., MD Anderson Cancer Center

Fig. 18.13 *Top*: Noncontrast T1-weighted axial (*left*) and coronal (*right*) images. On the axial image, the focal area of decreased signal (*arrow*) overlying the frontal sinus indicates the surgical site. On the coronal image, thickening of the left ophthalmic nerve is demonstrated (*arrow*). *Bottom*: Contrast enhanced, fat-saturated T1-weighted coronal images through the orbit (*left*) and orbital apex (*right*). Thickening and enhancement of the nerve is seen within the orbit and superior orbital fissure (*arrows*). More posterior images (*not shown*) demonstrated no involvement of Meckel's cave

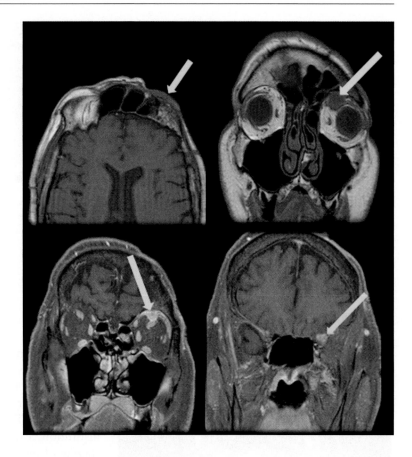

Illustrative Case 18.3

A 67-year-old man with a 5-year history of a tumor on the left temple was referred for excision (Fig. 18.14). CT was obtained preoperatively to evaluate for bone

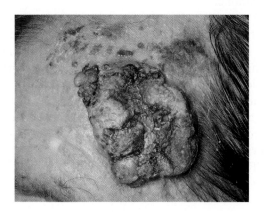

Fig. 18.14 A 6 × 4.5-cm tumor not attached to bone was apparent was on the left temple

involvement and nodal metastasis (Fig. 18.15). Seven months after his initial surgery, a follow-up CT demonstrated a new left preparotid lymph node suspicious for metastasis (Fig. 18.16). Ultrasound-guided fine needle aspiration (FNA) (Fig. 18.17) demonstrated metastatic squamous cell carcinoma. The patient had a left parotidectomy, confirming nodal metastasis. Left neck dissection on the same date demonstrated no cervical nodal metastases.

Illustrative Case 18.4

A 70-year-old man presented to Mohs surgery with a biopsy-proven SCC recurrence within a radial forearm flap on his left temple, which had been performed 6 months prior (Fig. 18.18). A CT was obtained as part of his preoperative work up (Fig. 18.19).

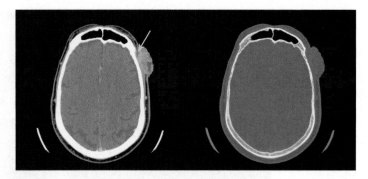

Fig. 18.15 *Left*: Axial postcontrast CT image through the frontal sinus demonstrates invasion of the temporalis musculature. *Right*: Bone window of the same CT image demonstrates no cortical erosion. No adenopathy was seen. Wide local excision was performed by Head and Neck surgery and the patient underwent a further flap repair by Plastic Surgery. Follow-up CT obtained 5 months later is shown in Fig. 18.16

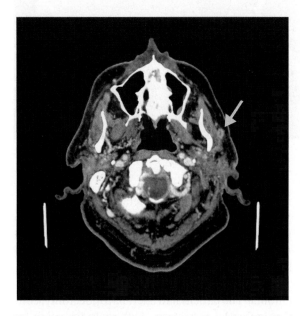

Fig. 18.16 Axial postcontrast CT image through the level of the parotid gland demonstrates a subcentimeter, enhancing, centrally necrotic preparotid lymph node suspicious for metastasis (*arrow*)

Melanoma

We will consider only cutaneous, not mucosal, melanomas in this chapter. Patients with American Joint Committee on Cancer (AJCC) stage I or II melanoma do not generally need routine imaging.[16] Imaging is indispensable for M staging and for following response to treatment for systemic disease. Patients with stages III and IV disease undergo regular MRI of the brain with contrast and PET/CT or CT with contrast at our institution. PET and PET/CT are indicated for staging of melanoma with multiple studies showing increased sensitivity and specificity compared to CT alone.[10] Lung and brain metastases are not reliably detected by PET due to factors discussed previously. Furthermore, PET cannot be used to identify locoregional nodal disease, especially axillary nodes. However, its ability to reveal extranodal metastasis is a strength of PET imaging in melanoma.

Preoperatively, lymphoscintigraphy (along with intraoperative blue dye) is frequently used to locate sentinel lymph nodes for sampling (Chapter 15). Cross-sectional imaging may help to identify locoregional nodal metastases. In the head and neck, detection of parotid adenopathy is critical to surgical planning. The presence of parotid adenopathy may steer the surgeon toward neck dissection even if the neck is clinically negative.[17]

Fig. 18.17 Ultrasound-guided biopsy of the suspected nodal metastasis in Case 18.3. The needle (*straight arrow*) approaches the rounded, hypoechoic lymph node (*curved arrow*)

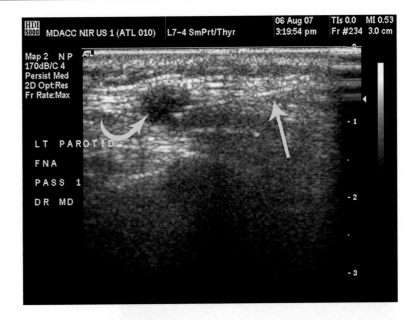

Fig. 18.18 Recurrent SCC is seen within the left forehead flap. Photograph courtesy of Roman Skoracki, M.D., MD Anderson Cancer Center

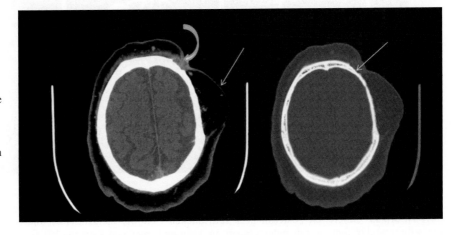

Fig. 18.19 *Left*: Axial postcontrast CT image at the level of the recurrence demonstrates an enhancing soft tissue mass (*curved arrow*) at the anterior margin of the flap (*straight arrow*). *Right*: The same image displayed in a bone window more clearly shows cortical erosion (*straight arrow*)

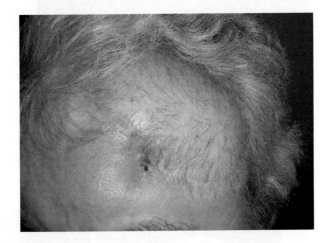

Illustrative Case 18.5

A 68-year-old man with a primary melanoma on the left occiput underwent radiation and excision at another hospital. One year later, the lesion recurred (Fig. 18.20). CT of the neck with contrast was obtained for restaging (Fig. 18.21).

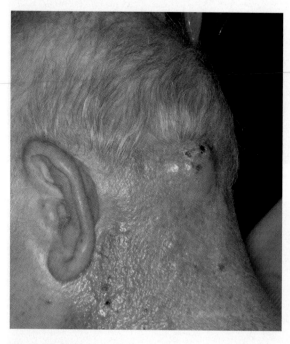

Fig. 18.20 Primary melanoma at the left occiput and dermal metastases over the angle of the jaw were apparent clinically

Dermatofibrosarcoma Protuberans

The deep extension and actual size of this spindle cell tumor can be difficult to determine based on physical examination. In cases of residual or recurrent tumor, or large fixed masses, imaging may be helpful to define the involvement of adjacent or possibly un-resectable structures. Imaging can also be helpful in planning wound closure and in follow-up.

Kransdorf in 1994 first reported the use of imaging, including CT, MRI, and arteriograms, to evaluate the extent of dermatofibrosarcoma protuberans (DFSP).[18] In 2002, Torreggiani et al. described the MRI signal characteristics of 10 cases of histologically proven DFSP.[19] These tumors demonstrated hypointensity compared to fat, and iso- or hypointensity compared to muscle on T1-weighted images. Thornton et al. in 2005 described a series of 10 pediatric patients with DFSP, 5 of whom were imaged with MR.[20] Of these 5 patients, 2 had MR evidence of deep extension, which increased the extent of surgical resection. Thus, MR has proven useful in determining subclinical extension, especially in large tumors and difficult locations. Thornton also reported the use of MRI in follow-up after surgery, for a limited period. Clinical surveillance is usually lifelong.

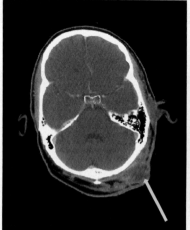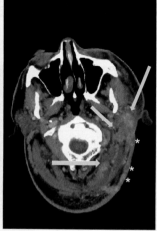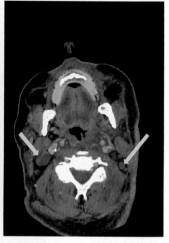

Fig. 18.21 *Left*: Primary site of melanoma in the scalp, extending from the skin almost to the periosteum (*arrow*). *Middle*: Severe left posterior neck skin thickening with nodular foci of rim enhancement in keeping with dermal metastases (*asterisks*). Deeper metastatic foci are seen within the left neck musculature and left parotid gland (*arrows*). *Right*: Appearance of a necrotic nodal metastasis on the right and subcentimeter nodal metastasis on the left (*arrows*)

Illustrative Case 18.6

A 49-year-old man presented to the ER with a 5-year history of a growing mass on his back (Fig. 18.22). MR was obtained to evaluate the extent of the mass prior to resection (Fig. 18.23).

Histology demonstrated DFSP and the patient underwent excision. Fourteen months after the surgery the patient developed a painful mass over the left clavicle, as seen on the MR in Fig. 18.24.

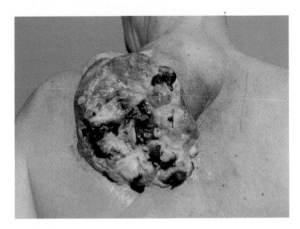

Fig. 18.22 A large tumor occupies the left upper back. Photograph courtesy of Matthew M. Hanasono, M.D., MD Anderson Cancer Center

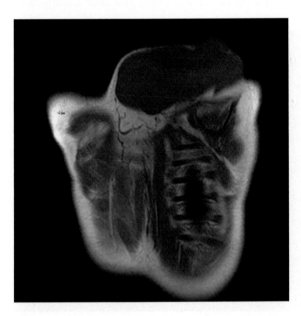

Fig. 18.23 T1-weighted noncontrast MR image of the chest. A large mass, iso-intense to muscle, involves the skin of the upper back and extends into the subcutaneous fat over the posterior chest wall

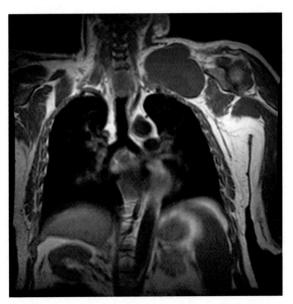

Fig. 18.24 Coronal T1-weighted noncontrast image through the chest. A new mass is seen at the *left* thoracic inlet, again iso-intense to muscle but anterior to the initial site of DFSP and no longer involving the skin. The patient underwent resection of the recurrence, followed by radiation treatment

Merkel Cell Carcinoma

This rare, aggressive neuroendocrine carcinoma is known to have a high risk of nodal metastasis, distant metastasis, and recurrence.[21] Imaging can be very helpful in evaluating the extent of spread. Gupta in 2006 recommended lymphoscintigraphy and sentinel lymph node biopsy for Merkel cell carcinoma (MCC) because it was much more sensitive than CT in their series.[22] See Fig. 18.6 for an example of the use of ultrasound-guided FNA to diagnose a nodal metastasis from Merkel cell carcinoma.

Although not all Merkel cell carcinomas are FDG avid, cases that are positive on PET have been reported.[23–25] The technique may also be helpful in predicting response to treatment and detecting progression.[23] Belhocine explored the correlation of FDG avidity with MIB-1 labeling in MCC and found that patients whose tumors were FDG-avid had a labeling index of 10–75%, with a mean of about 50%. The tumors that were not FDG-avid demonstrated a labeling index of 4–13%.[24] While some authors have suggested that nuclear medicine scans using octreotide may be highly specific for imaging of MCC, octreotide scanning in two recent studies did not demonstrate a clinical benefit in detection of metastases.[26,27]

Illustrative Case 18.7

A 51-year-old man had undergone excision of an MCC on his right thigh. A few months later, CT scan demonstrated peripancreatic adenopathy. During chemoradiation, progressive lymphadenopathy was noted. PET/CT was obtained as part of restaging prior to investigational therapy (Fig. 18.25).

Sebaceous Carcinoma

Sebaceous carcinoma may involve the periorbital region. If there is orbital involvement, orbital exenteration may be considered.[28] Orbital CT can then be helpful for preoperative planning. In a series of 21 patients, six out of seven who developed regional metastases had a T4 primary lesion,[29] so surveillance CT scanning should be useful only in the most aggressive of these cancers. In one sample of four cases of metastatic eyelid sebaceous carcinoma, a patient developed metastases almost 5 years out from initial diagnosis.[30] However, it is not known how often or for how long surveillance imaging should be obtained. In cases of suspected Muir-Torre syndrome, further evaluation of GI malignancies may be best accomplished by a combination of colonoscopy and CT.

Angiosarcoma

Scalp angiosarcoma may spread rapidly through the skin.[31] The extent of deep and superficial invasion may be assessed by imaging. When imaging the scalp, the postcontrast images should be fat saturated to null the signal from the subcutaneous fat, and to allow visualization of contrast enhancement. At MDACC, we typically include images of the neck as well as the scalp, as angiosarcoma may metastasize to cervical lymph nodes.

Isoda et al. in 2005 reviewed the MRI in eight cases of angiosarcoma. In all eight, the tumor was lower in signal intensity than subcutaneous fat and enhanced intensely. Of the seven cases for which clinical findings were available, in four the extent of tumor was greater by MR than was suspected by clinical evaluation. Only one of these patients had calvarial involvement on MR.[32]

Illustrative Case 18.8

An 80-year-old man presented to the ER with a rapidly growing scalp mass (Fig. 18.26). On exam, a 5-cm scalp tumor was noted and later confirmed by

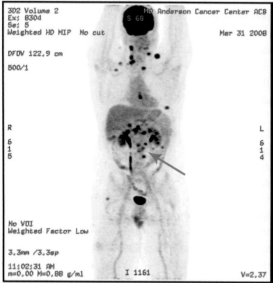
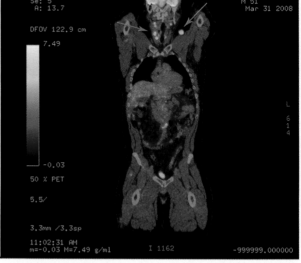

Fig. 18.25 *Left*: Maximum intensity projection reconstructed PET image. *Arrow*, one of several abdominal nodal metastases. *Right*: Fused PET/CT images, coronal plane through the clavicular heads and pubic symphysis. *Arrows* indicate the patient's palpable left supraclavicular subcutaneous metastasis, as well as unsuspected right neck nodal metastases

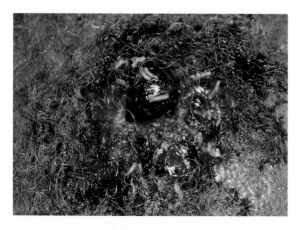

No one imaging modality is best for all purposes. Ultrasound is useful for evaluation of superficial nodes and for biopsy. Lymphoscintigraphy defines the sentinel nodes for biopsy and is most helpful in patients with melanoma. CT is also helpful for the assessment of nodes, cortical bone involvement, and for definition of the primary tumor. MR is by far the best modality for the evaluation of perineural involvement, and is also more sensitive than CT for defining marrow involvement. PET/CT is best for the imaging of distant metastases.

Fig. 18.26 Large hemorrhagic scalp tumor

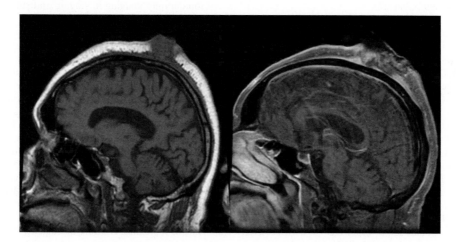

Fig. 18.27 *Left*: Sagittal T1 noncontrast MR image of the brain. The subtle *gray line* over the hyperintense subcutaneous fat represents normal skin. The angiosarcoma involves the skin and galea aponeurotica, and demonstrates signal iso-intense to muscle.[33] *Right*: sagittal postcontrast fat-saturated T1 image of the brain. The angiosarcoma demonstrates intense but heterogeneous enhancement. Enhancement in the periosteum likely represents tumor involvement. The bone cortex is not well evaluated by MR, but no bone marrow extension is identified. The patient underwent a course of chemoradiation with little effect and died shortly thereafter

biopsy to be an angiosarcoma. MRI was obtained to evaluate the extent of the lesion (Fig. 18.27).

Summary

Imaging in skin cancer can be useful for preoperative planning and to assess for perineural involvement, bony involvement, and nodal metastasis. It can help to define tumor size and depth and identify orbital involvement of tumor.

References

1. Beckmann EC. CT scanning the early days. *Br J Radiol.* 2006;79:5–8.
2. Broome DR, Girguis MS, Baron PW, Cottrell AC, Kjellin I, Kirk GA. Gadodiamide-associated nephrogenic systemic fibrosis: why radiologists should be concerned. *Am J Roentgenol* 2007;188(2):586–592.
3. U.S. Food and Drug Administration. Public health advisory and information for health care professionals: gadolinium-containing contrast agents for magnetic resonance imaging (marketed as Magnevist, Multihance, Omniscan, OptiMARK, Prohance). www.fda.gov. Accessed December 15, 2008.

4. Cowper SE. Nephrogenic Fibrosing Dermopathy [NFD/ NSF Website]. 2001–2007. http://www.icnfdr.org. Accessed December 15, 2008.

5. Shellock FG. *Pocket Guide to MR Procedures and Metallic Objects: Update 2001.* Philadelphia, PA: Lippincott Williams & Wilkins; 2001.

6. Nazarian S, Roguin A, Zviman MM, et al. Clinical utility and safety of a protocol for noncardiac and cardiac magnetic resonance imaging of patients with permanent pacemakers and implantable-cardioverter defibrillators at 1.5 tesla. *Circulation.* 2006;114(12): 1232–1233.

7. Parker GD, Harnsberger HR. Clinical-radiologic issues in perineural tumor spread of malignant diseases of the extracranial head and neck. *Radiographics.* 1991;11(3):383–399.

8. De Bondt RB, Nelemans PJ, Hofman PA, et al. Detection of lymph node metastases in head and neck cancer: a meta-analysis comparing ultrasound, ultrasound-guided fine needle aspiration, CT and MR imaging. *Eur J Radiol.* 2007;64(2):266–272.

9. Branstetter BF, Blodgett TM, Zimmer LA, Snyderman CH, Johnson JT, Raman S, Meltzer CC. Head and neck malignancy: is PET/CT more accurate than PET or CT alone? *Radiology* 2005;235(2):580–586.

10. Fletcher J, Djulbegovic B, Soares H, et al. Recommendations on the use of 18F-FDG PET in oncology. *J Nucl Med.* 2008;49(3):480–508.

11. Even-Sapir E, Lerman H, Lievshitz G, et al. Lymphoscintigraphy for sentinel node mapping using a hybrid SPECT/CT system. *J Nucl Med.* 2003;44(9):1413–1420.

12. Kienstra M, Padhya T. Head and neck melanoma. *Cancer Control.* 2005;12(4):242–247.

13. Leibovitch I, McNab A, Sullivan T, Davis G, Selva D. Orbital invasion by periocular basal cell carcinoma. *Ophthalmology.* 2005;112(4):717–723.

14. Adams S, Baum R, Stuckensen T, Bitter K, Hör G. Prospective comparison of 18F-FDG PET with conventional imaging modalities (CT, MRI, US) in lymph node staging of head and neck cancer. *Eur J Nucl Med.* 1998;25(9):1255–1260.

15. Wagner J, Evdokimow D, Weisberger E, et al. Sentinel node biopsy for high-risk nonmelanoma cutaneous malignancy. *Arch Dermatol.* 2004;140:75–79.

16. Huang CL, Halpern AC. Management of the patient with melanoma. In: Rigel D, ed. *Cancer of the Skin.* Philadelphia, PA: Elsevier Saunders; 2005:265.

17. Pathak I, O'Brien CJ, Petersen-Schaeffer K, et al. Do nodal metastases from cutaneous melanoma of the head and neck follow a clinically predictable pattern? *Head Neck.* 2001;23(9):785–790.

18. Kransdorf MJ, Meis-Kindblom JM. Dermatofibrosarcoma protuberans: Radiologic appearance. *Am J Roentgenol.* 1994;163(2):391–394.

19. Torreggiani W, Al-Ismail K, Munk P, Nicolaou S, O'Connell J, Knowling M. Dermatofibrosarcoma protuberans: MR imaging features. *Am J Roentgenol.* 2002;178:989–993.

20. Thornton S, Reid J, Papay F, Vidimos A. Childhood dermatofibrosarcoma protuberans: role of preoperative imaging. *J Am Acad Dermatol.* 2005;53(1):76–83.

21. Medina-Franco H, Urist MM, Fiveash J, Heslin MJ, Bland KI, Beenken SW. Multimodality treatment of Merkel cell carcinoma: case series and literature review of 1024 cases. *Ann Surg Oncol.* 2001;8(3):204–208.

22. Gupta SG, Wang LC, Peñas PF, Gellenthin M, Lee SJ, Nghiem P. Sentinel lymph node biopsy for evaluation and treatment of patients with Merkel cell carcinoma: the Dana-Farber experience and review of the literature. *Arch Dermatol.* 2006;142: 685–690.

23. Yao M, Smith R, Hoffman H, Funk G, Graham M, Buatti J. Merkel cell carcinoma: two case reports focusing on the role of fluorodeoxyglucose positron emission tomography imaging in staging and surveillance. *Am J Clin Oncol.* 2005;28(2):205–210.

24. Belhocine T, Pierard G, Frühling J, et al. Clinical added-value of 19FDG PET in neuroendocrine-Merkel cell carcinoma. *Oncol Rep.* 2006;16:347–352.

25. Iagaru A, Quon A, McDougall IR, Gambhir SS. Merkel cell carcinoma: is there a role for 2-deoxy-2-[F-18]fluoro-D-glucose-positron emission tomography/computed tomography? *Mol Imaging Biol.* 2006;8:212–217.

26. Durani BK, Klein A, Henze M, Haberkorn U, Hartschuh W. Clinical and laboratory investigations: somatostatin analogue scintigraphy in Merkel cell tumors. *Br J Dermatol.* 2003;148(6):1135–1140.

27. Guitera-Rovel P, Lumbroso J, Gautier-Gougis M, et al. Indium-111 octreotide scintigraphy of Merkel cell carcinomas and their metastases. *Ann Oncol.* 2001;12: 807–811.

28. Shields J, Demirci H, Marr B, Eagle R, Shields C. Sebaceous carcinoma of the ocular region: a review. *Surv Ophthalmol.* 2005;50(2):103–122.

29. Saito A, Tsutsumida A, Furukawa H, Saito N, Yamamoto Y. Sebaceous carcinoma of the eyelids: a review of 21 cases. *J Plast Reconstr Aesthet Surg.* 2008;61(11):1328–1331.

30. Husain A, Blumenschein G, Esmaeli B. Treatment and outcomes for metastatic sebaceous cell carcinoma of the eyelid. *Int J Dermatol.* 2008;47(3):276–279.

31. Rosai J, Sumner HW, Kostianovsky M, Perez-Mesa C. Angiosarcoma of the skin: a clinicopathologic and fine structural study. *Hum Pathol.* 1976;7(1):83–109.

32. Isoda H, Imai M, Inagawa S, Miura K, Sakahara H. Magnetic resonance imaging findings of angiosarcoma of the scalp. *J Comput Assist Tomogr.* 2005;29(6): 858–862.

33. Hayman L, Shukla V, Ly D, Taber K. Clinical and imaging anatomy of the scalp. *J Comput Assist Tomogr.* 2003;27(3):454–459.

Chapter 19
Radiation Oncology in Skin Cancer Treatment

Susan L. McGovern and Matthew T. Ballo

Radiation was first used to treat a patient with squamous cell carcinoma of the nose in 1900. Following the development of improved dermatologic and surgical techniques in the 1950s, the role for radiation in the treatment of skin cancer gradually decreased.[1] However, there remain certain settings in which radiation offers advantages over other currently available modalities. The goals of this chapter are to review the current indications for the use of radiation in the treatment of skin cancer, the techniques commonly employed in modern radiotherapy, the role of radiation in the treatment of specific skin malignancies, and the complications that arise from the use of radiation to treat skin cancers.

Indications for Radiation

The general advantages and disadvantages of external beam radiation are summarized in Table 19.1.[1] Broadly, external beam radiation is a painless outpatient procedure. It can be used in patients who are not surgical candidates due to medical reasons, particularly the elderly. It also allows for preservation of uninvolved structures adjacent to the lesion. This is especially important in the head and neck, where the cosmetic and functional consequences of treatment can be significant.

Practically, radiation requires a longer investment of time than surgery; typical regimens require daily treatments for 3–6 weeks.[1] Although the side effects of radiation are usually limited to the treated field, they can persist or worsen over time. For instance, the doses required for adequate tumor kill also usually cause permanent alopecia within the treated field.[2] The cosmetic sequelae of radiation, including dermatitis and telangiectases, also worsen over the decades following treatment.[3,4] Because radiation is a known carcinogen, there is also a risk of a second malignancy within the treated field. Due to these late effects, we typically do not recommend radiation for patients younger than 50 years of age if an equally effective, alternative method is available.[5]

These issues, as well as several patient-specific ones, are generally addressed during the patient's initial consultation with a radiation oncologist. Table 19.2 lists some of the factors that will be considered during that first visit; many of these questions are ideally addressed prior to the patient's arrival in the radiation clinic. One of the most important issues to discuss is the patient's expectation of radiation. Many patients have an inaccurate perception of the process and sequelae of radiation; this should be addressed up front and clearly during the initial visit.

Prior to the delivery of any radiation treatment, confirmation of the diagnosis with biopsy is necessary.[1] This establishes the histology of the lesion, which dictates subsequent decisions about the applicability and technique of radiation treatment. As shown in Table 19.3, the indications for radiation depend on the histology and location of the lesion. For instance, some cutaneous lymphomas, including mycosis fungoides, are highly radiosensitive lesions, and radiation can offer a unique therapeutic advantage.[1]

D.F. MacFarlane (ed.), *Skin Cancer Management*, DOI 10.1007/978-0-387-88495-0_19,
© Springer Science+Business Media, LLC 2010

Table 19.1 Advantages and disadvantages of radiation therapy[1]

Advantages	Disadvantages
Outpatient procedure	Typically requires a treatment course of 3–6 weeks
Treatment is painless	Can cause permanent alopecia
Can be used in patients that are medically inoperable, particularly the elderly	Long-term cosmetic sequelae of radiation, including dermatitis and telangiectases, worsen over the decades following treatment
Allows for preservation of uninvolved structures	Risk of second malignancy within the treated field

Table 19.2 Some questions that will typically be considered during the initial interview with a radiation oncologist. Communication between the referring physician and the radiation oncologist prior to the initial interview can address many of these issues

Typical radiation oncology questions
Has the histologic diagnosis been adequately established?
Has appropriate staging been completed?
Has this lesion occurred before?
Has the patient had any treatment for this lesion? If so, what? Have these treatments helped or not?
What treatments, if any, are planned?
What are the anticipated goals of radiation treatment—primary or adjuvant therapy? Definitive or palliative?
Has the patient undergone any previous radiation? If so, what site was treated? What was the duration (or, more ideally, dose) of the treatment? What facility performed the treatment? How long ago was treatment completed?
Does the patient have any other cancer diagnoses? If so, how were those conditions treated?
What is the patient's overall medical condition?
What are the patient's comorbidities?
Does the patient have a history of any conditions that may be exacerbated by radiation, such as CREST syndrome, dermatofibrosis, lupus, or scleroderma?
What are the patient's expectations regarding radiation?

Table 19.3 Indications for radiation therapy[1]

Highly indicated	• Cutaneous T-cell lymphoma • Some B-cell lymphomas • Kaposi's sarcoma
Good indication	• Basal cell carcinoma • Squamous cell carcinoma • Merkel cell tumors
Sometimes indicated	• Angiosarcoma • Melanoma
Rarely indicated	• Carcinoma of the scrotum, palms, soles • Fibrosarcoma

Most basal and squamous cell carcinomas are successfully addressed with surgical methods. Primary radiotherapy is preferred for the treatment of tumors that cannot be excised without causing a significant cosmetic or functional deformity, such as lesions on or near the nose, ears, and eyelids.[6,7] Similarly, lesions of the cheek, lip, or oral commissure that would require a full-thickness resection can also be effectively managed with radiotherapy.[5] For carcinomas that have been excised, postoperative radiation can be used to treat positive surgical margins, perineural invasion, bone or cartilage invasion, or extensive skeletal muscle involvement at the primary site.[5,8] Radiation can also address disease that has spread to the lymph nodes, particularly if there is extranodal extension or multiple positive lymph nodes.[5,8]

Radiation Modalities Used to Treat Skin Tumors

Early-stage skin lesions are ideally treated with orthovoltage or electron-beam radiation. Orthovoltage generators can provide beam energies in the

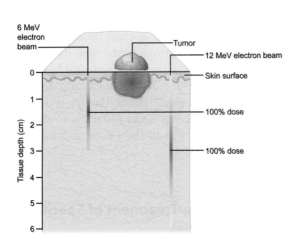

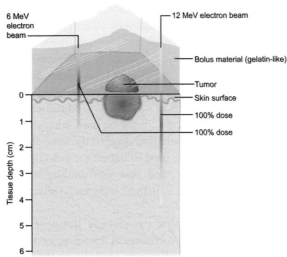

Fig. 19.1 Depth dose of electron beams and the influence of bolus.[1] (**a**) Depth doses of 6-MeV and 12-MeV electron beams without bolus. (**b**) Depth doses of 6-MeV and 12-MeV electron after passing through bolus placed on the skin. The bolus pulls up the dose to improve tumor coverage and spare underlying tissue (Illustration by Alice Y. Chen)

range of 75–125 kV and offer beam characteristics that are favorable for the treatment of lesions less than 5 mm in thickness.[2] Because of their limited applicability, orthovoltage units have almost completely disappeared from treatment centers in the United States. They have generally been replaced by linear accelerators that can produce both high energy photon and electron beams.

Electron beams are well-suited for the treatment of skin lesions.[9] The depth dose behavior of electron beams is illustrated in Fig. 19.1a, b. The energy of a given electron beam determines the depth of tissue it will adequately cover. For instance, a 6-MeV beam will cover approximately 2-cm depth and a 20-MeV beam will cover approximately 6-cm depth.[1] Generally, electron beams homogeneously cover a region of tissue to a specific depth and then dissipate rapidly.[8] This beam profile makes electrons almost ideal for the treatment of skin malignancies where critical normal structures such as the brain are often immediately below the lesion.

To improve the coverage of certain lesions, a bolus of 0.3–2-cm thickness is often applied to the skin (Fig. 19.1a, b). Bolus is a gelatinous tissue-equivalent material that effectively pulls the dose toward the skin, thereby enhancing coverage of more superficial lesions and allowing for increased sparing of underlying normal structures.[10] An example of the use of bolus is presented in Fig. 19.2, which

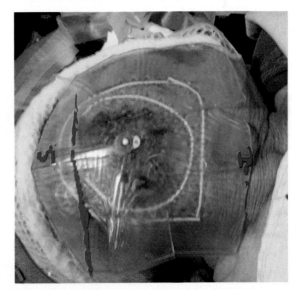

Fig. 19.2 Setup for electron beam treatment of a 93-year-old man with a locally advanced squamous cell carcinoma of the right preauricular region. The head and neck are immobilized with a custom-made mask. The lesion and the desired treatment field are outlined with radiopaque wire, which allows for visualization of the area on the planning CT scan. The external auditory canal is filled with Domeboro drops and TX-151, a pink tissue-equivalent putty, to alleviate dose inhomogeneities caused by the irregular surface of the ear. The entire field plus a wide margin are covered with 3-mm bolus to produce a homogenous dose distribution throughout the treated field. Not shown here, an additional piece of bolus 2-cm thick was applied to the superior aspect of the treatment field to further pull the dose away from the underlying temporal lobe

shows the setup used for treatment of a locally advanced preauricular squamous cell carcinoma.

Shielding is often required to protect the lens of the eye, which is an exceptionally radiosensitive tissue. Treatment of an eyelid tumor can easily expose the lens to more than 5–10 Gy, the threshold dose for the formation of cataracts.[2] Consequently, lead or tungsten shields[11] must be used when indicated to reduce the radiation dose to the lens. Similarly, lead can also be used to define the field limits and shape the beam such that surrounding uninvolved tissues are further spared radiation exposure.

Certain skin cancers, particularly those of the nose, are amenable to treatment by an interstitial technique in which radioactive sources are directly inserted into the tumor (Fig. 19.3a, b, c). This form of radiation is called brachytherapy. For the treatment of skin tumors, iridium-192 is the most commonly used source.[2] The dose of radiation decreases with the inverse square of the distance from the source, allowing for high doses close to the source

and a rapid drop-off in dose with distance.[2] The clinical advantage of this is that it enables us to deliver a high dose to the tumor while sparing much of the surrounding normal tissues. The disadvantages of this approach are that it requires general anesthesia for the placement of the radiation sources and a 4–6-day inpatient stay for the completion of treatment.[2] Brachytherapy is usually combined with external beam radiation to deliver an adequate dose both to the tumor and the surrounding tissue at risk.

Radiation in the Treatment of Specific Skin Malignancies

Basal and Squamous Cell Carcinomas

Basal and squamous cell carcinomas are the skin tumors most commonly treated with radiation, and the general approach to them is similar. Although

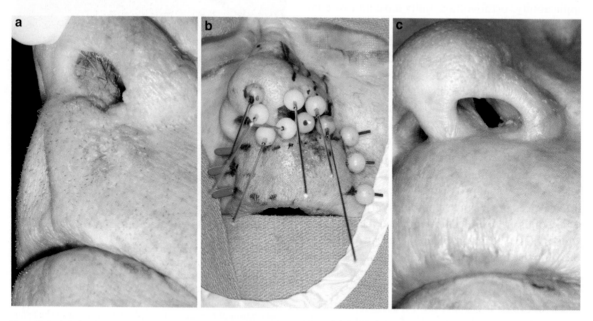

Fig. 19.3 (a) A 65-year-old man with squamous cell carcinoma of the left nasal vestibule that extended to the skin inferior to the nasal vestibule and ala. Because the patient had a history of hypertension, hyperlipidemia, and heart disease requiring coronary artery bypass grafting, he was dispositioned to receive treatment with definitive radiation alone. (b) The left nasal ala and nasolabial skin were initially treated with brachytherapy. Catheters were placed intraoperatively as shown.

Following recovery from anesthesia, iridium-192 sources were placed in the catheters to deliver a dose of 25 Gy over 51 h. After catheter removal and discharge from the hospital, the region was then treated with external beam radiation at 2 Gy per fraction to 50 Gy in 25 fractions, delivered over 5 weeks. (c) Four months after the completion of radiation, the lesion was completely resolved and he had no sign of recurrent disease. Note the expected alopecia within the treated field

surgery effectively manages most lesions, carcinomas that cannot be resected without a significant cosmetic or functional deficit can often be treated with definitive radiation. These include lesions of the nose, eyelid, ear, lip, and cheek, as described previously.[8]

Orthovoltage X-rays or, more commonly, electron beam radiation may be used for the treatment of carcinomas. The radiation portal typically encompasses the visible or palpable tumor plus an additional margin of 0.5–1.0 cm for lesions less than 1 cm and up to 2.0 cm for larger or poorly defined lesions.[12] When low-energy electrons will be used for treatment, an additional 0.5-cm margin is added to the field at the skin surface because the beam constricts with depth.[13] The final margins may be reduced when regions close to the eye are treated.[5]

The approach to postoperative radiation is similar. In the case of perineural invasion, the target volume is extended to include the potential route of perineural spread. For instance, the patient shown in Fig. 19.4a, b had a multiply recurrent squamous cell carcinoma of the right lower eyelid. Pathology from her surgical resection revealed invasion of the infraorbital nerve; she then received adjuvant radiation that treated the nerve all the

way to the skull base. For pathologically positive lymph nodes, the treatment field is extended to include regional lymphatics.[8] After a sufficient dose has been delivered to these regional areas, the field may be reduced to cover the primary lesion.[5]

A variety of dose and fractionation regimens have been used to treat skin carcinomas. Obviously, a shorter treatment course allows the patient to complete treatment more rapidly, but a more protracted course generally yields the best cosmetic results. The choice of a treatment schedule depends on the size of the lesion and its location.[8] Some commonly used treatment schemes are shown in Table 19.4. Because of the large treatment fields required, radiation for positive nodes is delivered at 2 Gy per fraction.[5] Postoperative radiation is also given at 2 Gy per fraction to minimize radiation-related sequelae in a healing operative bed.[5]

Almost all treatment modalities result in 5-year recurrence rates of 1–10% for previously untreated cutaneous basal or squamous cell carcinomas.[14,15] The primary determinant of local control after radiation is the size of the primary lesion.[5] In a series of 646 patients with basal cell, squamous cell, or mixed carcinomas of the face treated with radiation, the 8-year local control rate for lesions larger than

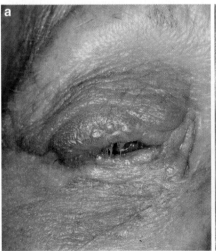 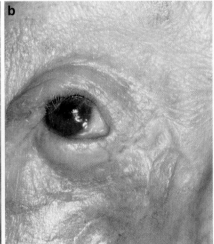

Fig. 19.4 (a) A 77-year-old woman with multiply recurrent squamous cell carcinoma of the right lower eyelid. The lesion had previously been resected three times. She underwent extensive surgical resection and reconstruction, with a right partial maxillectomy, right intraorbital nerve resection, and dissection of the pterygopalatine fossa to the skull base. Pathologic review revealed invasion of the infraorbital nerve. She then received adjuvant radiation to 60 Gy in 30 fractions, which covered the operative bed as well as the infraorbital nerve path to the skull base and the ipsilateral neck nodes. (b) Two months after the completion of radiation, she had recovered well from the acute radiation changes and was without sign of recurrent disease

Table 19.4 Common radiation schedules for the treatment of basal and squamous cell carcinoma[5]

Clinical scenario	Possible fractionation schemes	Total dose (Gy)	Total duration (days)
Most patients, most tumors	4 Gy × 10 fractions	40	12–14
	3 Gy × 15 fractions	45	19–21
	2.5 Gy × 20 fractions	50	26–28
Large treatment field and a good cosmetic outcome is desired[2] or near the eye[14]	2 Gy × 30 fractions	60	42–44
	2 Gy × 35 fractions	70	49–51
Elderly patient with ≤ 1-cm tumor	5 Gy × 8 fractions	40	10–12
Elderly patient in poor health	8 Gy × 4 fractions	32	4–7
	20 Gy × 1 fraction	20	1

5 cm was 53%, whereas the 10-year local control rate for lesions less than 2 cm was 98%.[14] After accounting for size of the primary lesion, basal cell carcinomas have slightly better local control rates than squamous cell carcinomas.[7] Because basal cell carcinomas rarely metastasize,[8] elective nodal irradiation is not performed for basal cell carcinomas of the skin.[5] It is indicated for large, infiltrative cutaneous squamous cell carcinomas, which have a much higher rate of lymphatic spread. Generally, nodal disease up to 3 cm without extracapsular spread can be addressed by either surgery or radiation alone.[12]

Carcinomas that recur after radiation are more difficult to control than previously untreated lesions;[13] These lesions may be most appropriately addressed by surgical resection. The current experience with re-irradiation to address recurrent disease is quite limited.[16]

Melanoma

Melanoma has long been labeled a radioresistant cancer. Many patients are not considered candidates for radiation simply because of this stigma. Indeed, radiation is unlikely to improve overall survival. However, several studies suggest that adjuvant radiation may increase locoregional control, particularly when high-risk features are present.[17] Because locoregional failures can carry significant morbidity, especially in the head and neck, we advocate the use of radiation in appropriately selected patients. In this section, we will review the role of

radiation in the treatment of melanoma, with a particular emphasis on the indications for radiation that should trigger a referral to a radiation oncologist (Table 19.5).

Wide local excision is the standard of care for localized (stage I or II) cutaneous melanoma.[5,8] Radiation alone is seldom indicated for treatment of primary disease, except in the case of large facial lentigo maligna melanomas that would require extensive reconstruction after wide excision.[18] Patients with close or positive margins after excision should ideally be taken back to the operating room so that adequate margins can be obtained. In cases where additional excision is cosmetic or functionally undesirable, adjuvant radiation to address the close or positive margin should be considered.[17,19]

Patients with known lymph node metastases (stage III) are typically treated with wide local excision and therapeutic lymph node dissection. Patients found to have four or more involved nodes, lymph nodes larger than 3 cm, nodal extra-capsular

Table 19.5 Indications for referral to a radiation oncologist for patients with stages I–III melanoma[9]

Positive or close surgical margins that cannot be re-excised
Large lentigo maligna melanomas of the face that would require extensive reconstruction after wide local excision
Positive lymph nodes larger than 3 cm
Lymph node extra-capsular extension
Four or more positive lymph nodes
Recurrent nodal disease after previous therapeutic lymph node dissection

extension, or recurrent nodal disease after a previous therapeutic nodal dissection are candidates for nodal radiation to improve regional control (Table 19.5).[20] This recommendation is supported by the observation that 5-year regional control for such patients can be as high as 89% with nodal radiation,[21] compared to 50–70% for patients who do not receive adjuvant radiation.[22,23] Although radiation does not have an impact on overall survival, the potential regional control benefit for patients with the above-risk factors should prompt consideration of adjuvant radiation.

Disagreement continues to exist regarding the management of regional lymph nodes in melanoma.[8] Before the development of sentinel lymph node biopsy, elective nodal radiation was routinely performed for patients with melanomas of the head and neck at least 1.5-mm thick or Clark level IV or V.[24] This is no longer our typical practice; we now reserve elective nodal radiation for elderly patients who are not candidates for surgery or clinical trial.[5]

Based on our experience and the pervasive belief that melanoma is radioresistant, we continue to recommend a hypofractionated schedule for the treatment of melanoma.[25–27] This means giving a higher dose of radiation per fraction but fewer total fractions. For melanoma, we prescribe 30 Gy divided into five fractions over 2½ weeks. Practically, this means treatment is either delivered every Monday and Thursday or every Tuesday and Friday. The maximum allowed dose to the brain or spinal cord is 24 Gy in four fractions over 2 weeks; if this is problematic, a more conventional schedule should be used.[5]

For adjuvant treatment of the primary site, the radiation field encompasses the surgical bed plus at least an additional 2-cm margin. Treatment is typically delivered with an electron beam using a bolus of appropriate thickness.[28]

For nodal radiation, the treatment portal is tailored to the appropriate nodal basin such that it encompasses the draining lymphatics and spares adjacent critical structures. The cervical nodes are usually treated with an appositional electron beam field that covers the ipsilateral nodes down to the clavicle.[28] The axilla is treated with anterior–posterior fields using megavoltage photons from a linear accelerator.[5] Similarly, inguinal nodes are treated with anterior–posterior photon fields, with matched electron fields as needed to entirely cover the surgical scar.[5]

Merkel Cell Carcinoma

Merkel cell carcinoma is an aggressive tumor. Lymph node metastases occur in two-thirds of patients, and distant metastases occur in approximately one-third of patients.[29] Furthermore, patients with nodal involvement at presentation have a much poorer prognosis compared to node negative patients.[30] Fortunately, Merkel cell carcinoma is radiosensitive. It has been established that gross disease can be controlled with surgery and adjuvant radiation with low rates of recurrence within the irradiated field.[31,32] However, in a series of 31 patients who received radiation at MD Anderson, three developed recurrences on the edge of the radiation field,[30] suggesting that an appropriate treatment field should encompass large margins around the surgical bed.

Therefore, our current recommendations for treatment of the primary site of disease are surgical excision followed by adjuvant radiation. The surgical procedure need not be extensive, as postoperative radiation should always be given and should include a generous 4–5-cm margin, except when limited by the tolerance of adjacent critical structures.[8] When the primary site is in the head and neck, we recommend treatment of the entire ipsilateral neck.[5]

Given the propensity of Merkel cell carcinoma to spread to regional lymph nodes, routine elective nodal irradiation was previously advised. However, current guidelines support the use of sentinel node biopsy;[13] if the sentinel node is positive, nodal irradiation is preferred over lymphadenectomy. For patients who present with involved lymph nodes, we recommend excision of the primary disease and therapeutic lymphadenectomy, followed by radiation of the primary surgical bed and draining lymphatics.[5]

Radiation is typically delivered in 2-Gy fractions using electrons with an appropriate bolus. The elective region is treated to 46–50 Gy, followed by an additional 10-Gy boost in five fractions to a smaller volume encompassing the microscopic or gross residual disease. Large, bulky tumors should receive a total dose of 66 Gy.[5]

Adnexal Carcinoma

Carcinomas of the adnexal structures of the skin are uncommon. Sebaceous carcinomas are typically treated with wide local excision and lymphadenectomy if lymph nodes are involved.[33] Because of the rarity of this tumor, recommendations for postoperative radiation are not well-described, but general indications for adjuvant radiation can be suggested based on the behavior of other carcinomas. These indications include positive margins, perineural invasion, bone or cartilage invasion, extensive muscle invasion, an involved lymph node larger than 3 cm, extracapsular extension, and multiple positive lymph nodes.[5]

Eccrine and apocrine carcinomas are addressed by wide local excision and postoperative radiation.[5] Adjuvant radiation is particularly important for eccrine tumors, which tend to recur locally when treated with surgery alone.[34] Patients with adenopathy should undergo therapeutic nodal dissection and postoperative radiation to the nodal basin.

For all adnexal carcinomas, the radiation target is the surgical bed plus 2–3-cm margins and the draining lymphatics. The typical postoperative dose is 60 Gy administered at 2 Gy per fraction.[5]

Mycosis Fungoides

The first documented use of radiation to treat mycosis fungoides, a low-grade cutaneous T-cell lymphoma, was in 1902.[35] Because lymphocytes are extremely radiosensitive, dramatic responses could be obtained with early methods of radiation, but achieving a sustained response was practically impossible due to the difficulty of safely treating the entire skin surface.[36] Improvements in radiation technology over the last several decades have lead to the development of total-skin electron irradiation (TSEI) as a safe and highly effective treatment for mycosis fungoides.

TSEI can be used in the management of almost all stages of mycosis fungoides.[37] The target is the entire skin surface, including the epidermis, adnexal structures, and dermis.[37] The goal of treatment is to provide sufficient dose to the skin so that a durable remission is obtained, while ensuring patient comfort and minimizing toxicity.

TSEI is technically complex. At MD Anderson, we use a modified Stanford technique[36] in which patients are typically placed in a standing position at least 3.5 m from the linear accelerator source. A Lucite plate is placed between the patient and the linear accelerator to scatter and degrade the electron beam, which has a nominal energy of 9 MeV. Over the entire course of treatment, the patient is positioned in six different positions relative to the linear accelerator (anterior, posterior, and four oblique stances) to ensure that the entire skin surface is exposed to the electron beam.[38] In each position, the patient is treated with the beam angled 18° above and then again with the beam angled 18° below the central axis. This technique and the use of a Lucite plate results in the production of a homogeneous dose distribution in which 80% of the dose is located at 0.7-cm depth. This is almost ideal coverage, as the malignant infiltrates are generally limited to the epidermis and upper dermis.[36]

The total skin surface is treated to at least 32 Gy in 2-Gy fractions. Sites of gross disease may be boosted with appositional electron fields for an additional 8–16 Gy as clinically indicated. The soles of the feet, which are shielded from the radiation while the patient is standing, are boosted with additional appositional fields so that they receive at least 22 Gy. If the scalp has gross disease, it will also be boosted to ensure adequate coverage. Appositional fields are usually treated with 1-cm bolus to ensure adequate dose is delivered to the skin. To protect the lens of the eye, specialized lead shields are placed in the eye during treatment. The feet are also shielded with lead boots for half of the treatment. Treatments are delivered 2–4 days per week such that the entire treatment course takes 9–10 weeks.

The initial response occurs over the first few weeks of treatment. Figure 19.5a shows a representative lesion on the arm of a 71-year-old woman with stage IB mycosis fungoides that showed a good response after the first 20 Gy of treatment (Fig. 19.5b). Although the treatment effect is often durable, TSEI may be repeated for recurrent disease, especially if the patient had a good response to the first course.

With good supportive care, many patients can tolerate the entire treatment course without an

Fig. 19.5 Representative lesion on the arm of a 71-year-old woman with progressive stage IB mycosis fungoides unresponsive to medical therapy. (**a**) The lesion prior to total skin electron irradiation. (**b**) The lesion 1 month later, after 20 Gy of total skin electron irradiation. After 32 Gy total skin irradiation, her residual lesions received an additional 8–24 Gy each. She completed the treatment in 9 weeks, with resolution of all of her lesions

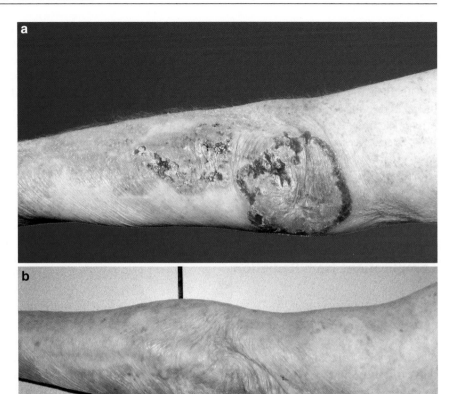

unscheduled break. However, the side effects of TSEI require diligent management. Table 19.6 shows acute and chronic side effects of TSEI, which must be clearly communicated to the patient prior to the beginning of treatment.

Radiation for Advanced Disease and for Palliation

For patients with locally advanced inoperable skin cancers, radiation can often provide local control and symptomatic relief.[5] The outcome depends on the tumor size, location, and expected toxicity of the treatment. Doses up to 60–70 Gy delivered over 6–8 weeks can provide local control,[39] although the likelihood of such control is decreased by adverse features such as bone involvement and perineural spread.[39]

Table 19.6 Side effects of total skin electron irradiation[1,37,41]

Acute side effects
• Erythema and hyperpigmentation, greater in areas of previous ultraviolet exposure
• Desquamation, particularly in tissue folds
• Pruritus
• Bullae, typically over hands and feet
• Fatigue
• Xerosis
• Temporary, complete alopecia
• Temporary loss of fingernails and toenails
• Hypohidrosis/anhidrosis

Chronic side effects
• Dyspigmentation
• Telangiectases
• Atrophy of the skin
• Xerosis
• Alopecia
• Hypohidrosis/anhidrosis
• Skin cancer development

The fractionation schedule used for palliation of inoperable or metastatic disease depends on the patient's life expectancy and the tumor location. For carcinomas, the most commonly used regimens are 30 Gy in 10 fractions over 2 weeks or 45–50 Gy in 18–25 fractions over 4–5 weeks.[5] For melanoma, a hypofractionated schedule of 36 Gy in six fractions over 3 weeks may be used for metastatic disease outside the brain. For melanoma patients with brain metastases but otherwise good disease control, stereotactic radiosurgery should be considered.[40]

Complications from Radiation

Even with modern methods, the doses of radiation necessary to control tumors cause acute and chronic side effects that should be reviewed in detail with the patient prior to the initiation of treatment. One of the earliest responses to treatment is erythema within the treated field,[8] which constitutes the first stage of acute radiation dermatitis.[40] This usually progresses to dry then moist desquamation, especially as tumoricidal doses are reached. When this occurs, the affected area should be treated with mild, low pH cleansing agents that do not exacerbate the existing dermatitis and may reduce the bacterial load. Petrolatum-based emollients with or without hydrogel dressings may also be used to maintain a moist environment, which will enhance re-epithelialization. Topical or oral antibacterial agents should be considered in wounds that are at high risk for infection or are already infected (see Fig. 19.6). Additionally, silver-based dressings are antibacterial and may also be helpful. Consultation with a multidisciplinary wound care team should be considered for radiation-related dermatitis that does not respond to these measures.

Depending on the individual, the skin reaction peaks at about 3–6 weeks, then resolves. The skin should be shielded from additional injury during and after treatment.[8] This includes protection from sunlight, heat, cold, and friction.[5,41] Patients should be advised to apply sunscreens with protection factors of at least 15 to the treated area.[5] When the head or neck has been treated, patients should wear a hat when outdoors. These habits should continue throughout and after the completion of treatment.

Additional specific acute effects depend on the size and location of the treated lesion. These include mucositis of the oral and nasal mucosa, dryness of the nasal passages, synechiae, conjunctivitis, and alopecia.[5] These reactions generally worsen over the treatment course and typically resolve over the days to weeks following the completion of treatment; they can usually be managed conservatively.

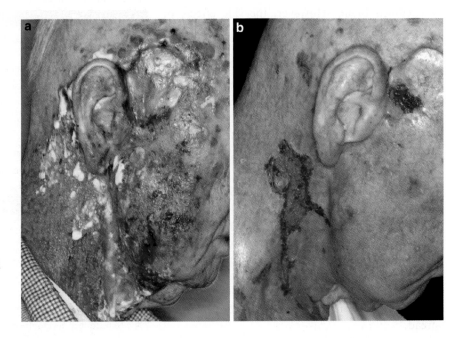

Fig. 19.6 (a) Radiation dermatitis and superinfection in the irradiated field in a patient receiving radiation for a metastatic SCC. (b) Marked improvement following topical emollients, antibacterial cream, and antibiotics

Long-term complications can develop over the months to years following radiation and are generally limited to the irradiated field. The likelihood of late effects increases with larger fraction sizes, higher total doses, and larger volumes of irradiated tissue. Common long-term effects include fibrosis, hyperpigmentation, hypopigmentation, telangiectases, and atrophy of the skin.[5] To reduce the risk of chronic fibrosis, physical therapy as well as active and passive range of motion exercises can help maintain mobility and prevent contractures.[41] Dryness of the skin due to loss of sweat gland function and alopecia are usually permanent. Because of vascular changes, irradiated skin may heal more poorly from surgery.[8] Additional long-term effects also depend on the location of the irradiated field. For instance, radiation near the eye can cause ectropion, cataracts, or epiphora.[5]

The risk of tissue necrosis from modern therapeutic radiation is much lower than commonly believed. Using contemporary methods, the rate of soft tissue necrosis should be less than 3%,[2] while the risk of bone necrosis is approximately 1%.[5]

Ionizing radiation also increases the risk of skin cancers within the treated field. In particular, an increased incidence of BCC has been observed following radiation and this risk is greater for radiation exposure at young ages[42,43] (Fig. 19.7).

The occurrence of other tumors including radiation keratoses, SCC, and melanoma is not as well documented[41] (Fig. 19.8). Of interest, it appears from available evidence that the excess risk of skin cancer lasts 45 years or more following treatment.[44]

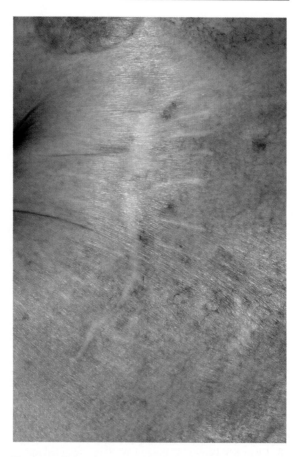

Fig. 19.7 Telangiectases and superficial BCC have developed in the irradiation field of this 66-year-old female who received irradiation for breast cancer some 30 years previously. The superficial BCC responded well to imiquimod

Summary

In appropriately selected skin cancer patients, radiation can be a useful primary or adjunctive therapy that allows for the preservation of adjacent normal tissues. A variety of techniques are available that can provide good tumor coverage while minimizing the exposure of critical normal structures. With attentive patient care during treatment, most side effects can be managed conservatively. Long-term follow-up of irradiated patients is important to monitor for the development of late effects and new, metachronous tumors.

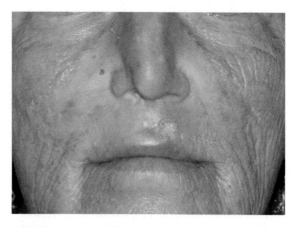

Fig. 19.8 Development of SCC on the lip in this 53-year-old patient who underwent irradiation for SCC of the nasal cavity 6 months previously

Acknowledgments Many thanks to William Morrison, M.D., for valuable discussions and to Sherry Garcia, M.P.A.S., PA-C for providing patient cases.

References

1. Wilson L, Panizzon RG. Radiation Treatment. In: Bolognia JL, Jorizzo JL, Rapini RP, eds. *Dermatology*. 1st ed. London: Elsevier Ltd.; 2003:2185–2195.

2. Morrison WH, Garden AS, Ang KK. Radiation therapy for nonmelanoma skin carcinomas. *Clin Plast Surg*. Oct 1997;24(4):719–729.

3. Silverman MK, Kopf AW, Gladstein AH, Bart RS, Grin CM, Levenstein MJ. Recurrence rates of treated basal cell carcinomas. Part 4: X-ray therapy. *J Dermatol Surg Oncol*. Jul 1992;18(7):549–554.

4. Silverman MK, Kopf AW, Grin CM, Bart RS, Levenstein MJ. Recurrence rates of treated basal cell carcinomas. Part 1: overview. *J Dermatol Surg Oncol*. Sep 1991;17(9):713–718.

5. Guadagnolo AB, Ang KK, Ballo MT. The Skin.In: Cox JD, Ang KK, eds. *Radiation Oncology*. 9th ed. Philadelphia: Mosby; In press.

6. Petsuksiri J, Frank SJ, Garden AS, et al. Outcomes after radiotherapy for squamous cell carcinoma of the eyelid. *Cancer*. Jan 1 2008;112(1):111–118.

7. Lovett RD, Perez CA, Shapiro SJ, Garcia DM. External irradiation of epithelial skin cancer. *Int J Radiat Oncol Biol Phys*. Aug 1990;19(2):235–242.

8. Chao KS, Perez CA, Brady LW. Skin, Acquired immunodeficiency syndrome, and kaposi's sarcoma. In: Chao KS, Perez CA, Brady LW, eds. *Radiation Oncology: Management Decisions*. 2nd ed. Philadelphia: Lippincott Williams & Wilkins; 2002:111–121.

9. Griep C, Davelaar J, Scholten AN, Chin A, Leer JW. Electron beam therapy is not inferior to superficial x-ray therapy in the treatment of skin carcinoma. *Int J Radiat Oncol Biol Phys*. Jul 30 1995;32(5):1347–1350.

10. Perez CA, Lovett RD, Gerber R. Electron beam and x-rays in the treatment of epithelial skin cancer: dosimetric considerations and clinical results. In: Vaeth JM, Meyer JL, eds. *Frontiers of Radiation Therapy And Oncology: The Role of High Energy Electrons in the Treatment of Cancer*. Vol 25. Basel: S. Karger; 1991:90–106.

11. Shiu AS, Tung SS, Gastorf RJ, Hogstrom KR, Morrison WH, Peters LJ. Dosimetric evaluation of lead and tungsten eye shields in electron beam treatment. *Int J Radiat Oncol Biol Phys*. Jun 1 1996;35(3):599–604.

12. Ang KK. Altered fractionation trials in head and neck cancer. *Semin Radiat Oncol*. Oct 1998;8(4):230–236.

13. Wilder RB, Margolis LW. Skin cancer. In: Leibel SA, Phillips TL, eds. *Textbook of Radiation Oncology*. Philadelphia: WB Saunders; 1998:1165–1182.

14. Petrovich Z, Kuisk H, Langholz B, et al. Treatment results and patterns of failure in 646 patients with carcinoma of the eyelids, pinna, and nose. *Am J Surg*. Oct 1987;154(4):447–450.

15. Rowe DE, Carroll RJ, Day CL, Jr. Long-term recurrence rates in previously untreated (primary) basal cell carcinoma: implications for patient follow-up. *J Dermatol Surg Oncol*. Mar 1989;15(3):315–328.

16. Chao CK, Gerber RM, Perez CA. Reirradiation of recurrent skin cancer of the face. A successful salvage modality. *Cancer*. May 1 1995;75(9):2351–2355.

17. Mendenhall WM, Amdur RJ, Grobmyer SR, et al. Adjuvant radiotherapy for cutaneous melanoma. *Cancer*. Mar 15 2008;112(6):1189–1196.

18. Harwood AR. Conventional fractionated radiotherapy for 51 patients with lentigo maligna and lentigo maligna melanoma. *Int J Radiat Oncol Biol Phys*. Jul 1983;9(7):1019–1021.

19. Stevens G, Thompson JF, Firth I, O'Brien CJ, McCarthy WH, Quinn MJ. Locally advanced melanoma: results of postoperative hypofractionated radiation therapy. *Cancer*. Jan 1 2000;88(1):88–94.

20. Solan MJ, Brady LW, Binnick SA, Fitzpatrick PJ. Skin. In: Perez CA, Brady LW, eds. *Principles and Practice of Radiation Oncology*. 3rd ed. Philadelphia: Lippincott-Raven Publishers; 1998:723–744.

21. Ballo MT, Ross MI, Cormier JN, et al. Combined-modality therapy for patients with regional nodal metastases from melanoma. *Int J Radiat Oncol Biol Phys*. Jan 1 2006;64(1):106–113.

22. Lee RJ, Gibbs JF, Proulx GM, Kollmorgen DR, Jia C, Kraybill WG. Nodal basin recurrence following lymph node dissection for melanoma: implications for adjuvant radiotherapy. *Int J Radiat Oncol Biol Phys*. Jan 15 2000;46(2):467–474.

23. Monsour PD, Sause WT, Avent JM, Noyes RD. Local control following therapeutic nodal dissection for melanoma. *J Surg Oncol*. Sep 1993;54(1):18–22.

24. Ang KK, Peters LJ, Weber RS, et al. Postoperative radiotherapy for cutaneous melanoma of the head and neck region. *Int J Radiat Oncol Biol Phys*. Nov 15 1994;30(4):795–798.

25. Ballo MT, Zagars GK, Gershenwald JE, et al. A critical assessment of adjuvant radiotherapy for inguinal lymph node metastases from melanoma. *Ann Surg Oncol*. Dec 2004;11(12):1079–1084.

26. Ballo MT, Garden AS, Myers JN, et al. Melanoma metastatic to cervical lymph nodes: can radiotherapy replace formal dissection after local excision of nodal disease? *Head Neck*. Aug 2005;27(8):718–721.

27. Ballo MT, Strom EA, Zagars GK, et al. Adjuvant irradiation for axillary metastases from malignant melanoma. *Int J Radiat Oncol Biol Phys*. Mar 15 2002;52(4):964–972.

28. Ballo MT, Ang KK. Radiotherapy for cutaneous malignant melanoma: rationale and indications. *Oncology (Williston Park)*. Jan 2004;18(1):99–107; discussion 107–110, 113–104.

29. Yiengpruksawan A, Coit DG, Thaler HT, Urmacher C, Knapper WK. Merkel cell carcinoma. Prognosis and management. *Arch Surg*. Dec 1991;126(12):1514–1519.

30. Morrison WH, Peters LJ, Silva EG, Wendt CD, Ang KK, Goepfert H. The essential role of radiation therapy in securing locoregional control of Merkel cell

carcinoma. *Int J Radiat Oncol Biol Phys.* Sep 1990;19(3):583–591.

31. Meeuwissen JA, Bourne RG, Kearsley JH. The importance of postoperative radiation therapy in the treatment of Merkel cell carcinoma. *Int J Radiat Oncol Biol Phys.* Jan 15 1995;31(2):325–331.

32. Pacella J, Ashby M, Ainslie J, Minty C. The role of radiotherapy in the management of primary cutaneous neuroendocrine tumors (Merkel cell or trabecular carcinoma): experience at the Peter MacCallum Cancer Institute (Melbourne, Australia). *Int J Radiat Oncol Biol Phys.* Jun 1988;14(6):1077–1084.

33. Tan KC, Lee ST, Cheah ST. Surgical treatment of sebaceous carcinoma of eyelids with clinico-pathological correlation. *Br J Plast Surg.* Feb–Mar 1991;44(2):117–121.

34. Voutsadakis IA, Bruckner HW. Eccrine sweat gland carcinoma: a case report and review of diagnosis and treatment. *Conn Med.* May 2000;64(5):263–266.

35. Scholtz W. Ueber den einfluss der rontgenstrahlen auf die haut in gesunden und krankem zustande. *Arch Dermat U Syph.* 1902;59:421.

36. Hoppe RT. Mycosis fungoides: radiation therapy. *Dermatol Ther.* 2003;16(4):347–354.

37. Jones GW, Kacinski BM, Wilson LD, et al. Total skin electron radiation in the management of mycosis fungoides: consensus of the European Organization for Research and Treatment of Cancer (EORTC) Cutaneous Lymphoma Project Group. *J Am Acad Dermatol.* Sep 2002;47(3):364–370.

38. Hoppe RT, Fuks Z, Bagshaw MA. Radiation therapy in the management of cutaneous T-cell lymphomas. *Cancer Treat Rep.* Apr 1979;63(4):625–632.

39. Lee WR, Mendenhall WM, Parsons JT, Million RR. Radical radiotherapy for T4 carcinoma of the skin of the head and neck: a multivariate analysis. *Head Neck.* Jul-Aug 1993;15(4):320–324.

40. Chang EL, Selek U, Hassenbusch SJ 3rd, et al. Outcome variation among "radioresistant" brain metastases treated with stereotactic radiosurgery. *Neurosurgery.* May 2005;56(5):936–945; discussion 936–945.

41. Hymes SR, Strom EA, Fife C. Radiation dermatitis: clinical presentation, pathophysiology, and treatment 2006. *J Am Acad Dermatol.* 2006;54;28–46.

42. Karagas MR, McDonald JA, Greenburg ER et al. Risk of basal cell and squamous cell skin cancers after ionizing radiation therapy. For The Skin Cancer Prevention Study Group. *J Natl Cancer Inst.* 1996;88:1848–1853.

43. Perkins JL, Liu Y, Mitby PA, et al. Nonmelanoma skin cancer in survivors of childhood and adolescent cancer: a report from the childhood cancer survivor study. *J Clin Oncol.* 2005;23:3733–3741.

44. Shore RE. Radiation-induced skin cancer in humans. *Med Pediatr Oncol.* 2001;36:549–554.

Chapter 20
When to Refer Out

Daniel M. Siegel, Laura T. Cepeda, and Deborah F. MacFarlane

As physicians treating skin cancers, our training and experience vary. Regardless, many of us have the need and opportunity to perform varying degrees of skin surgery. The procedures we perform will be based on our experiences and particular areas of expertise, but for even the most experienced practitioner, there are patients whom one should refer out instead of treating. Deciding just which patients to refer out may be difficult and is a skill that is often acquired painfully through experience. It is our hope to provide some guidelines to aid in the decision to refer out so that one may avoid some potential medical, surgical, psychological, or legal headaches. The following will be written from the viewpoint of the Mohs surgeon, but hopefully there will be insights to be gleaned by anyone treating skin cancers.

Reasons to Refer Out

The Lesion

Some lesions are simply too large to be excised under local anesthesia. While one can perform appendectomies under local anesthetic in certain dire situations, there is no reason why they should not be performed under general anesthetic; and the same applies to certain large skin cancers. Morbidity, patient discomfort, and operative time may all be reduced in such procedures. Very large skin cancers near anatomically vital structures can be referred out. While Frederick Mohs, for instance,

successfully treated two cases of carcinoma of the larynx under local anesthesia, there is no reason to perform such procedures under local anesthetic.[1]

Similarly, extensive skin cancers of the genital and/or rectal area can often more easily be treated under general anesthesia, but cure rates may be lower.

The patient who presents with a multiply recurrent skin cancer following several Mohs procedures is probably best referred on to a head and neck surgeon to have the area excised under general anesthetic with the same concern regarding cure rates.

The Patient

While very elderly patients with various comorbidities can safely undergo Mohs surgery,[2] some patients of any age are simply too frail physically and/or mentally to withstand the challenges of prolonged conscious surgery plus possible revisions.

Other patients will mention up front that they are extremely nervous about having procedures performed under local anesthetic. Listen to them and explore their past surgical experiences. Nothing is to be gained by trying to convince such a patient that an excision performed under local will be easy. It is better to spell out the entire procedure at length to the patient and their family members and/or caregivers. Patients who are unable to communicate, for example those who have had prior cerebral events, may be better managed with excision under general

D.F. MacFarlane (ed.), *Skin Cancer Management*, DOI 10.1007/978-0-387-88495-0_20,
© Springer Science+Business Media, LLC 2010

anesthetic if the risks of the anesthesia do not out-weigh its benefits.

> Listen to your patients' esthetic concerns.

Even though they may be paralyzed and in a wheel-chair, do not assume that their facial appearance will be less important to them; often quite the reverse is true.

Psychological Referrals

This is probably the most difficult area for the majority of physicians to deal with. Successful management requires that the surgeon first consider the patient's psychological needs and put aside the knowledge that their skills may be entirely adequate to treat the patient. This relates both to oncologic and cosmetic procedures.

Screening these sorts of patients can at times be difficult, but over the years we have noticed that there are certain features that many of these patients share:

1. The patient will often be hostile and unpleasant on the phone with staff members, but especially pleasant when in the room with the physician.

> Take note if your staff comments on a patient's belligerent attitude toward them.

2. The patient spontaneously, during the course of the consultation, blurts out, "Shouldn't this be done by a plastic surgeon?"
3. The patient has unrealistic expectations and is most concerned with maintaining their appearance from their premorbid state regardless of how large a tumor may be.
4. The patient has very distinct anatomy whereby obtaining the desired outcome can be rendered difficult. Examples include individuals with petite, pert noses where even the smallest distortion would be noticeable. Similar anatomic issues could be raised with regard to lips and eyelids in some individuals. Ears are a less common cause of this concern as one can generally only see one ear at a time, and slight to significant asymmetry of ears is often the norm even in the premorbid state.

5. Other warning signs include the patient in whom you preoperatively point out that they have a deviated septum or other abnormality of symmetry and the patient expresses a complete unawareness of the problem. Although it sounds a bit paranoid, the physician must be aware that sometimes this asymmetry, if not well documented in the premorbid state, can be used in legal claims postoperatively as something that was done to the patient.

> The importance of photography, pre- and post-operatively cannot be overemphasized.

Dermatologic surgeons not infrequently see patients with body dysmorphic disorder (BDD).[3] Also known as dysmorphobia, this is a psychiatric condition that consists of a distressing and/or impairing preoccupation with a nonexistent or slight defect in appearance.[4] The outcome with surgery is often poor with complications including dissatisfaction, litigation, violence toward the surgeon, depression, or suicide.[5] While any area of the body may be the focus of concern, the most common areas are the skin, hair, and the nose.[6,7] Bear this in mind when evaluating patients with nasal skin cancers. We have encountered several patients with coarse rhinophymatous noses who perseverated postoperatively upon small surgical scars left on their noses. This was despite extensive preoperative education that surgery upon sebaceous skin does not produce fine scars. Such patients may push for numerous surgical revisions.

Recognition of this disorder is essential to avoid unnecessary and often unsatisfying surgical outcomes. However, this disorder often goes unrecognized.[8] Dufresne et al. designed a brief screening questionnaire for BDD in a cosmetic dermatology surgery practice, which has a sensitivity of 100% and a specificity of 93%.[9] Practitioners may copy the questionnaire for use in their practices. Of the 46 subjects upon whom they used this questionnaire, 15.2% had current BDD. Interestingly, one of these patients demonstrated symptoms of BDD in the postoperative period, although BDD had not been apparent at the time of the consultation. BDD has also been observed to occur postoperatively in other patients.[10] These observations should be borne in mind by anyone performing reconstruction following cancer surgery.

The dermatologic surgeon can provide education about the diagnosis of BDD and refer the patient to a psychiatrist or other qualified mental health professional familiar with this disorder. Serotonin-reuptake inhibitors and cognitive-behavioral therapy are often effective.[11]

The Doctor

As we progress in our medical careers we find that we may not be as current with newer therapies as those who have specialized in particular areas. In such instances, we should not hesitate to share patients who need these therapies with those in our communities who are most enthusiastic about their use, skilled in their application, and best equipped to handle these patients. These are often easy decisions to make. We see a patient who has an obvious disease of a severity beyond which we are comfortable managing, and we simply refer that person on. Alternatively, we see some patients, scratch our heads, and in a state of slightly embarrassed confusion, send these patients on to someone in the community for diagnosis and management of their conditions. Sometimes we refer these patients with the intent of having the accepting consultant take over the care of the patient, while other times we simply want their wisdom and advice so that we may continue to manage the patient. A decision as to which way to proceed here becomes an individual one.

Our threshold for referral out for reconstruction after a Mohs procedure tends to be low. Our philosophy is that if the patient requests to have a plastic surgeon perform the reconstruction, we are more than happy to arrange this. To try to argue the patient out of their decision may cause them to be ultimately unhappy with the result. Some patients are not pleased no matter who performs the reconstruction. Although our skills may be perfectly adequate with regard to achieving that outcome, if there is any doubt, we prefer to sleep well that night knowing that while we have cleared the tumor, someone else will deal with the less absolute process of helping this patient regain or develop the appearance they wish to have.

The Doctor's Colleagues

This is important so that you may work together not only for the unexpected disaster, but also for the less complex cases where their skills will enhance the patient's final outcome. Ideally, get to know your surgical colleagues on a first-name basis and learn what their particular interests and areas of expertise are. This is helpful for those times when you may wish to have uncensored conversations with them about difficult or complex patients.

> Developing relationships with your colleagues in the other surgical disciplines is vital.

Remember, what you put in the chart lasts forever, but what you say on the phone only reverberates between the two of you. These relationships are also very helpful for facilitating emergent situations, such as when a "simple" Mohs excision evolves into a much more complex process involving vital structures and necessitating general anesthesia to complete the tumor removal or undertake reconstruction. Similarly, be available to treat their patients as soon as possible once you receive the request. If you are in a position to do so, offer to have their fellows rotate with you, agree to lecture at their rounds, write or coauthor chapters with them, and participate in their research. These same tenets are applicable to developing relationships with your neuroradiologists, radiation oncologists, medical oncologists, and indeed anyone whose expertise you may seek while caring for your skin cancer patients.

It is advantageous to find colleagues to refer to whose approach to esthetics and to handling patients mirrors your own. Not uncommonly, one may have a patient with a small wound, for which second intention healing would be optimal, but who demands to see a plastic surgeon. It can be reaffirming when the patient returns the following week saying that the plastic surgeon suggested letting the wound heal on its own first before doing anything. Having your recommendations reinforced by colleagues not only validates your knowledge in a patient's eyes, but can also be reassuring to a patient who initially has difficulty accepting a diagnosis or necessary treatment option.

Specialists to Whom You May Need to Refer

Medical Oncology

The management of basal cell and squamous cell carcinoma has not changed dramatically in the past few decades. However, the medical oncologist can be a valuable adjunct for the patient with the rare metastatic basal cell carcinoma or the less rare patient with metastatic squamous cell carcinoma.

Geneticists

These colleagues are especially useful for the management of those genodermatoses associated with skin cancer. Muir-Torre is one notable example and it is particularly helpful to have a geneticist perform the necessary diagnostic tests and to take over the medical management of these patients and their relatives.

Surgical Oncology

A head and neck surgeon with expertise and interest in oncology can be your most valuable ally in the management of aggressive head and neck cancers that may invade the ear canal or nasal cavity. Remember that they have specialized equipment that allows them to better visualize these areas. Fiber-optic telescopes are used for intranasal illumination and magnification, and microscopic visualization is available for the ear canal.

Similarly, an oculoplastic surgeon is especially helpful when it comes to infiltrative carcinomas involving the medial canthal area.[12] Lesions suspected to invade the lacrimal drainage system are probably best investigated preoperatively by an oculoplastic surgeon by cannulating and irrigating the drainage system combined with an intranasal examination from the middle meatus to the inferior meatus. In addition, lesions known to extend down the lacrimal drainage system beyond the common canaliculus should be referred on for consideration of a partial maxillectomy (either direct external or endoscopic internal) and eventual tear drain reconstruction via either a dacryocystorhinostomy or conjunctivodacryocystorhinostomy once disease is clearly eradicated. Oculoplastic surgeons also have access to instruments that may be useful in skin cancer management. Slit lamp examinations for instance, coupled with special vital stains, such as Rose Bengal, may be helpful in identifying the extent of conjunctival and corneal lesions.

> Err on the side of over-involving your surgical colleagues preoperatively.

Who knows if the skin cancer you are planning on excising will reach a level of invasion that either/both you and/or the patient is not comfortable with excising further under local anesthesia. It is far better to refer patients out liberally and to send on the occasional patient whom you might have handled well, than to be overly possessive and conservative with regard to referrals out and to then have long and deep regrets over the one that should have gotten away, but did not.

Radiation Oncology

The most costly way to treat skin cancer in the United States today is by radiation oncology. The cost of a fractionated course of radiation therapy may run more than $10,000 for even a very small skin cancer. Linguistically, the radiation oncologist uses the term "control" of cancer with treatment instead of "cure" that is preferred for most tumors. While radiation is not the preferred primary therapy for most skin cancers, it can be used as an adjunct for certain patients (see Chapter 19). Squamous cell carcinomas that exhibit aggressive histologic patterns such as perineural, perivascular, intravascular, or intraneural invasion may benefit from an adjunctive course of radiation to potentially treat a field even if negative margins are achieved with excision. One must consider the downside of radiation, which, depending on the site, can result in permanently dry eyes, dry mouth, and other alterations of activities of daily living, in addition to esthetic deformities such as hair loss.

For the younger patient, we do not, in general, advocate radiation therapy, as the margin is blind and the recurrences are often more technically challenging than the primary tumor might have been.

For the nursing home-bound patient with multiple comorbidities who might be a radiation candidate, consider as an alternative cryosurgery with well-measured halo-thaw times or a thermocouple (see Chapter 7). While the same limitation exists here as for radiotherapy (blind margin), the cost, not only in dollars but also in terms of time, is far less to the patient and health care system. An oozing and weeping, but infection-resistant, wound for 10–20 days is the only appreciable side effect.

Prosthetics

Significant advances in the field of material science has resulted in the production of new silicones with improved characteristics and improved methods of prosthesis coloration.[13] One major change has been the increased use of extraoral endosseous implants, resulting in the improved retention and stability of maxillofacial prostheses.[14] Wearing such prostheses has been found to lessen the psychological impact of the facial defect.[15] A maxillofacial prosthodontist or anaplastologist can create silicone and rubber replicas of noses, ears, lips, and other body parts that look as good as the patient's own. It is important, however, that patients (and physicians) realize that the mean lifespan of a prosthesis is approximately 14 months.[16] If a patient has a tumor that you suspect will be extensive and the patient is not a candidate for reconstruction, it is advantageous to involve maxillofacial prosthodontists preoperatively, so that they may observe the patient's pre-morbid appearance. They may need to perform imaging and measurements preoperatively as well as postoperatively to create the best prosthesis in an appropriate time frame. Indeed, the physical and mental well-being of these patients demands good organization and communication among the health professionals involved in their treatments.[16] It is not uncommon for a patient who initially considers a prosthesis to be a "temporary" solution, to keep it, often avoiding multiple prolonged reconstructive procedures and allowing easier surveillance of the defect frequently associated with an aggressive tumor[17] (Figs. 20.1a, b and 20.2a, b).

Given the ever-increasing number of nonmelanoma skin cancers, it is increasingly important that as physicians we educate ourselves not only as to the best techniques to manage our patients with skin cancers, but also to be knowledgeable of the various skill sets of our medical and surgical colleagues who are addressing the same problem.

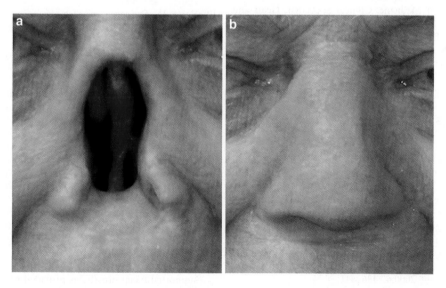

Fig. 20.1 (**a**) A 73-year-old female with history of adenoid basal cell carcinoma of the right nasal region, following surgical resection of right nasal ala. (**b**) Nasal defect restored with silicone nasal prosthesis characterized to patient's unique skin tones. Medical grade liquid adhesive is used to retain the prosthesis but must be removed daily to avoid irritation of the bearing tissue. Photographs courtesy of Patricia C. Montgomery Anaplastologist, Section of Dental Oncology and Prosthodontics Department of Head and Neck Surgery, MDACC

Fig. 20.2 (**a**) A 76-year-old male with a history of a squamous cell carcinoma of the nasal dorsum, following surgical resection with partial rhinectomy and septectomy. (**b**) Total nasal defect restored with silicone nasal prosthesis. Photographs courtesy of Patricia C. Montgomery Anaplastologist, Section of Dental Oncology and Prosthodontics Department of Head and Neck Surgery, MDACC

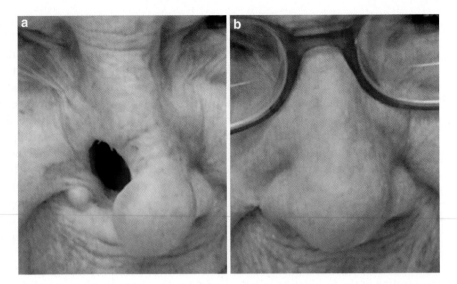

As detailed previously, there will always be patients who should be referred out and it is our hope that this discussion has provided the practitioner with a few points as to how to identify and manage such patients.

Acknowledgments University of Wisconsin School of Medicine and Public Health for access to F.E. Mohs text, Chemosurgery in Cancer, Gangrene and Infections 1956. Charles N.S. Sopakar, M.D., Ph.D. occuloplastic surgeon, Clinical Associate Professor Ophthalmology and Plastic Surgery, Baylor College of Medicine, Clinical Specialist, Head and Neck Surgery. M.D. Anderson Cancer Center; Mark S. Chambers, D.M.D., M.S. Professor, Chief, Section of Oncologic Dentistry and Prosthodontics, Department of Head and Neck Surgery, University of Texas M.D. Anderson Cancer Center.

References

1. F.E. Mohs Chemosurgery in Cancer, Gangrene and Infections, Charles C. Thomas publisher, Springfield, IL 1956, LCCC#56-6397, p. 136–137.
2. MacFarlane DF, Pustelny BL, Goldberg LH. As assessment of the suitability of mohs micrographic surgery in patients aged 90 years and older. *Dermatol Surg.* 1998 Oct;24(10);1085–1086.
3. Philips KA, Dufresne RG Jr, Wilkel C, et al. Rate of body dysmorphic disorder in dermatology patients. *J Am Acad Dermatol.* 2000;42:436–441.
4. American Psychiatric Association Diagnostic and Statistical Manual of Mental Disorders (DSM-IV), 4th ed. Washington, DC: American Psychiatric Association, 1994.
5. Phillips KA. Body dysmorphic disorder: the distress of imagined ugliness. *Am J Psychiatry.* 1991;148:1138–1149.
6. Philips KA, McElroy SL, Keck PE Jr, et al. Body dysmorphic disorder: 30 cases of imagined ugliness. *Am J Psychiatry.* 1993:150:302–308.
7. Amodeo CA. The central role of the nose in the face and the psyche: review of the nose and the psyche. *Aesth Plast Surg.* 2007:31:406–410.
8. Hanes KR. Body dysmorphic disorder: an underestimated entity? (letter) *Australas J Dermatol.* 1995;36: 227–229.
9. Dufresne R Jr, Phillips KA, Vittorio CC. A screening questionnaire for body dysmporphic disorder in a cosmetic dermatologic surgery practice. *Dermatol Surg.* 2001;27:457–462.
10. Veale D. Outcome of cosmetic surgery and 'D.I.Y.' surgery in patients with body dysmorphic disorder.' *Psychiatr Bull.* 2000;24:218–221.
11. Phillips KA, Dufresne RG. Body dysmorphic disorder: a guide for primary care physicians. *Prim Care.* 2002 March;29(1):99vii.
12. Boynton JR, Rounds MF, Quatela VC et al. The significance of positive margins (known and unknown) at the conclusion of mohs surgery in the orbital region. *Ophthalmic Plast Reconstr Surg.* 1996;12:51–57.
13. Aziz T, Waters M, Jagger R. Surface modification of an experimental silicone rubber maxillofacial material to improve wettability. *J Dent.* 2003 Mar;31(3):213–216.
14. Arcuri MR, Rubenstein JT. Facial Implants. *Dent Clin North Am.* 1998;42(1):161–175.
15. Honda MJ, Hatanaka T, Okazaki Y, et al. Long-term results of osseointegrated implant-retained facial prostheses: a 5-year retrospective study. *Nagoya J Med Sci.* 2005 Jun;67(3–4):109–116.
16. Hooper SM, Westcott T, Evans PLL, et al. Implant—supported facial prostheses provided by a maxillofacial unit in a UK regional hospital: longevity and patient options. *J Prosthodont.* 2005:14:32–38.
17. Bou C, Pomar P, Miguel JL, et al. Maxillo-facial prostheses: an issue in public health. *Odontostomatol Trop.* 2006 Mar;29(113):34–40.

Chapter 21
Chemoprevention of Skin Cancer

Fiona Zwald and David Lambert

This chapter focuses on the use of systemic and topical retinoids in the chemoprevention of skin cancer and will aim to demystify their use in the clinical arena. The use of nonsteroidal anti-inflammatory agents, antioxidants, and tea polyploids will also be addressed. Topical imiquimod, 5-fluorouracil, and photodynamic therapy have been detailed elsewhere (see Chapters 2 and 4).

Retinoids have been used in dermatology for many years. Their mechanism of action has been suggested to include induction of apoptosis, cell cycle modulation, and effects on keratinocyte differentiation.[1–3]

At high doses, oral retinoids have proven effective in reducing the incidence of basal cell carcinoma (BCC) and squamous cell carcinoma (SCC) in patients with xeroderma pigmentosum (XP) and basal cell nevus syndrome (BCNS).[4] In patients with psoriasis and a history of extensive psoralen ultraviolet-A treatment, oral retinoids reduce the occurrence of SCC. Systemic retinoids have also been used to suppress the explosive development of SCC in solid organ transplant recipients.[5,6]

The use of systemic retinoid therapy has fallen out of favor in recent years due to the adverse events experienced by patients and abnormal laboratory tests that may require dose reduction. Therefore, use of oral retinoid therapy requires experience and education of the patient prior to commencing therapy.

Topical retinoids provide only modest benefit. Studies have examined the use of topical 0.1% tretinoin and 0.3% adapalene and found some reduction in keratotic lesions, but only after 6 months of use.[7] Therefore, the role of topical retinoid therapy is limited to adjunctive use with other modalities or in conjunction with oral retinoid therapy.

This chapter offers a practical approach to chemoprevention with oral and topical retinoid therapy and aims to demystify their use to optimize clinical benefits and patient compliance. The approach outlined below should be considered a basic guide and should be individualized for each patient. More complete prescribing information should be consulted for additional detail.

Systemic Retinoid Therapy

Oral retinoids include isotretinoin 0.5–1.0 mg/kg/day, etretinate 50 mg/day (now off the market), and acitretin 25–50 mg/day. Isotretinoin has been used primarily in XP and in BCNS. Acitretin and its predecessor etretinate have been used for solid organ transplant recipients and patients with psoriasis. There is a wealth of information in the literature on the use of acitretin as a chemopreventative in the solid organ transplant population.[8–13] There is no comparative study of acitretin and isotretinoin in organ transplant recipients. Isotretinoin is a preferred option in organ transplant patients of childbearing age because of its shorter half-life and concerns for the potential teratogenicity of the systemic retinoids (Table 21.1). None of these agents is currently approved by the US Food and Drug Administration (FDA) for cancer chemoprevention.

D.F. MacFarlane (ed.), *Skin Cancer Management*, DOI 10.1007/978-0-387-88495-0_21,
© Springer Science+Business Media, LLC 2010

Table 21.1 Systemic retinoids used for Nonmelanoma Skin Cancer prevention

Agent	Indication	Chemoprevention	Comments
Acitretin	Severe psoriasis	Several studies	Most commonly used chemopreventive agent in transplant patients
Isotretinoin	Recalcitrant acne	Xeroderma pigmentosum	Preferred in women of childbearing potential

Indications

Before considering chemoprevention with systemic retinoids, the physician must first balance the morbidity and inconvenience of surgery for nonmelanoma skin cancer (NMSC) and risk of progression of NMSC versus adverse effects of systemic therapy. Retinoids should be considered as chemoprevention only in patients with significant NMSC development or who are at risk for future catastrophic NMSC development. It must be emphasized that systemic retinoid therapy is chemopreventive and augments, but does not completely replace, surgical therapy because therapeutic improvement does not prevent all new skin cancers. In patients who are not surgical candidates, systemic retinoid therapy may also be offered to reduce morbidity and mortality associated with the high-risk tumor. Systemic retinoid therapy may also be offered in cases of metastatic disease.

> Coordinate all care with the primary care physician, or, in the case of solid organ transplant recipients, the primary transplant physician.

Indications for chemoprevention with systemic retinoid therapy are outlined in Table 21.2. Systemic retinoid therapy should be considered if a patient develops, on average, five to ten nonmelanoma skin cancers per year.[14] This threshold may be set lower in organ transplant recipients, who have developed field actinic keratoses with increasing frequency of aggressive nonmelanoma skin cancer (NMSC) development. Another group of patients who deserve special mention are those who are immunosuppressed due to lymphoma/leukemia. Emerging literature reports increased metastasis and mortality from development of NMSC in this group of patients.[15]

Table 21.2 When to consider systemic retinoids for chemoprevention

Consider systemic retinoids
Field actinic keratoses
Multiple skin cancers per year (5–10 years)
Multiple NMSC in high-risk locations, e.g., head and neck
Multiple NMSC in high-risk patient, e.g., solid organ transplant recipient
Explosive SCC development
Eruptive keratoacanthomas
Single skin cancer with high metastatic risk
Metastatic squamous cell carcinoma
In transplant recipients in conjunction with decreased immunosuppression
Patient with lymphoma/leukemia with NMSC
Patient undergoing prolonged UV phototherapy with a history of NMSC

High-risk SCC is another indication for chemoprevention with systemic retinoids and is described as a lesion that develops in a high-risk location (i.e., ear, perioral, periorbital area) and is of large size, poorly differentiated, and may be recurrent in nature with perineural involvement.[16,17]

Contraindications

Acitretin is a known teratogen (pregnancy category X) and should not be used in women who are pregnant. Another contraindication would include the presence of severe hyperlipidemia refractory to standard treatments and markedly elevated liver function enzymes, prior to the commencement of oral retinoid therapy. Chemoprevention with oral retinoids is a continuous lifelong treatment,

Table 21.3 Contraindications for systemic retinoids for chemoprevention

Pregnancy and lactation
Women of childbearing potential who cannot guarantee adequate contraception during and up to 3 years following discontinuation of acitretin
Moderate to severe liver dysfunction
Severe kidney dysfunction
Hyperlipidemia, especially hypertriglyceridemia, which cannot be controlled
Concomitant medications that interfere with retinoids
Concomitant hepatotoxic drugs
Alcohol abuse

therefore, further elevation of hyperlipidemia or liver function enzymes—should this occur despite standard therapy—would be considered injurious to the patient, especially in the setting of solid organ transplantation (Table 21.3). Detail will be provided below as to the required laboratory testing in advance of therapy (Table 21.4) and the management of adverse events (Table 21.5). The package insert for acitretin provides details on the required safeguards. Readers are encouraged to consult the package insert prior to commencement of systemic therapy.

Dosing Recommendations

Table 21.4 Laboratory monitoring for patients on systemic retinoid therapy

Laboratory monitoring
Baseline labs every 2 to 4 weeks until stable, then every 3 months ○ fasting lipids ○ LFTs
As indicated ○ glucose ○ CBC ○ Spinal radiograph or bone densitometry for patients at risk for osteoporosis or calcification
Every 2 weeks for 1 month if dose elevation, then every 3 months ○ fasting lipids ○ LFTs
Women of childbearing potential (teratogenicity) ○ acitretin cannot be used in women who intend to become pregnant for at least 3 years after stopping therapy ○ isotretinoin is preferred therapy

To minimize side effects, acitretin is started at a low dose of 10 mg/day and increased by 10-mg increments at 2- to 4-week intervals to achieve the desired effect. Most patients will begin to experience mucocutaneous symptoms at 20 mg/day. The target dose is 20–25 mg/day (Tables 21.6 and 21.7).[18] In general, adverse side effects are dose related (Table 21.8).

Patients must be maintained on systemic retinoids to achieve chemosuppression. If the medication is discontinued, a rebound effect occurs, which is often very difficult to control.[6] Patients experience multiple aggressive SCCs over a relatively short period of time. Therefore, it is imperative that, when at all possible, the drug is not discontinued but the dosage reduced should the adverse effects of the medication preclude a higher dose. Dosage reduction often allows for a tolerable maintenance dose for each patient.

Table 21.5 Management of laboratory adverse events of systemic retinoid therapy

Laboratory value	Recommended therapy	Comments
Hypercholesterolemia	Statins, diet modification, exercise	Monitor LFTs every 3 months on statin therapy
Elevated triglycerides	Lifestyle changes	Fenofibrate, niacin
Decreased HDL cholesterol	Gemfibrozil	
Elevated LFTs	Reduce dose or discontinue depending on level Consider reintroduction at 25% dosage Discontinue alcohol, acetaminophen Recheck at 2 weeks	

Table 21.6 The realities of systemic retinoid therapy

Response and side effects are dose dependent
Low-dose and slow-dose increments may decrease side effects
Start at 10 mg/day (or 10-mg QOD)
Advance by 10-mg increments at 2–4-week intervals to desired effect
Manage mucocutaneous side effects aggressively
Target dose: 20–25 mg/day
Some patients may tolerate only average of 10–15 mg/day
A few patients will tolerate 35–50 mg/day
Some patients may develop "tolerance" after having been at a suppressive level; may require and tolerate an increased dose

Table 21.7 Suggested dose escalation schedule of acitretin

Gradual dose escalation improves adherence
Beginning dose: 10 mg daily or every other day
Intermediate dose: 20 mg/day
Desired dose: 25 mg/day; may increase to 50 mg if tolerated (uncommon)
Most common tolerated dose: 25 mg/day or 25 mg four to five times per week

Table 21.8 Management of mucocutaneous side effects of systemic retinoid therapy

Hair loss can be a problem at higher doses and is variable between patients
Cheilitis, dry skin, and hair loss may cause many to discontinue therapy

Use emollients frequently from start of low-dose therapy
  ○ Cheilitis/rhinitis: apply Aquaphor® or petrolatum to lips five to ten times daily and inside nose at bedtime
  ○ Xerosis/pruritus: tepid showers/bath, apply moisturizer after bathing and multiple times during the day
  ○ Xerophthalmia: artificial tears; avoid contact lenses

Pyogenic granulomas – reduce dose

Rebound will occur in all patients if retinoid is discontinued, therefore, plan on long-term/life-long therapy.

To allow for better tolerance of the medication, gradual dose escalation to the effective dose is recommended (Table 21.6). Starting with 10-mg acitretin tablets allows for easier dose adjustments, which then allows for a daily treatment regimen. Once the patient is comfortable at 20 mg daily, the 25-mg tablet may be prescribed. Every dose escalation requires laboratory monitoring and instruction and education as to the prevention of mucocutaneous side effects. Few patients tolerate dosages of more than 25 mg/day. In some patients who are highly motivated, dosages of 50 mg/day or alternating 25 and 50 mg/day have been used. The goal of chemoprevention with retinoid therapy is reduction in NMSC development to a more manageable level. The goal is not complete elimination of NMSC, as this would require higher doses than patients can often tolerate, which then results in discontinuation of therapy and noncompliance. Patients with NMSC at high risk for metastasis and those with inoperable metastatic disease deserve special mention. To prevent clinical metastases in tumors at high risk for metastases, further dose elevation may be warranted. In those patients with inoperable metastatic disease, retinoids are used as adjunctive therapy with chemotherapeutic agents. In this clinical scenario, more aggressive retinoid therapy may be necessary to achieve chemosuppressive effects.

Adverse Effects

Early studies with systemic retinoid therapy involved the use of higher doses of isotretinoin and etretinate than current therapy, resulting in many adverse events that negatively affected tolerance.

Routine Monitoring and Management of Adverse Effects

Mucocutaneous Side Effects

Mucocutaneous side effects such as cheilitis and dry skin are the most troublesome for patients, especially at higher doses, and can be managed proactively with emollient therapy (Table 21.8)[18,19] (Figs. 21.1 and 21.2). As therapy continues, patients

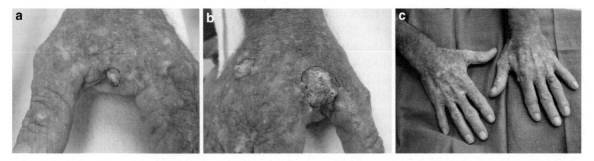

Fig. 21.1 Dorsal hands prior to treatment with systemic retinoids (**a**) left hand (**b**) right hand. (**c**) Improved dorsal hands and forearms after 14 months of acitretin 25 mg/day. Photographs courtesy of Dr. Thomas Stasko, Vanderbilt University

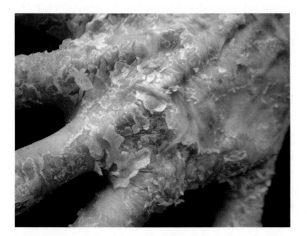

Fig. 21.2 Marked desquamation of the hands. Dose reduced to 25 mg, alternating with 50-mg acitretin per day. Photograph courtesy of Dr. Thomas Stasko, Vanderbilt University

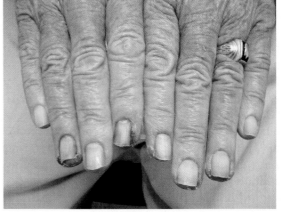

Fig. 21.3 Periungal pyogenic granulomas in a patient being treated with acitretin 25 mg/day. Photograph courtesy of Dr. Thomas Stasko, Vanderbilt University

are often better able to tolerate the mucocutaneous side effects. Alopecia and paronychia may occur at higher doses and may often reverse with dose reduction. Periungual pyogenic granulomas have been observed (Fig. 21.3).

> Consider decreasing retinoid dose by 25% for severe mucocutaneous adverse events.

Laboratory Monitoring

A baseline fasting lipid panel, liver function tests (LFTs), serum creatinine and glucose, and complete blood count should be performed before commencing therapy. These values are rechecked at 2–4 weeks and monthly thereafter for the first 3 months. If laboratory tests remain stable, the dose may be increased to achieve maximum therapeutic efficacy. Laboratory tests may be rechecked at 2 weeks after every dose elevation. If the dose is not increased, laboratory tests should be checked every 3 months.

Management of laboratory abnormalities requires communication with the transplant medical team. Treatment of hypercholesterolemia and hypertriglyceridemia, usually with lipid-lowering agents, should be in conjunction with the patient's primary care and/or transplant physician. The lipid elevation associated with oral retinoids is reversible upon cessation of therapy. Because elevated lipids can increase cardiac risk, hyperlipidemia should be aggressively managed in consultation with the transplant physician.

Elevation of LFTs of two or three times normal requires reduction of retinoid dose by 50% and reevaluation in 2 weeks. Alcohol use should be discontinued and may convert acitretin to etretinate.[18] If persistent elevation or elevation of LFTs more than three times normal occurs, the drug should be discontinued. Repeat LFTs should be checked every 2 weeks until resolved and re-introduction of retinoid therapy can be considered at 25% of prior maintenance dose (Tables 21.4, 21.5 and 21.8).

Pregnancy Testing

Retinoids are well-known teratogens; a pregnancy test should be performed in women of childbearing potential. Retinoid chemoprevention is only for nonpregnant women who are severely affected by NMSC and are unresponsive to other therapies, or when no alternative therapy is available. Two negative pregnancy tests must be recorded before beginning the treatment and two forms of contraception must be used for at least 1 month prior to starting acitretin, during therapy, and for at least 3 years after discontinuing therapy.

Calcification

Controversy exists regarding the development of calcification while on retinoid therapy. Bone radiographs are not routinely ordered prior to therapy, but may be necessary if the patient describes symptoms that could suggest calcification, or in a pediatric patient or if the patient is at high risk for skeletal abnormalities. Before starting long-term therapy, patients at risk of developing osteoporosis may benefit from preventive agents, e.g., calcium, vitamin D, or bisphosphonates.

Use in Organ Transplant Recipients

Murphy et al. first investigated the use of low-dose acitretin (0.3 mg/kg/day) as chemoprophylaxis in organ transplant recipients.[10,12] A significant reduction in NMSC occurred, which was sustained over a

5-year period and this dose of acitretin was well tolerated. However, as noted with many other studies, a rebound in tumor development occurred once the drug was discontinued.

There has been some discussion regarding a potential immunostimulatory effect of systemic retinoid therapy and consequent organ rejection. One study demonstrated that etretinate enhanced natural killer cell activity whereas isotretinoin did not have such an effect.[20] However, other studies, did not report any change in cell-mediated immunity in renal transplant patients treated with etretinate.[8] In essence, there have been no reports of increased organ rejection due to systemic retinoid therapy in over 20 years of use in the solid organ transplant population.

Wound Healing

There is also concern regarding the effect of systemic retinoid therapy on wound healing. Healing of repaired wounds is generally not impeded by systemic retinoids. However, existing lesions are often inflamed. Retinoid-induced xerosis may predispose to increased colonization by bacteria on the skin, increasing the risk of infection to recent surgical sites. For secondary intention healing, retinoid therapy has been associated with the formation of hypertrophic granulation tissue. A recent study demonstrated that there was no difference in the incidence of infection, dehiscence, hypertrophic granulation tissue, or hypertrophic scarring in organ transplant recipients treated with oral acitretin following surgical excision and treatment for skin cancer.[21]

Chemoprevention of Nonmelanoma Skin Cancer: Other Agents

Those patients with actinic damage who do not develop NMSC, or who develop less than five NMSC lesions per year, may be considered at low or moderate risk. For those patients, use of topical agents for NMSC chemoprevention may be appropriate. A variety of topical therapies are effective for the treatment of AK and for topical NMSC chemoprevention. Topical retinoids, the use of non-steroidal anti-inflammatory agents, and tea polyploids will be discussed below. Other antioxidants and T4 endonuclease will be briefly mentioned. Topical imiquimod, 5-fluorouracil, and photodynamic therapy will be detailed elsewhere (Chapters 2 and 4).

Topical Retinoid Therapy

The use of topical retinoids to improve the appearance of sun-damaged skin has been well documented. Topical retinoids, which include tretinoin, adapalene, and tazarotene, are also effective in the prevention and treatment of early actinic keratoses (AKs).[22,23]

> Always recommend sun protection when prescribing retinoids.

Topical Tretinoin

Topical tretinoin has been used to treat AKs in a number of studies. Among nonimmunosuppressed patients, a 50% decrease in AKs has been reported using tretinoin 0.05% cream.[24] Topical tretinoin in combination with topical 5-fluorouracil—a regimen of topical tretinoin 5 days per week and 5-fluorouracil topically 2 days per week—has also been proven as effective treatment for AKs.[25] The efficacy of topical tretinoin as a chemopreventive in the setting of solid organ transplantation in patients with AKs and SCC has been evaluated.[26] Combined therapy with low-dose etretinate (10 mg daily) and topical tretinoin cream (0.025% nightly for 1 month, then 0.05% nightly) demonstrated greater than 50% reduction in SCC at 6 months (three of four patients). Patients treated with topical tretinoin only demonstrated improvement in AKs and verrucae (two of three patients). In this high-risk risk group, the combination of low-dose systemic retinoid therapy with topical retinoids achieved improvement with minimal side effects,[27] whereas topical tretinoin alone may be better reserved for the management of AKs and verrucae.[28,29]

Adapalene

Adapalene is a synthetic retinoid used topically for indications similar to those of tretinoin. A trial of adapalene 0.1% gel nightly for 9 months is well tolerated. Following treatment, 13% of patients demonstrated clearance or marked improvement in AKs, while 49% showed only moderate improvement.[30] Overall, topical tretinoin and adapalene may be utilized primarily for improvement of the appearance of photodamaged skin, with moderate improvement of AKs.

> Adapalene may be good choice for patients with sensitive skin.

Tazarotene

Tazarotene, another topical retinoid, has been studied for improvement of actinic damage and as a chemopreventive agent. A large study of patients applying once-daily applications of tazarotene 0.1% cream documented improvement of fine wrinkling, mottled hyperpigmentation, and photodamage.[31] Topical tazarotene therapy has also been shown to be effective against superficial NMSC. Complete clinical responses of 50–70% of superficial BCC lesions have been reported.[32–35] Topical tazarotene therapy has been shown in preliminary studies to induce resolution in squamous cell carcinoma in situ lesions.[36]

Application of Topical Retinoids

Topical retinoids are used once-daily at night and require on average 6–12 months for significant benefit to occur. Adverse events include irritant retinoid dermatitis and prolonged redness, which often limits frequency of application.

> Advocate mild cleansing and use of emollients along with therapy

Alternate nightly application may be necessary for successful long-term use. Both formulation and strength of the topical retinoid may be altered to accommodate patient skin type. Adapalene is reportedly less irritating than tretinoin and may be more suitable for sensitive skin than tretinoin. Tazarotene may be better suited for patients with hyperkeratotic AKs. Additionally, topical retinoids may be combined with topical 5-FU for the treatment of hyperkeratotic AKs of the extremities. Topical retinoid use is outlined in Tables 21.9 and 21.10.

Table 21.9 Indications for use of topical retinoid therapy

Mild to moderate sun-damaged skin
Fine rhytides, mottled hyperpigmentation
Actinic keratoses
Superficial NMSC (tazarotene, investigational)
Contraindicated in pregnancy

Table 21.10 How to use a topical retinoid for the treatment of actinic keratoses

Start every other night, apply sparingly to freshly cleaned skin
Advance to nightly as tolerated over weeks to months
Initial agent is tretinoin cream 0.05%
Apply a pea-sized amount to the affected areas and smooth in gently without scrubbing the skin
Moisturize the skin after application
Use sunscreen SPF >30 daily before going outdoors, and avoid strong sunlight if unprotected
Increase the amount of cream applied as tolerated
If irritation develops, stop treatment for 2 days, apply plenty of moisturizer, and restart with smaller amounts of cream initially at alternate day usage
If no improvement after 2 months of use, switch to a stronger agent
Milder agents include tretinoin emollient cream 0.02%, adapalene cream 0.1%. Stronger agents include tretinoin cream 0.1%, tazarotene cream or gel 0.1%
Combine therapy with oral retinoids for immunosuppressed patients

Nonsteroidal Anti-inflammatory Drugs

Nonsteroidal anti-inflammatory drugs (NSAIDs) have been suggested to have anti-cancer activity in both animal and human studies. It has been observed that acute exposure of human keratinocytes to UVB irradiation resulted in an increase in cyclooxygenase-2 (COX-2) and in production

of prostaglandin E2.[37] Oral celecoxib (a specific COX-2 inhibitor) and indomethacin (a nonspecific NSAID) blocked UV-induced prostaglandin synthesis and reduced tumor formation in mice.[38–40]

A case-control study in Australia assessed human subjects with SCC and control subjects with AKs with regard to oral NSAIDs use.[41] Regular aspirin use was defined as one full tablet (e.g., 200-mg aspirin) eight or more times per week for at least 1 year. Longer durations of use were associated with lower risk of NMSC. Those subjects who regularly ingested low-dose preparations of NSAIDs showed no risk reduction. Infrequent or shorter-term use of NSAIDs also showed no benefit. Control subjects were assessed for the prevalence of AKs based on their NSAID use. Regular users of full-dose NSAIDs had AK counts approximately half that of subjects who never used NSAIDs. Regular users of low-dose NSAIDs were observed to have significantly fewer AKs. While preliminary, the data suggests that regular NSAID use may be beneficial in the prevention of SCC and AKs. No statistically significant effect has been found using oral celecoxib in patients with the basal cell nevus syndrome.[36] It should be noted that selective COX-2 inhibitory drugs have been associated with a higher risk of adverse cardiovascular events, therefore whether NSAIDs are universally appropriate preventive agents for NMSC and AKs remains to be confirmed.[42]

Diclofenac

Diclofenac is an NSAID that works by inhibition of the enzymes COX-1 and COX-2. Diclofenac formulated in 3% hyaluronic acid (hyaluronan) is indicated for the treatment of AKs and is most commonly used as a field treatment for multiple AKs. Diclofenac has been approved by the FDA for twice-daily treatment of AKs for 60–90 days (Table 21.11). Topical diclofenac was initially observed to induce clinical regression of AKs when used as a topical inflammatory agent for arthritis.[43]

Further studies have shown that it can be an effective agent without serious side effects.[44,45] There have been many studies evaluating the efficacy of diclofenac in the treatment of AK. All

Table 21.11 How to use topical diclofenac

Apply twice-daily for 60–90 days to the affected areas
Treatment times are on average 75 days
Apply sunscreen during treatment to minimize photosensitivity
Diclofenac is contraindicated in patients with a known allergy to aspirin or other NSAIDs
Therapeutic benefit is maintained for more than 1 month after cessation of therapy

studies involved diclofenac 3% in 2.5% hyaluronic acid. None have involved organ transplant patients. Nelson treated 76 patients twice-daily for 90 days with follow-up 30 days later.[44] The distribution of AKs was predominantly in the head and neck area. Complete clearance was observed in 41% at day 90 and 58% at day 120. The efficacy of diclofenac appears to be dependent on the dosage or amount of gel used, which might explain the lower response rate by Gebauer where 0.25 g of diclofenac was used daily.[45] In comparison, 0.5 g[46] or 1 g[43] twice-daily has been used in other studies.

> There is some evidence to suggest that diclofenac is more effective on the face, but it is also more effective on the arms and hands, especially if a greater amount of gel is used.

Diclofenac causes much less skin inflammation and erosion than 5-FU (Chapter 2), and less dryness and peeling than topical tretinoin. The most common adverse effects are pruritus, erythema, crusting, and irritant dermatitis, which resolve within 1–2 weeks after stopping treatment (Table 21.11).

> Although side effects are less for diclofenac than 5-FU, the longer duration of therapy may be a disadvantage. However, for some patients, who cannot tolerate the significant side effects of 5-FU, diclofenac may be a useful alternative

Polyphenolic Antioxidants: Green Tea

Green tea is consumed as a popular beverage worldwide. It contains polyphenolic compounds, epicatechins, which are antioxidants. Topical or oral consumption of green tea polyphenols (GTP) has been proven to inhibit ultraviolet radiation-induced skin tumorigenesis in human and mouse models.[47] The major chemopreventive constituent in green tea responsible for these photoprotective effects is epigallocatechin-3-gallate (EGCG).[48] Studies on human skin have demonstrated that green tea polyphenols prevent ultraviolet B-induced cyclobutane pyrimidine dimers (CPD), which are considered to be mediators of UVB-induced immune suppression and skin cancer induction.[49] GTP-treated human skin prevented penetration of UV radiation, demonstrated by the absence of immunostaining for CPD in the reticular dermis. In mice, EGCG treatment also results in reduction of the UVB-induced immunoregulatory cytokine interleukin IL-10 in skin as well as draining lymph nodes and an elevated amount of IL-12 in draining lymph nodes.[49] These in vivo observations suggest that GTPs are photoprotective and can be used for the prevention of UVB-induced photodamage. However, as yet, there have been no clinical trials in humans and further studies are necessary to demonstrate whether EGCG can inhibit skin cancer development in vivo.

Other Promising Chemopreventive Agents

T4 endonuclease V is a bacterial enzyme that repairs UV-induced DNA damage. Recent studies have utilized a liposomal formulation of the enzyme delivered topically to murine skin and to patients with xeroderma pigmentosum (XP) before and after UV exposure. In mice, the incidence of UV-induced skin tumors were reduced in the treated mice; and it was discovered that the liposomal formulation of the repair enzyme localized to the epidermis and stimulated the repair of UV-induced cyclobutane pyrimidine dimers.[50] In patients with XP, who have a defect in nucleotide excision repair of DNA, topical T4 endonuclease reduced the rate of development of AKs and BCCs. The study group was not large enough to evaluate the impact on SCC development in this group of patients. Further investigation of T4 endonuclease is underway and so far it appears to be safe for topical application.[51]

Other agents under investigation include difluoromethylornithine (DFMO) and other antioxidants, e.g., grape seed, silymarin, genistein, curcumin, and lycopene (Table 21.12).[52] DFMO has been shown to be chemopreventive in mouse models.[53] Silymarin and genistein have been found to dose-dependently inhibit skin carcinogenesis in mice when applied topically.[54,55] Curcumin has been studied in arsenic-induced Bowen's disease and found to be nontoxic when taken at 8,000 mg/kg/d for 3 months, but trials are yet to be performed to determine whether the same chemopreventive effects are observed in humans.[56]

Table 21.12 Proposed preventive agents for NMSC

Agent	Source(s)
Curcumin	Curcuma longa (spice)
DFMO	Polyamine biosynthetic pathway enzyme
EGCG	Green tea
Genistein	Soy (isoflavone)
GSP	Grape seed
Lycopene	Tomatoes, fruits (carotenoid)
Silymarin	Milk thistle
Vitamin C	Fruits, vegetables

Summary

Nonmelanoma skin cancer is the single most commonly diagnosed malignancy in the Caucasian population with an estimated 1 million new cases reported each year.[57] Skin cancer, especially SCC, behaves more aggressively in the solid organ transplant population. The first step in chemoprevention is the application of sunscreen, sun avoidance, protective clothing, education of the patient, and regular skin screening and surveillance for new lesions. Effective chemoprevention with oral retinoids requires ongoing communication between the patient and dermatologist. While topical retinoids and NSAIDs are of proven benefit in the treatment of AKs, their use as monotherapy is best reserved for those patients at less risk for NSMC development. They are, however, more effective in combination with oral retinoids for those patients at higher risk. Other agents such as difluoromethylamine, T4 endonuclease, curcumin, and genistein appear safe; however, further studies are necessary to establish their efficacy in humans.

References

1. Class of retinoids with selective inhibition of AP-1 inhibits proliferation. *Nature*. 1994:372:107–110.
2. Rudkin GH, Carlsen BT, Chung CY, et al. Retinoids inhibit squamous cell carcinoma growth and intercellular communication. *J Surg Res*. 2002;103:183.
3. Verma AK. Retinoids in chemoprevention of cancer. *J Biol Regul Homeost Agents*. 2003;17:92.
4. Kraemer KH, DiGiovanna JJ, Moshell AN, Tarone RE, Peck GL. Prevention of skin cancer in xeroderma pigmentosum with the use of oral isotretinoin. *N Engl J Med*. 1988;318:1633–1637.
5. Euvrard S, Kanitakis J, Claudy A. Skin cancers after organ transplantation. *N Engl J Med*. 2003;348;1681–1691.
6. Bavinck JN, Tieben LM, Van der Woude FJ, et al. Prevention of skin cancer and reduction of keratotic skin lesions during acitretin therapy in renal transplant recipients: a double-blind, placebo controlled study. *J Clin Oncol*. 1995;13:1933–1938.
7. Euvrard S, Verschoore M, Touraine J, et al. Topical retinoids for warts and keratoses in transplant recipients. *Lancet*. 1992;340(8810):48–49.
8. Shuttleworth D, Marks R, Griffin PJ, Salaman JR. Treatment of cutaneous neoplasia with etretinate in renal transplant recipients. *QJ Med*. 1988:68:717–725.
9. Kelly JW, Sabto J, Gurr FW, et al. Retinoids to prevent skin cancer in organ transplant recipients. *Lancet*. 1991:338:1407.
10. Gibson GE, O'Grady A, Kay EW, et al. Low-dose retinoid therapy for chemoprophylaxis of skin cancer in renal transplant recipients. *J Eur Acad Dermatol Venereol*. 1998:10:42–47.
11. DiGiovanna JJ. Retinoid chemoprevention in the high-risk patient. *J Am Acad Dermatol*. 1998:39:S82–S85.
12. McKenna DB, Murphy GM. Skin cancer chemoprophylaxis in renal transplant recipients: 5 years of experience using low-dose acitretin. *Br J Dermatol*. 1999:140:656–660.
13. George R, Weightman W, Russ GR, et al. Acitretin for chemoprevention of non-melanoma skin cancers in renal transplant recipients. *Australas J Dermatol*. 2002; 43:269–273.
14. Kovach BT, Sams HH, Stasko T. Systemic strategies for chemoprevention of skin cancers in transplant recipients. *Clin Transplant*. 2005;19:726–734.
15. Mehrany K, Weenig RH, Lee KK, et al. Increased metastasis and mortality from cutaneous squamous cell carcinoma in patients with chronic lymphocytic leukemia. *J Am Acad Dermatol*. 2005;53:1067–1071.
16. Stasko T, Brown MD, Carucci JA, et al. Guidelines for the management of squamous cell carcinoma in organ transplant recipients. *Dermatol Surg*. 2004;30:642.
17. Martinez JC, Otley CC, Stasko T, et al. Transplant Skin Cancer Collaborative. Defining the course of metastatic skin cancer in organ transplant recipients: a multicenter collaborative study. *Arch Dermatol*. 2003;139:301.
18. Otley CC, Stasko T, Tope WD, et al. Chemoprevention of nonmelanoma skin cancer with systemic retinoids: practical dosing and management of adverse effects. *Dermatol Surg*. 2006;32:562–568.

19. Neuhaus IM, Tope WD. Practical retinoid chemoprophylaxis in solid organ transplant recipients. *Dermatol Ther*. 2005;18(1):28–33.

20. McKerrow KJ, MacKie RM, Lesko MJ, Pearson C. The effect of oral retinoid therapy on the normal human immune system. *Br J Dermatol*. 1988;119:313–320.

21. Tan SR, Tope WD. Effect of acitretin on wound healing in organ transplant recipients. *Dermatol Surg*. 2004; 30:667–673.

22. Sekula-Gibbs S, Uptmore D, Otillar L. Retinoids. *J Am Acad Dermatol*. 2004;50:405–415.

23. Yaar M, Gilchrest BA. Photoaging: mechanism, prevention and therapy. *Br J Dermatol*. 2007;157:874–887.

24. Odom R. Managing actinic keratoses with retinoids. *J Am Acad Dermatol*. 1998;39:S74–S78.

25. Bercovitch L. Topical chemotherapy of actinic keratoses of the upper extremity with tretinoin and 5-fluorouracil: a double-blind controlled study. *Br J Dermatol*. 1987; 116:549–552.

26. Euvard S, Kanitkas J, Claudy A. Topical retinoids for the management of dysplastic epithelial lesions. In: *Skin Diseases after Organ Transplantation*. Montrouge: John Libby Eurotext; 1998:P175–P182.

27. Rook AH, Jaworsky C, Nguyen T, et al. Beneficial effect of low-dose systemic retinoid in combination with topical tretinoin for the treatment and prophylaxis of premalignant and malignant skin lesions in renal transplant recipients. *Transplantation*. 1995;59:714–719.

28. Smit JV, Cox S, Blokx WAM, van de Kerkhof PCM, deJongh GJ, deJong EMGJ. Actinic keratoses in renal transplant recipients do not improve with calcipotriol cream and all-trans retinoic acid cream as monotherapies or in combination during a 6-week treatment period. *Br J Dermatol*. 2002;147:816–818.

29. Brenner S, Wolf R, Dascalu DI. Topical tretinoin treatment in basal cell carcinoma. *J Dermatol Surg Oncol*. 1993;19:264–266.

30. Kang S, Goldfarb MT, Weiss JS, et al. Assessment of adapalene gel for the treatment of actinic keratoses and lentigenes: a randomized trial. *J Am Acad Dermatol*. 2003;49:83–90.

31. Phillips TJ, Gottlieb AB, Leyden JJ, et al. Efficacy of 0.1% tazarotene cream for treatment of photodamage. *Arch Dermatol*. 2002;138:1486–1493.

32. Peris K, Fargnoli MC, Chimenti S. Preliminary observations on the use of topical tazarotene to treat basal cell carcinoma. *N Engl J Med*. 1999;341:1767–1768.

33. Bianchi L, Orlandi A, Campione E, et al. Topical treatment of basal cell carcinoma with tazarotene: a clinicopathological study on a large series of cases. *Br J Dermatol*. 2004;151:148–156.

34. Peris K, Ferrari A, Fargnoli MC, Piccolo D, Chimenti S. Dermoscopic monitoring of tazarotene treatment of superficial basal cell carcinoma. *Dermatol Surg*. 2005; 31:217–220.

35. Duvic M, Ni X, Talpur R, et al. Tazarotene-induced gene 3 is suppressed in basal cell carcinomas and reversed in vivo by tazarotene application. *J Invest Dermatol*. 2003; 121:902–909.

36. Bardazzi F, Bianchi F, Parente G. A pilot study on the use of topical tazarotene to treat squamous cell carcinoma in situ. *J Am Acad Dermatol*. 2005;52:1102–1104.

37. Buckman SY, Gresham A, Hale P, et al. COX-2 expression is induced by UVB exposure in human skin: implications for the development of skin cancer. *Carcinogenesis*. 1998;19:723–729.

38. Fischer SM, Lo HH, Gordon GB, et al. Chemopreventive activity of celecoxib, a specific cyclooxygenase-2 inhibitor, and indomethacin against ultraviolet light-induced skin carcinogenesis. *Mol Carcinog*. 1999;25:231–240.

39. Wilgus TA, Koki AT, Zweifel BS, Kusewitt DF, Rubal PA, Oberyszyn TM. Inhibition of cutaneous ultraviolet light B-mediated inflammation and tumor formation with topical celecoxib treatment. *Mol Carcinog*. 2003; 38:49–58.

40. Tripp CS, Blomme EA, Chinn KS, Hardy MM, LaCelle P, Pentland AP. Epidermal COX-2 induction following ultraviolet irradiation: suggested mechanism for the role of COX-2 inhibition in photoprotection. *J Invest Dermatol*. 2003;121(4):853–861.

41. Butler GJ, Neale R, Green AC, Pandeya N, Whiteman DC. Nonsteroidal anti-inflammatory drugs and the risk of actinic keratoses and squamous cell cancers of the skin. *J Am Acad Dermatol*. 2005;53:966–972.

42. Farooq M, Haq I, Qureshi AS. Cardiovascular risks of COX inhibition: current perspectives. *Expert Opin Pharmacother*. 2008;9:1311–1319.

43. Rivers JK, Mclean DI. An open study to assess the efficacy and safety of topical 3% diclofenac in a 2.5% hyaluronic acid gel for the treatment of actinic keratoses. *Arch Dermatol*. 1997;133:1239–1242.

44. Nelson C, Rigel D, Smith S, Swanson N, Wolf J. Phase IV, open label assessment of the treatment of actinic keratoses with 3.0% diclofenac sodium topical gel. *J Drugs Dermatol*. 2004;3(4):401–407.

45. Gebauer K, Brown P, Varigos G. Topical diclofenac in hyaluronan gel for the treatment of solar keratoses. *Aust J Dermatol*. 2005;44:40–43.

46. Rivers JK, Arlette J, Shear N, et al. Topical treatment of actinic keratoses with 2.5% diclofenac in 2.5% hyaluronic acid gel. *Br J Dermatol*. 2002;146:94–100.

47. Katiyar SK, Perez A, Mukhtar H. Green tea polyphenol treatment to human skin prevents formation of ultraviolet light B-induced pyrimidine dimers in DNA. *Clin Cancer Res*. 2000 Oct;6(10):3864–3869.

48. Katiyar SK, Elmets CA. Green tea polyphenolic antioxidants and skin photoprotection. *Int J Oncol*. 2001 Jun;18(6):1307–1313.

49. Katiyar SK, Bergamo BM, Vyalil PK, Elmets CA. Green tea polyphenols: DNA photodamage and photoimmunology. *J Photochem Photobiol B*. 2001 Dec 31;65(2–3): 109–114.

50. Yarosh D, Alas LG, Yee V, et al. Pyrimidine dimer removal enhanced by DNA repair liposomes reduces the incidence of UV skin cancer in mice. *Cancer Res*. 1992;52:4227–4231.

51. Yarosh D, Klein J, O'Connor A, et al. Effect of topically applied T4 endonuclease V in liposomes on skin cancer in xeroderma pigmentosum: a randomized study. Xeroderma Pigmentosum Study Group. *Lancet*. 2001;357:926–929.

52. Wright TI, Spencer JM, Flowers FP. Chemoprevention of non-melanoma skin cancer. *J Am Acad Dermatol*. 2006;54:933–946.

53. Arbeit JM, Riley RR, Huey B, et al. Difluoromethylornithine chemoprevention of epidermal carcinogenesis in K14-HPV16 transgenic mice. *Cancer Res.* 1999;59: 3610–3620.

54. Ahmad N, Gali H, Javed S, et al. Skin cancer chemopreventive effects of a flavinoid silymarin are mediated via impairment of receptor tryosine kinase signaling and perturbation in cell cycle progression. *Biochem Biophys Res Commun.* 1998;247: 294–301.

55. Shyong EQ, Lu Y. Effects of genistein on PUVA induced photodamage. *Carcinogenesis.* 2002;23: 317–321.

56. Cheng AL, Hsu CH, Lin HK, et al. Phase 1 clinical trial of curcumin, a chemopreventive agent, in patients with high-risk or pre-malignant lesions. *Anticancer Res.* 2001; 21:2895–2900.

57. Greenlee RT, Murray T, Bolden S, et al. Cancer statistics. *CA Cancer J Clin.* 2000;50:7–33.

Index

D.F. MacFarlane (ed.), *Skin Cancer Management*, DOI 10.1007/978-0-387-88495-0,
© Springer Science+Business Media, LLC 2010